Diseases of Swine

Diseases of Swine

Edited by Anne Martin

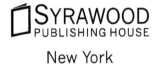

SYRAWOOD
PUBLISHING HOUSE
New York

Published by Syrawood Publishing House,
750 Third Avenue, 9th Floor,
New York, NY 10017, USA
www.syrawoodpublishinghouse.com

Diseases of Swine
Edited by Anne Martin

International Standard Book Number: 978-1-64740-409-3 (Hardback)

Cataloging-in-publication Data

Diseases of swine / edited by Anne Martin.
    p. cm.
Includes bibliographical references and index.
ISBN 978-1-64740-409-3
1. Swine--Diseases. 2. Swine--Diseases--Treatment. I. Martin, Anne.
SF971 .D57 2023
636.408 96--dc23

TABLE OF CONTENTS

Preface...VII

Chapter 1   **Cellular Innate Immunity against PRRSV and Swine Influenza Viruses**.. 1
Elisa Crisci, Lorenzo Fraile and Maria Montoya

Chapter 2   **A Serological Survey on Swine Brucellosis using Standard Procedures, Dot Blot, and Western Blot in Finisher Pigs**...27
Fabrizio Bertelloni, Mario Forzan, Barbara Turchi, Simona Sagona,
Maurizio Mazzei Antonio Felicioli, Filippo Fratini and Domenico Cerri

Chapter 3   **Evaluation of the Efficiency of Active and Passive Surveillance in the Detection of African Swine Fever in Wild Boar**.. 33
Vincenzo Gervasi, Andrea Marcon, Silvia Bellini and Vittorio Guberti

Chapter 4   **Development of a High-Throughput Serum Neutralization Test using Recombinant Pestiviruses Possessing a Small Reporter Tag**..43
Madoka Tetsuo, Keita Matsuno, Tomokazu Tamura, Takasuke Fukuhara,
Taksoo Kim, Masatoshi Okamatsu, Norbert Tautz, Yoshiharu Matsuura and
Yoshihiro Sakoda

Chapter 5   **Rapid Spread of Classical Swine Fever Virus among South Korean Wild Boars in Areas Near the Border with North Korea**.. 56
SeEun Choe, Ra Mi Cha, Dae-Sung Yu, Ki-Sun Kim, Sok Song, Sung-Hyun Choi,
Byung-Il Jung, Seong-In Lim, Bang-Hun Hyun, Bong-Kyun Park and Dong-Jun An

Chapter 6   **Comparison of the Pathogenicity of Classical Swine Fever Virus Subgenotype 2.1c and 2.1d Strains**...67
Genxi Hao, Huawei Zhang, Huanchun Chen, Ping Qian and Xiangmin Li

Chapter 7   **In Vivo Demonstration of the Superior Replication and Infectivity of Genotype 2.1 with Respect to Genotype 3.4 of Classical Swine Fever Virus by Dual Infections**.. 78
Yu-Liang Huang, Kuo-Jung Tsai, Ming-Chung Deng, Hsin-Meng Liu,
Chin-Cheng Huang, Fun-In Wang and Chia-Yi Chang

Chapter 8   **Dynamics of Classical Swine Fever Spread in Wild Boar in 2018–2019**.........................91
Norikazu Isoda, Kairi Baba, Satoshi Ito, Mitsugi Ito,
Yoshihiro Sakoda and Kohei Makita

Chapter 9   **Serodynamic Analysis of the Piglets Born from Sows Vaccinated with Modified Live Vaccine or E2 Subunit Vaccine for Classical Swine Fever**.............................102
Yi-Chia Li, Ming-Tang Chiou and Chao-Nan Lin

Chapter 10   **Foetal Immune Response Activation and High Replication Rate during Generation of Classical Swine Fever Congenital Infection**.................................112
José Alejandro Bohórquez, Sara Muñoz-González, Marta Pérez-Simó, Iván Muñoz, Rosa Rosell, Liani Coronado, Mariano Domingo and Llilianne Ganges

Chapter 11   **Pathogenicity and Genetic Characterization of Vietnamese Classical Swine Fever Virus: 2014–2018**.................................130
SeEun Choe, Van Phan Le, Jihye Shin, Jae-Hoon Kim, Ki-Sun Kim, Sok Song, Ra Mi Cha, Gyu-Nam Park, Thi Lan Nguyen, Bang-Hun Hyun, Bong-Kyun Park and Dong-Jun An

Chapter 12   **Classical Swine Fever Virus Biology, Clinicopathology, Diagnosis, Vaccines and a Meta-Analysis of Prevalence**.................................142
Yashpal Singh Malik, Sudipta Bhat, O. R. Vinodh Kumar, Ajay Kumar Yadav, Shubhankar Sircar, Mohd Ikram Ansari, Dilip Kumar Sarma, Tridib Kumar Rajkhowa, Souvik Ghosh and Kuldeep Dhama

Chapter 13   **Impact of a Live Attenuated Classical Swine Fever Virus Introduced to Jeju Island, a CSF-Free Area**.................................160
SeEun Choe, Jae-Hoon Kim, Ki-Sun Kim, Sok Song, Wan-Choul Kang, Hyeon-Ju Kim, Gyu-Nam Park, Ra Mi Cha, In-Soo Cho, Bang-Hun Hyun, Bong-Kyun Park and Dong-Jun An

Chapter 14   **Adverse Effects of Classical Swine Fever Virus LOM Vaccine and Jeju LOM Strains in Pregnant Sows and Specific Pathogen-Free Pigs**.................................174
SeEun Choe, Jae-Hoon Kim, Ki-Sun Kim, Sok Song, Ra Mi Cha, Wan-Choul Kang, Hyeun-Ju Kim, Gyu-Nam Park, Jihye Shin, Hyoung-Nam Jo, In-Soo Cho, Bang-Hun Hyun, Bong-Kyun Park and Dong-Jun An

Chapter 15   **Apoptosis, Autophagy and Pyroptosis: Immune Escape Strategies for Persistent Infection and Pathogenesis of Classical Swine Fever Virus**.................................188
Sheng-ming Ma, Qian Mao, Lin Yi, Ming-qiu Zhao and Jin-ding Chen

Chapter 16   **Role of Wild Boar in the Spread of Classical Swine Fever**.................................201
Satoshi Ito, Cristina Jurado, Jaime Bosch, Mitsugi Ito, José Manuel Sánchez-Vizcaíno, Norikazu Isoda and Yoshihiro Sakoda

Chapter 17   **Recent Advances in the Diagnosis of Classical Swine Fever and Future Perspectives**.................................213
Lihua Wang, Rachel Madera, Yuzhen Li, David Scott McVey, Barbara S. Drolet and Jishu Shi

Permissions

List of Contributors

Index

PREFACE

I am honored to present to you this unique book which encompasses the most up-to-date data in the field. I was extremely pleased to get this opportunity of editing the work of experts from across the globe. I have also written papers in this field and researched the various aspects revolving around the progress of the discipline. I have tried to unify my knowledge along with that of stalwarts from every corner of the world, to produce a text which not only benefits the readers but also facilitates the growth of the field.

Swine refers to a type of omnivorous mammal that belongs to suidae family. They have thick bodies and short legs. Commercial breeds of domestic swine raised for meat production are easily accessible throughout the world. Diseases among swine can be caused by protozoa, bacteria, viruses, noxious substances, dietary deficiencies, and internal and external parasites. The diseases associated with swine include coccidiosis, swine dysentery, exudative dermatitis, porcine parvovirus, respiratory diseases and mastitis. Some of the safety measures that can be helpful in preventing diseases of swine include careful observation, nutritious pig feed, providing a clean environment for the animals, and quarantining infected animals. This book is a detailed explanation of the various diseases of swine. A number of latest researches have been included to keep the readers up-to-date with the global concepts in this area of study. The book will prove to be immensely beneficial to students and researchers involved in the field of veterinary science and medicine.

Finally, I would like to thank all the contributing authors for their valuable time and contributions. This book would not have been possible without their efforts. I would also like to thank my friends and family for their constant support.

Editor

Cellular Innate Immunity against PRRSV and Swine Influenza Viruses

Elisa Crisci [1,2], Lorenzo Fraile [3] and Maria Montoya [4,*]

1   Department of Population Health and Pathobiology, College of Veterinary Medicine,
     North Carolina State University, Raleigh, NC 27607, USA; ecrisci@ncsu.edu
2   Comparative Medicine Institute, North Carolina State University, Raleigh, NC 27607, USA
3   Universitat de Lleida, 25198 Lleida, Spain; lorenzo.fraile@ca.udl.cat
4   Centro de Investigaciones Biológicas, Consejo Superior de Investigaciones Científicas (CIB-CSIC),
     28040 Madrid, Spain
*   Correspondence: maria.montoya@cib.csic.es

Abstract: Porcine respiratory disease complex (PRDC) is a polymicrobial syndrome that results from a combination of infectious agents, such as environmental stressors, population size, management strategies, age, and genetics. PRDC results in reduced performance as well as increased mortality rates and production costs in the pig industry worldwide. This review focuses on the interactions of two enveloped RNA viruses—porcine reproductive and respiratory syndrome virus (PRRSV) and swine influenza virus (SwIV)—as major etiological agents that contribute to PRDC within the porcine cellular innate immunity during infection. The innate immune system of the porcine lung includes alveolar and parenchymal/interstitial macrophages, neutrophils (PMN), conventional dendritic cells (DC) and plasmacytoid DC, natural killer cells, and γδ T cells, thus the in vitro and in vivo interactions between those cells and PRRSV and SwIV are reviewed. Likewise, the few studies regarding PRRSV-SwIV co-infection are illustrated together with the different modulation mechanisms that are induced by the two viruses. Alterations in responses by natural killer (NK), PMN, or γδ T cells have not received much attention within the scientific community as their counterpart antigen-presenting cells and there are numerous gaps in the knowledge regarding the role of those cells in both infections. This review will help in paving the way for future directions in PRRSV and SwIV research and enhancing the understanding of the innate mechanisms that are involved during infection with these viruses.

Keywords: pig; innate immunity; PRRSV; swine influenza virus

1. The Porcine Respiratory Complex: General Features and PRRSV and SwIV Involvement

The term porcine respiratory disease complex (PRDC) was used in the past to describe the pneumonia of multiple etiologies that cause clinical disease with negative consequences on productive parameters during the finishing process. Nowadays, the term delineates a more general term describing a polymicrobial syndrome that results from a combination of infectious agents, environmental stressors, population size, management strategies, age, and genetics that causes reduced performance, together with increase mortality rates and production costs in the pig industry worldwide. The etiology of the PRDC has been in continuous progression due to pathogen evolution as well as in management and stressor changes in pig farming [1–3].

The respiratory disease complex is the consequence of impairment of the normal respiratory immune system due to pathogens that are able to harm these defenses and establish infection on their own. Those microorganisms are normally considered to be the primary etiological agents and only, subsequently, other opportunistic agents appear in order to take advantage of the virulence mechanisms of the primary ones [1–3].

Porcine primary agents include viruses, like porcine reproductive and respiratory syndrome virus (PRRSV), swine influenza virus (SwIV), porcine circovirus type 2, pseudorabies virus, and bacteria, like *Mycoplasma hyopneumoniae*, *Bordetella bronchiseptica*, and *Actinobacillus pleuropneumoniae* [4–6]. Minor viral pathogens that are associated with respiratory implication are also the result of *paramyxoviridae* family viruses (such as porcine rubulavirus and Nipah virus), porcine cytomegalovirus, porcine respiratory coronavirus, porcine parvovirus, and porcine torque tenovirus [7]. *Pasteurella multocida*, *Haemophilus parasuis*, *Streptococcus suis*, and *Trueperella pyogenes* are other common minor bacterial agents that are only linked with respiratory manifestations [8], although this latter one can also cause primary respiratory disease, likely through a blood-borne route [1–3].

In this review, we will focus, in particular, on two enveloped RNA viruses, PRRSV and SwIV, as major etiological agents that contribute to PRDC and on the recent discoveries in porcine cellular innate immunity during PRRSV and/or SwIV infection.

1.1. Porcine Reproductive and Respiratory Syndrome Virus

Porcine reproductive and respiratory syndrome virus (PRRSV) is a member of the family *Arteriviridae*, which also includes the simian hemorrhagic fever virus (SHFV) and equine arterivirus (EAV). It is an enveloped, positive-stranded RNA virus and the viral genome, packed by nucleocapsid proteins, contains 11 known open reading frames (ORFs). The replicase gene consists in ORFs 1a and 1b regions that encode two large nonstructural polyproteins, pp1a and pp1ab, which are processed into at least 14 non-structural proteins (nsps). The other genes, ORF2-7, encode for four membrane-associated glycoproteins (GP2a, GP3, GP4, and GP5), three unglycosylated membrane proteins (E, ORF5a, and M), and a nucleaocapsid protein (N) [9,10]. PRRSV exists as two species, type 1 (European origin, PRRSV-1) and type 2 (North American origin, PRRSV-2), which share only 55–70% nucleotide identity, but its replication and recombination properties have led to the extraordinary phenotype and genotype diversity worldwide [11,12].

Swine are the only natural host of PRRSV and the virus has a very restricted tropism for cell of the monocytic lineage. The fully differentiated porcine alveolar macrophages have been considered as the cell target for PRRSV [13], but more recently parenchyma macrophage-like/pulmonary intravascular macrophages (PIM) have been described as also supporting PRRSV replication [14].

On the macrophages, CD163 has been determined to be the major receptor that mediates viral internalization and disassembly. CD169 (sialoadhesin or siglec-1) can also serve as a virus receptor via interaction with GP5/M ectodomains, but it is considered to be not essential for attachment and/or internalization. Other cellular receptors are heparan sulphate, vimentin, CD151, DC-SIGN (CD209), and, lately, siglec-10, has been shown to be involved in the entry process of PRRSV [15]. Recently, CD163 has been edited in pig zygotes using CRISPR/Cas9, so as to remove the viral interaction domain while maintaining protein expression and biological function. These "edited" pigs were resistant to PRRSV-1 as well as PRRSV-2 infection in vitro. Moreover, when these animals were challenged with a highly virulent PRRSV-1 subtype 2 strain, the edited pigs showed no signs of infection or viremia or antibody response indicative of a productive infection, which is in contrast to the wild-type control group. Thus, "edited" pigs are fully resistant to infection by PRRSV and confirm CD163 as major PRRSV receptor [16,17].

1.2. Swine Influenza Virus

Influenza viruses (IVs) are enveloped, single stranded RNA viruses belonging to the family *Orthomyxoviridae*. This family comprises different genera; in particular A, B, and C. Influenza A viruses are further classified into subtypes based on the antigenicity of their hemagglutinin (HA) and neuraminidase (NA) molecules. Currently, 18 HA (H1-H18) and 11 NA subtypes (N1-N11) have been described [18,19].

Influenza A and B viruses possess the segmented genome of eight single-stranded negative-sense RNA molecules that typically encode 11 or 12 viral proteins [20]. The viral envelope consists of a lipid bilayer that contains transmembrane proteins on the outside and matrix protein (M1) on the inside. The lipids that compose the envelope derived from the host plasma membrane and are selectively enriched in cholesterol and glycosphingolipids. The three transmembrane envelope proteins—HA, NA, and M2 (ion channel)—are anchored in the lipid bilayer of the viral envelope. HA is the major envelope protein forming the spikes [21]. HA provides the receptor-binding site and elicits neutralizing antibodies. It binds to a host cell receptor that contains terminal α-2,6-linked or α-2,3-linked sialic acid (α-2,6-SA or α-2,3-SA) moieties.

IVs infect different animal species and pigs (*Sus scrofa*) and they are one of the natural hosts of these viruses. Swine influenza is a highly important respiratory swine disease and the main causative viruses are type A IVs H1N1, H1N2, and H3N2 subtypes [22], which are antigenically related to human IVs. Pigs are susceptible to infection with avian and human IVs [23,24] and they are supposed to play an important role in human influenza ecology. In fact, genetic reassortment between human and/or avian and/or swine IVs can occur. The potential to generate novel IVs has resulted in swine being labelled "mixing vessels". There are three facts that support the mixing vessel hypothesis: (1) swine are susceptible to avian and human viruses; (2) reassortment of swine/avian/human viruses occurs in pigs; and, (3) pigs can transmit reassortant IVs to humans [25]. Infection in pigs with IVs results in an acute respiratory infection that resolves within a week if no other complications are present with the activation of the immune system [26].

2. Porcine Innate Immune System

2.1. Dendritic Cells

Dendritic cells (DC) are key antigen presenting cells that prime naïve T cells and drive the adaptive immune response. They are very effective in sensing viruses through a wide range of surface, cytosolic, and endosomal receptors, and Toll-like receptors (TLR) are crucial DC pattern recognition receptors between those.

Summerfield and McCullough firstly reviewed the Porcine DC family in 2009. In vitro, DC can be divided in monocyte-derived DC (moDC) and bone marrow derived DC (BMDC, considered conventional DC). In vivo, besides moDC and the conventional DC (cDC), we also have the plasmacytoid DC (pDC) and both are located in the blood and the mucosa of the different biological tracts.

In vitro, moDC and BMDC generally express CD172a, CD1, CD14 low/+, CD16, SLAII +/hi, and CD80/86, while blood cDC normally present CD14−, low CD172a, and variable CD1 and CD16 expressions (Table 1). In all cases, cDC are CD4− and they predominantly express TRL2, TLR4, and TLR3 and TLR8. On the other side, pDC are generally CD172a low/−, CD123+, CD135+, CD1+/−, CD16+/−, CD4+, SLAII+, CD80/86low, and CD14− (Table 1), and they predominantly express TLR7 and TLR9 [27,28]. moDC have been extensively used in the last decade as an in vitro strategy to study the effect of different viruses on pivotal cells driving adaptive immunity. Generally, moDC have been generated after PBMC isolation, CD14+ selection, or PBMC plastic culture to isolate adherent monocytes. Using different amounts of GMCSF and IL4, moDC were harvested after 5–7 days of culture and immature or mature moDC were used for PRRSV infection [29].

In vivo, cDC have been mainly studied from peripheral blood mononuclear cells (PBMC) following different sorting strategies, given the low percentage of these cells in a normal pig (between 0.1–1%). Their phenotype is as stated above, but other markers have been used to define different subsets as cDC1 or cDC2 using CD1, CADM1, or XCR1 [30]. Mucosal DC present a similar basic phenotype to cDC and pDC, but the surface marker expressions showed different profiles, depending on the biological tract considered. Pulmonary and tracheal DC have been characterized into three distinctive populations according to their phenotype and functional capacities: cDC1, cDC2, and inflammatory DC [31]. Given the respiratory tropism of PRRSV and SwIV, in this review we will only focus on results that were obtained using in vitro derived-DC and primary DC present in the respiratory tract.

Table 1. Porcine innate immune cells phenotype and porcine reproductive and respiratory syndrome virus (PRRSV) and swine influenza viruses (SwIV) susceptibility.

Porcine Innate Immune Cells	Phenotype	PRRSV Susceptibility	SwIV Susceptibility
MoDC BMDC cDC	*In vitro* moDC and BMDC SLAII+, SLAI+, CD80/86low/+, CD16+, CD14low, CD172a+, CD1+	Yes	Limited replicationin BMDC *(Mussa et al. 2011)* Replication in GM-CSF derived DC *(Ocana-Macchi et al. 2012)*
	In vivo tracheal cDC1 and cDC2 *(Resendiz et al. 2018)* cDC1, CD163-, SLAIIhi, CADM1+, CD172a −, FLT3+, XCR1+ cDC2 CD163-, SLAIIhi, CADM1hi, CD172a+, FLT3+, FcεR1α+	No	N/A
	In vivo lung DC (density gradient separation and CD11c+) *(Loving et al. 2007)* SLAI+, CD80/86+, SLAII+, and CD16+, CD14low, CD172a+, CD1+	No	N/A
	In vivo lung DC *(Proll et al. 2017)* CD11c+, CD86+, CD80+, CD40+	Yes	N/A
	In vivo lung CDC1, CDC2, moDC *(Bordet et al. 2018)* cDC1 SLAIIhi, CD163-, CD172a-/low, CD11c+, CadM1+ XCR1+ cDC2 SLAIIhi, CD163-, CD172a+, CD11c+, Cadm1+, CD1+ FcεRIα+ moDC SLAIIhi, CD163low, CD172a+, CD11chi	No	*In vivo* moDC increase in number during SwIV *(Maisonnasse et al. 2016)*
pDC	*In vivo* CD4+/hi, CD172alow/+, CD1a+, CD11a+, CD11b-, CD11c-, CD16+, CD18+, CD29+, CD44+, SLAII+, CD123+, CD135+, CD14-	No	N/A
Macrophages	*In vivo* lung alveolar MΦ CD163+, CD169+, SWC9+ (CD203a), CD172a+, CD14+, CD16+, and SLAII+	Yes	*In vitro* transformed 3D/4 cells infected by H1N1 pdm 2009 *(Gao et al. 2012)*
	In vivo AM-like/PIM MΦ CD163+, CD169+, CD172a+, CD14+, CD16+, and SLAII+	Yes	
Neutrophils	*In vivo* SWC1+ or CD21+, SWC8+	No	Not clear
NK and γδ T cells	*In vivo* NK perforin+, CD2+, CD8α+, NKp46+, CD8β-, CD11b+, CD16+, CD3-, CD4-, CD5-/low, CD6-	No	No
	In vivo γδ T cells divided in 3 subsets: TCRγδ hi, CD2−CD8−, TCRγδ med CD2+CD8− and TCRγδ med CD2+CD8+	No	No

2.2. Macrophages

Some macrophage (MΦ) precursors differentiate in the bone marrow into monocytes, which enter the blood stream. They then migrate to the different tissues, where they further differentiate into specific macrophages. They constitute the so-called mononuclear phagocyte system (MPS). MΦ are considered to be antigen presenting cells and they have important regulatory and effector functions in the specific immune response and in the maintenance of tissue homeostasis [32].

Two MΦ subsets are recognized, being referred to as M1 and M2, which result from classical or alternative activation, respectively. Classical (M1) activation of MΦ requires two signals, namely IFNγ and TLR ligation, and they can be generated in vitro using IFNγ and LPS. M1 macrophages are able to kill intracellular pathogens infecting them, and then produce pro-inflammatory cytokines, including IL1β, TNFα, IL6, IL12, and IL23. Alternative (M2) activation of macrophages occurs via IL4 or IL13 and reflects increased mannose receptor expression (CD206) and are distinct from M1 MΦs by their limited killing ability. M2 MΦs are associated with wound repair, producing components for extracellular matrix synthesis [33–35].

Porcine macrophages express CD163, a scavenger receptor, CD169 (also known as sialoadhesin or siglec-1), and SWC9/CD203a (found in lung macrophages). Additionally, the other monocytic lineage markers are CD172a, CD14, CD16, and SLAII. They mainly express TLR2, TLR4, and TLR3, 7, 8 [32]. Porcine lung macrophages can be divided based on the microenvironment within the lung: alveolar macrophages (AM), pulmonary intravascular macrophages (PIM) and interstitial macrophages (IM) [36,37]. Swine PIM and IM have been recently included in the so-called AM-like macrophages [14].

2.3. Neutrophils

Neutrophils or polymorphonuclear neutrophils (PMNs) are the first line of specialized innate phagocytes during acute pathogens infection. They are an important component in the simulation of the inflammatory response, in some cases, causing detrimental collateral damage and killing pathogens through phagocytosis, degranulation, and extracellular traps (NETs) formation. During the NETs formation they release antimicrobial peptides, such as several neutrophil serine proteases (NSPs). Swine PMNs are SWC1+ or CD21+ and SWC8+ display the same morphology as those of humans, but are a smaller size, with lower granularity and higher activation threshold [27,38].

2.4. Natural Killer Cells

Circulating porcine lymphocyte population features are unusual when compared with human and mice populations, since they present abundant natural killer (NK) and γδ T cells [39,40]. NKT cells are not included in this section.

NK cells are a component of the innate immune system with the ability to spontaneously attack pathogen-infected and malignant body cells as well as to produce regulatory cytokines, such as IFNγ. They lyse virus-infected target cells and up regulate effector/activation molecules, like perforin and CD25. In some cases of activation, an additional SLAII DR expression was described. Porcine NK cells have been identified by a complex phenotype of perforin+, CD2+, CD8α+, CD8β-, CD11b+, CD16+, CD3−, CD4−, CD5−, CD6− [39,41–43], and for the expression of NKp46, an evolutionary conserved mammal receptor that belongs to the family of natural cytotoxicity receptors (NCRs). Studies considering NKp46 expression in pigs defined three distinct NK-cell subsets: NKp46−, NKp46+, and NKp46hi CD3− lymphocytes that display the phenotypic and functional properties of NK cells [42,43]. A distinct population of CD3+NKp46+ cells could also be identified where the majority of CD3+NKp46+ cells express CD8αβ heterodimer, comparable to porcine cytolytic T cells, while a minor subset belongs to the TCRγδ+ T cells. Nonetheless, the CD3+NKp46+ cells express NK-associated molecules, such as perforin, CD16, NKp30, and NKp44. Functionally, they respond to in vitro stimulation in a NK-like manner and they have the capacity of spontaneous cytolytic activity. Degranulation could be induced in CD3+NKp46+ lymphocytes by receptor triggering of both NKp46 and CD3 [42,43].

2.5. γδ T Cells

Swine, together with ruminants and birds, belongs to the group of γδ high species in which γδ T cells are not preferentially limited to epithelia and they may account for 25–85%, depending on the age of all circulating peripheral blood lymphocytes (PBL). T cells of γδ lineage are evolutionary conserved cells that develop in the thymus similarly to αβ T cells, but they do not need any selection for pre-antigen receptors and therefore mature faster than $\alpha\beta$ T cells. $\gamma\delta$ T share many features with $\alpha\beta$ T cells, such as potent cytotoxic activity, regulatory functions, including the ability to induce maturation of dendritic cell, the capacity to produce a variety of cytokines, and they also generate and retain immunologic memory. $\gamma\delta$ T respond rapidly to infection and they are probably involved mainly in mucosal immunity. They can act as antigen-presenting cells and their TCR recognizes a broad spectrum of unprocessed or non-peptide antigens without any requirement for MHC co-signalization. Due to their nature, the $\gamma\delta$ T cells are often categorized as unconventional T cells and probably form a unique link between innate and adaptive immune responses [40,41,44,45].

Traditionally, $\gamma\delta$ T cells in swine are subdivided into three subsets based on their expression of CD2 and CD8 and they include CD2−CD8−, CD2+CD8−, and CD2+CD8+ cells. These individual subsets differ in their homing characteristic and cytotoxic activities. Porcine $\gamma\delta$ T cells have two levels of TCR$\gamma\delta$ expression: TCR$\gamma\delta$med cells are mostly CD3+CD2+CD8− and CD2+CD8+, whereas TCR$\gamma\delta$hi cells are highly enriched for CD2−CD8−. Finally, many $\gamma\delta$ T cells can constitutively express CD25 and MHCII and the frequency of $\gamma\delta$ T cells that are positive for CD25, CD11b, SWC1, and SWC7 can be increased by stimulation [40,41,44,45].

3. Innate Cellular Immune Responses Triggered by PRRSV

PRRSV is capable of causing reproductive and respiratory disease, and PRRS has an estimated annual cost to the swine industry of 664 million dollars in the United States of America (USA) [46]. The innate immune system is the first line of defense against any infection and, in particular, for PRRSV, lung MΦ, and DC is critical in the prevention of viral invasion in the blood circulation and inducing protective adaptive immunity.

Generally, PRRSV elicits poor innate responses that are associated with incomplete viral clearance in most of the pigs, depending on their age and immune status [9,10]. Infection with certain PRRSV strains induces significant suppression of NK cytotoxic activity and the quantity of the innate cytokines secreted in PRRSV-infected pigs is significantly lower than other viral infections and it is strain dependent [9,10,47]. PRRSV infection is generally a poor inducer of type I IFNs and its level remains low throughout the course of infection, as noted in pigs that were infected with many field isolates. Thus, to establish clinical disease in pigs, PRRSV modulates the host innate immunity through the dysregulation of NK cell function and IFNs production [34]. A recent study has provided new insight by showing how new virulent strains can differently modulate the inflammatory response toward a Th1 response in the lung [48].

3.1. Macrophages

Porcine alveolar macrophages (PAMs) have been extensively studied during PRRSV infection as the primary cell target of the virus. In this section, we will only review the latest discoveries while focusing on recent advances that were achieved with genomics approaches in primary PAMs and in the new insights on lung interstitial macrophages. When compared to porcine AM, PIM are equally permissive to PRRSV infection [14,37]. Almost two decades ago, PRRSV-2 antigens and nucleic acids have been demonstrated in PIM both in vitro and in vivo [37]. Examination of cultured PIM infected with PRRSV revealed the accumulation of viral particles in vesicles and the infection induces either PIM apoptosis or cell lysis. The PIM in vitro bactericidal activity is decreased as the in vivo phagocytic activity, measured by pulmonary copper clearance in PRRSV-infected pigs [37]. Recently, AM-like cells have been defined as macrophages phagocytosing blood-borne particles, which is in agreement with the PIM identity [14]. PIM were described as the major producer of PRRSV-1 Lena virus and their infection correlated better with viremia in vivo than AM infection. Thus, AM-like cells were as permissive as AM to PRRSV infection in vitro and in vivo, and PIM-expressed genes were characteristic of an embryonic monocyte-derived macrophage population [14].

Macrophages that were infected with PRRSV are functionally compromised in many ways, including cytokine production [34,49] and polarization [50]. PRRSV-2 prototype virus VR-2332 is one of the most studied strains, and the reactomes of infected PAM have been described at different time points. 573 differentially expressed genes (DEGs) were assigned into six biological systems, 60 functional categories and 504 pathways. Cell growth and death, transcription processes, signal transductions, energy metabolism, immune system, and infectious diseases formed the major reactomes of PAMs responding to PRRSV infection [51].

Only recently, data using different PRRSV-2 isolates suggests that macrophages polarization modulates PRRSV infection. Anti-viral cytokine expression was significantly higher in M1 macrophages than in M2 macrophages or non-polarized controls and both highly pathogenic (HP)(HuN4) and classic PRRSV (CH-1a) replication was significantly impaired in M1 PAMs [50]. Additionally, in HP PRRSV PAM infection (JXwn06), genes that are involved in IFN-related signaling pathways, pro-inflammatory cytokines and chemokines, phagocytosis, and antigen presentation and processing were significantly downregulated, indicating the aberrant function of PAM during the infection [52]. In particular, during early HP infection, the IFNβ downregulation seems to be mediated by a post-transcriptional inhibition through cellular miRNAs upregulation. This inhibition is stronger in HP when compared to a low pathogenic (LP) strain [53]. Additionally, lncRNAs have been reported during PRRSV and, in particular, 299 novel lncRNAs were differentially expressed after 12–24 hpi. All of the lncRNAs were enriched in pathways related to viral infection and immune response, particularly lncRNA TCONS_00054158 was adjacent to the TRAIL gene that was involved in apoptosis induction [54]. Moreover, during early infection, PRRSV-2 has been reported to induce both IL1β mRNA expression and secretion in a time- and dose-dependent manner, as mediated by the TLR4/MyD88 pathway and by the NLRP3 pathway [55,56]. The inhibitory effect appeared only in the late infection, where levels of pro-IL1β and procaspase-1 mRNA and the mature IL1β protein decreased to mock level. An IL1β antagonist, nsp11, and its endoribonuclease activity, encoded by the virus to limit antiviral reponses, mediated the effected [55].

Transcriptome differences between breeds during high pathogenic PRRSV infection have also been highlighted. Previous studies showed that Large White (LW) breed are more susceptible to PRRSV than Chinese breed Tongcheng (TC). At 7 dpi, PRRSV-infected PAM from TC showed 1257 differentially expressed genes (DEGs) involved in hepatic fibrosis/hepatic stellate cell activation, phospholipase C, granulocyte adhesion, and diapedesis pathways. In particular, 549 specific DEGs, including VAV2, BCL2, and BAX, were enriched in activation of leukocyte extravasation and suppression of apoptosis. On the other hand, 898 specific DEGs were defined in LW pigs, including genes that are involved in the suppression of Gαq and PI3K-AKT signaling. In this study, the authors proposed that in TC, the promotion of extravasation, migration of leukocyte and suppression of apoptosis constitute the defense mechanism against PRRSV [57].

In summary, an aberrant antiviral response is induced in PAMs by PRRSV infection, suppressing IFN type I induction, and M1 polarization impair viral replication (Figures 1 and 2).

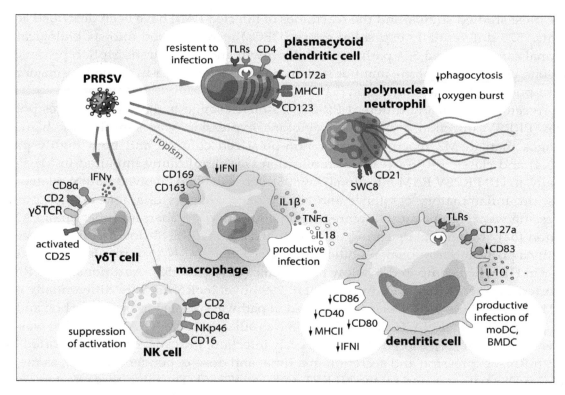

Figure 1. PRRSV interaction with cells from the innate immune system and the main effects reported.

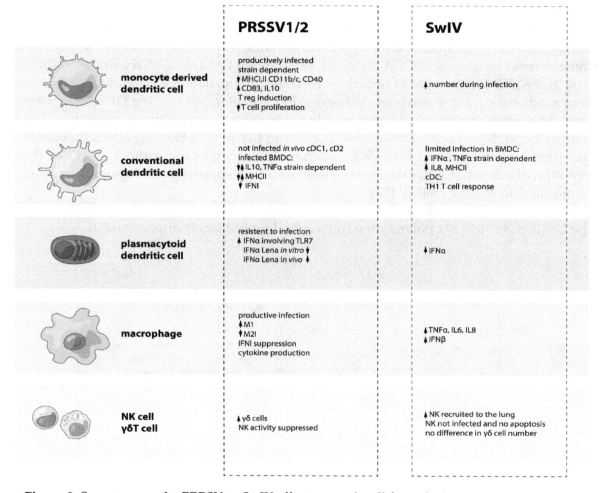

Figure 2. Summary on the PRRSV or SwIV effects on each cell from the innate immune system.

3.2. Dendritic Cells

The PRRSV infection of DC has been controversial in the last decade, which is mainly due to the different in vitro DC generation systems and the intrinsic variability of the virus. In this section, we will summarize the most common DC systems that are used when infecting with PRRSV, the most relevant discoveries, and the new knowledge in the field.

3.2.1. Conventional DC and Monocyte-Derived DC

Several PRRSV-1 and 2 viruses have been used when infecting DC, showing how the different outcomes are also related to the different strains and multiplicity of infection (MOI) used in the in vitro system. All in all, there is a clear agreement in the scientific community regarding the ability of PRRSV to productively infect moDC in vitro, despite the kinetics divergences that are related to the different MOI and time employed [58–63] and the variance between immature and mature moDC [64] or the proliferation levels of certain PRRSV strain [65].

Inconsistent data regarding PRRSV infection of other DC subsets are noticeable when primary lung and tracheal DC are considered. In fact, a recent publication [66] using primary lung DC, which was generated with enzymatic treatment and with an unclear DC phenotype (Table 1), showed that PRRSV-1 Lelystad (LV) virus was able to infect lung DC more efficiently in Duroc than in the Pietrain breed. On the other side, starting with Loving et al. in 2007 and finishing with recent results from both Resendiz et al. and Bordet et al. in 2018, it has been demonstrated that primary lung and tracheal DC are unable to support PRRSV-1 and 2 replication [48,60,67]. In Loving et al., lung DC were generated by density gradient separation and the selection of CD11c+ (Table 1), and PRRSV-2 NADC-8 did not infect them [60]. In Bordet et al., PRRSV-1 LV, Flanders13 and Lena did not infect, in vivo or in vitro, lung cDC1 cDC2 and moDC (only some residual infection in moDC) (Table 1) [48]. Following the same line of results, tracheal cDC1 and cDC2 (Table 1) were not susceptible to PRRSV-2 CIAD008 [67]. The scenario exhibits another layer of complexity when considering surface markers expression and T cell proliferation in studies where the outcomes differ when considering the PRRSV genotype, strains, and time points that are used in each experimental system.

PRRSV-2 generally reduced the antigen presenting functions of moDC by downregulating the expression of SLAI, SLAII, CD14, and CD11b/c, and by impairing their ability to activate both allogeneic and syngeneic T cell proliferation (PRRSV-2 SD-23983) [68]. Similar results were obtained with CNV-3 [69] and NVSL 97-7895 [59]. Liaoning et al. show unchanged SLAII but decreased SLAI, CD40, and CD80 [65], and other Chinese high and low pathogenic viruses that modulated CD83 [70,71]. DC-SIGN was not shown to be relevant during PRRSV-2 infection of moDC [61], and several PRRSV-2 isolates and commercial Ingelvac PRRS MLV vaccine showed no reduction in levels of T CD25+ or IFNγ+ or TNFα+ cells that were cultured with infected moDC. In primary lung, DC PRRSV-2 infection does not modify CD80/86 expression but downregulates SLAI, whereas PRRSV infected lung DC conserved their normal T proliferation ability [60].

When PRRSV-1 was used in the experiments, some strains reduce SLAI and increase T proliferation without the production of IFNγ in T cells [63] and others increase SLAII and CD80/86 in PRRSV N+ when compared with N− cells [62]. Prior infection moDC showed high expression levels of CD163 and low CD169 and replication was clearly restricted to a CD163+ CD169dim phenotype. There were no differences in the proliferation and frequency of Foxp3 after co-culturing with infected moDC [62]. PRRSV-1 LV, FL13, or Lena showed no differences in CD80/86, CD40, SLAII, SLAI expression on primary lung DC [48], and moDC showed different infection phenotype during dexamethasone and IL10 treatment [64].

Taking into account all of this variability, Rodríguez-Gómez et al. [62] considered the problem of the moDC markers expression, explaining the divergent outcomes to the use of different viral strains and virulence in the same genotype and to a suboptimal characterization of the experimental protocol that were used to generate moDC.

The production of cytokines is the most diverse aspect of infection. Strains, time points, and in vitro conditions showed disparate results, from no mRNA IL10 change [58] to high IL10 production [59,63,67,69] during PRRSV infection. Some strains do not promote the Th1 response [48,68] (PRRSV-2), whereas others do [48,61,69]. Additionally, disparity is found when considering antiviral factors, on one side moDC and lung DC responded to PRRSV with increased transcription of IFNβ, but there were no alterations in IFNα, MX, or PKR transcripts [60], and on the other side PRRSV infection activated IFNα, IFNβ transcription, but block of IFNα production [72]. In this last case, PRRSV-2 efficiently activated IFNα/β transcription in moDC in a time-dependent and transient manner, but little or no detectable IFNα was found in the supernatant and cell lysate of infected PRRSV DC. This effect was shown to be PI3K activation-dependent, but the post-transcriptional mechanism blocking IFNα production is still undefined [72].

An important and surprising finding was the role of Foxp3 Tregs during PRRSV infection. Hernendez group [59,63,73] added several pieces of the puzzle, which introduced a new role of IL10 and Tregs during PRRSV infection. In particular, first using PRRSV-2 NVSL 97-7895 [59] and then other European strains (2992, 2993) [63], they showed increased IL10 production during infection. An important outcome was the lack of Treg induction by PRRSV-1 infected moDC [63]. On the other side, with PRRSV-2 NVSL 97-7895 and CIAD008, they showed the induction of Foxp3+ CD25+ cells in PRRSV infected DCs, reversible by IFNα treatment, and upregulation of TGFβ expression in co-culture, but not IL10. Additionally, the upregulation of Foxp3 mRNA and the suppressor activity of Tregs on PHA stimulated lymphocytes were shown [73].

Finally, more recent studies on the interaction between DC and PRRSV have been focused on intracellular pathways and transcriptome. Chen et al. showed the involvement of different viral proteins on CD83 expression. CD83 is induced and viral proteins (N, nsp1, nsp10) affect the CD83 promoter in a time and dose dependent manner via the NFkB and Sp1 signaling pathways. PRRSV stimulates the expression of Sp1 and NFkB mRNA and NSp1α impairs moDC function releasing soluble CD83. PRRSV infection inhibits TAP1 and ERp57 expression (MHC complex proteins) by the induction of soluble CD83 and an impaired ability to stimulate T proliferation [70,71].

On the other hand, Proll et al. performed the first Gene Ontology (GO) analysis to determine the immune response to PRRSV LV infection in lung DC of two different breeds (Duroc and Pietrain). Although the phenotyping of DC was not very specific and lung DC probably included a macrophage component, the transcriptome profile showed breed specific differences in response to the infection. They identified key clusters and pathways as well as specific genes (SEC61β, SLA7) that play important roles in animal health. Finally, the up regulation of IL1β in Duroc could explain the better immune response of Duroc when compared to Pietrain [66].

3.2.2. Bone Marrow Derived DC

Mateu's group performed the first study in bone marrow derived DC (BMDC), which extensively used BMDC to study PRRSV pathogenesis. They tested 39 European isolates that were able to induce different patterns of IL10 and TNFα production and different surface markers regulation. BMDC were productively infected by PRRSV isolated and MHCII upregulation was observed in selected PRRSV-1 strains [74]. Between the PRRSV-1 strains, high pathogenic Lena, together with Belgium A and Lelystad, reflected a different pattern. Lena showed a higher replication rate and apoptosis in BMDC when compared with other PRRSV-1 strains (Lelystad and Belgium A), but controversially it induced SLAII down regulation together with CD14, SWC3, and CD163 [75].

A most recent publication from Mateu's group had characterized, in more detail, the interaction between PRRSV-1 strains and BMDC [76] when PRRSV-1 replication and attachment in immature (iBMDC) and mature BMDC (mBMDC) was studied. Replication kinetics showed that titres in iBMDC were significantly higher than mBMDC by 24 hpi and iBMDC were more efficient in the support of PRRSV-1 replication than mBMDC. iBMDC attachment by all of the strain was possible in cells that lack porcine CD163 or sialoadhesin (CD169) receptors or in cells with heparan sulfate (unspecific attachment receptor) removed. PRRSV-1 nucleocapsid could be observed in CD163− iBMDC and those cells were only infected when CD163low/hi cells were present, indicating that the susceptibility of CD163− cells derived as result of the milieu that was created by CD163+ infected BMDC, by receptor-independent mechanisms or that some cells expressed CD163 at levels that were below the technical sensitivity [76].

This study, together with most recent ones [64,77,78], questioned the notion of CD163 relevance during the infection. Nevertheless, the essential role of this receptor for viral uncoating and pathogenesis is still supported by the generation of genome edited pigs that lack the CD163 SRCR5 domain, which showed to be resistant to PRRSV infection [16,17].

As a whole, DC responses against PPRSV showed a general dysregulation of the IFN response, downregulation of activation and maturation markers with an induction of IL10 and Treg (Figures 1 and 2).

3.2.3. Plasmacytoid DC

Plasmacytoid dendritic cells (pDC) are the major source of type I IFNs and other inflammatory cytokines after exposure to viruses. Type I interferons are essential for direct antiviral activity and, despite pDC low frequency, they can produce around 100 times more IFNα than any other cell type and sense viruses in the absence of replication [79]. In pigs, these cells (Table 1) represent 0.1–0.3% of blood leukocytes and their role during PRRS was not clear until 2010 when few groups started to consider the involvement of these cells during the infection.

Zuckermann's group studied, for the first time, the exposure of pDC, much broadly defined as CD4hi CD172alow CD1a+ CD11a+ CD11b− CD11c− CD16+ CD18+ CD29+ CD44+ SLAII+, to several pig viruses and, among them, American PRRSV [80]. PRRSV-2 46448 was not able to induce the production of IFNα in pDCs, even when doses were 100-fold. PRRSV-2 was able to stimulate a low but detectable IL2 production, but it failed to induce detectable IL8, IFNγ, TNFα, IL12, and IRF7 production. PRRSV exposed pDC remained relatively inert, showing unaltered morphology and CD80/86 downregulation when compared with untreated cells [80]. Subsequently, the study was expanded with several PRRSV-2 strains that were used in combination with potent pDC stimulators as TGEV and ODN D19 [81]. Interestingly, prolonged incubation of porcine pDC with PRRSV-2 did not significantly alter cell viability and pDC were resistant to the infection. Additionally, pDC suppression occurred independent of virus viability and the acidification of pDC early endosomes, but correlated with diminished levels of IFNα mRNA. This change was attributed to an abrogation of transcription resulting from a decrease in IRF7 production, limited as a consequence of the nuclear translocation block of STAT1. PRRSV strains confirmed TNFα synthesis inhibition but promoted NFkB phosporilation, which is necessary for pro-inflammatory cytokines expression [81].

Zuckermann opened a new research direction in PRRSV that was subsequently taken over by the Summerfield group in the last five years. They started to explore interactions of both PRRSV genotypes with pDC using a broad spectrum of PRRSV-1 and 2 strains [82,83]. Controversially, Summerfield at al. demonstrated how several type 2 strains induced weak or no suppression of IFNα in CpG-stimulated pDC and stimulated IFN-α in CD172alow CD4hi CD14− pDC. Interestingly, a high percentage of pDC was observed after PRRSV stimulation when compared to mock, suggesting the promotion of pDC survival by the virus [82]. Additionally, in this study, PRRSV sensing by pDC did not require live virus and pDC were confirmed to not be permissive to PRRSV. IFNα response involved the activation of the TLR7 pathway and it was enhanced by IFNγ and IL4. A surprising finding was that moDC were protected from PRRSV infection and killing when cultured with enriched pDC [82]. The divergent outcomes that were obtained by Zuckermann and Summerfield may lead back to the different pig genetics and to the diverse pDC isolation method and virus strains that were adopted in the studies. The role of pig genetics in the different outcomes after PRRSV infection has been reported [84–86], but its relationship with innate immune responses and particularly with pDC remains to be elucidated [87].

Data from both groups and genotypes found agreement only when pDC were exposed to Lena, the recent virulent PRRSV-1.3 strain that showed not to be able to induce IFNα in pDC in vitro but pig infected in vivo with Lena showed a systemic IFNα response [83]. In particular, an exosome fraction of Lena-infected cells but not Lena virions themselves were able to activate pDC [83].

PRRSV infected macrophages were more potent in activating pDC independently of the viral strains. This activation required cell adhesion molecules mediating contacts between MΦ and pDC, intact cytoskeleton and sphingomyelinase activity, but it was not induced by free PRRSV virions released from infected macrophages. Additionally, ITGAL-mediated intercellular adhesion was required for efficient sensing of PRRSV-infected MΦ [83].

Taken together, all of the findings demonstrate that pDC respond to PRRSV-1 and 2 genotypes and suppressive activities are moderate and strain-dependent (Figure 1). They may be a source of IFNα responses reported in PRRSV-infected animals, further contributing to the puzzling immunopathogenesis of PRRS.

3.3. Neutrophils

Pigs that develop interstitial pneumonia in the lungs after PRRSV infection normally show the mononuclear infiltration of alveolar septae and accumulations with macrophages and cell debris in the alveoli. Generally, high pathogenic strains exhibited severe pathology with increased neutrophils, mast cells, and macrophages when compared with low virulent strains [75,88]. Additionally, PRRSV-2 (IAF-Klop) infection leads to a significant increase in proteolytic activity in pulmonary fluids. Maximal activity was found at 7 and 14 days pi, with a return towards normal levels at day 42. Zymographic analyses showed a significant increase in the secretion of matrix metalloproteases 2 and 9, which are two enzymes involved in tissue remodeling [89].

Neutrophils (PMNs) interact with opsonized immune complexes through Fcγ receptors, activating and inhibitory receptors, which bind the Fc domain of IgG. In a study using PRRSV-2 HN07-1 or BJ-4, viral infection downregulates PMNs antibody-dependent phagocytosis and also impaired PMNs ability to kill E. coli, thus confirming that PMNs were impaired during PRRSV infection. In infected animals, the expression of FcγRIIIA inhibitory receptor decreased and reached the lowest point at 5 dpi in both PRRSV strains, and together with the late upregulation of FcγRIIIB, both contribute to decreased PMNs phagocytosis. The oxygen burst function of the PMNs was also depressed, and generally the consequences of infection by the more pathogenic strain HN07-1 were greater [90].

In another study, the PMNs infiltration was determined by the measurement of myeloperoxidase and enzyme activity in the lung, together with qPCR. In the lung, IL8, which is chemoattractant for neutrophil recruitment, was upregulated, and ICAM-1, responsible for firm neutrophils adhesion and transendothelial migration, was high in naturally infected animals. Moreover, VCAM-1 displayed a high level in experimentally and naturally infected pig lungs [91]. The induction of IL8 by PRRSV was further confirmed in vivo and in vitro, and it is likely through the TAK-1/JNK/AP-1 pathway [92].

In summary, PRRSV infection mainly impairs PMNs antibody-dependent phagocytosis and bacteria killing ability, together with the depression of the oxygen burst function, but seem to induce IL8 production (Figures 1 and 2).

3.4. NK and γδ Tcells

It is surprising that very few works have studied NK and γδT cells during PRRSV infection. One of the first preliminary studies was performed in Spain, where the piglets were inoculated with PRRSV-1 5710. T cell cultures that were established by stimulating responding cells with PRRSV showed an increase of double positive memory CD8+CD4+ as well as CD4−CD8+ effector lymphocyte subsets within activated cells, whereas CD4+CD8− declined along the time. Within the activated cells, those expressing the TCRγδ receptor also increased, with most of them also being positive for CD8. In resting cells, the majority of γδ cells were CD8− [93]. Almost concomitant, the Bianchi's group studied the change in detailed CD8+ cells subpopulations in BAL fluid in pigs that were infected with PRRSV-1 TerHuurne. NK (Table 1) were the main cells present in the lung of gnotobiotic and SPF piglets during the first days of infection, whereas CD8+ γδ T cells presence was never relevant After day 7, the increase of CD8+ cells correlated with a rapid decrease of PRRSV in the BAL fluid and CD8+ γδ T cells disappeared in the CD8+ cells [94]. Nevertheless, the use of different European strains showed different patterns in BAL leucocyte populations at early and late time points. In fact, at day 3 pi a significantly higher percentage of CD8− γδ T cells was observed in pigs that were infected with Belgium A and Lelystad, but not in strain Lena. At day 35 pi, cytotoxic T cells were almost double in percentage in all infections and CD8− γδ T cells were significantly lower [95].

On the other side, in a Canadian study using a PRRSV-2 experimental infection (LHVA-93-3), Magar's group investigated the persistence of the virus in blood, spleen, lymph nodes, and tonsil. The authors discriminated between different CD8+ T cell subsets, and also between those NK cells. They defined NK cells as CD2+ CD8low and MIL4+, and they were not significantly modified in spleen and blood during infection in spite of a transient increase in the spleen at 3pi, followed by a gradual decrease up until 60 days pi. However, NK cells were rarely present in the tonsil and mediastinal lymph node, and they increased only at 3 days pi. Thus, it seemed that NK were not significantly modified during PRRSV-2 infection [96].

With the prototype VR-2332 in germ free piglets, the proportion γδT cells and NK decreased in BAL and only the CD2+CD8a+ γδ T subset increased. Tracheo-bronchial and mesenteric lymph nodes showed no differences in frequencies of NK and γδ T, but the CD2+CD8α+ subset increased together with a proportional decrease in the CD2-CD8α− subset [97].

An interesting study was performed in gilts, which were experimentally inoculated twice with PRRSV-2 MN-30100 and monitored for lymphocyte subpopulations, antigen specific proliferation, and IFNγ production. Following primary exposure to PRRSV, peripheral circulating γδ T cells percentage increased from day 14 to day 70, and then decreased to control at 120 days. γδ T cells responded to PRRSV infection significantly when compared to CD4 at an early stage and they were the major producer of IFNγ throughout the study [98]. Another study using different Minnesota strains, together with the prototype PRRSV-2 VR2332, showed an opposite outcome in tissues (PBMC, lung, tonsil, LN, bone marrow, spleen). PRRSV infection did not change the CD4+ or CD8+ population in any tissue, and by contrast, the γδ T cells were significantly decreased in lung and all LN and reduced non-significantly in every other tissue [99].

Seven-week-old nursery pigs in a commercial setting were injected with MN 1-18-2, and at day 2 pi, approximately 50% of viremic pigs had greater than 50% reduction in NK cell mediated cytotoxicity. Reduced frequency of CD4−CD8+ and CD4+CD8+ T cells and upregulated frequency of lymphocytes bearing natural Treg phenotype was detected in viremic pigs. All of the viremic contact pigs also had comparable immune cell modulation [100].

More recently, the interaction between NK and PRRSV-infected PAM was investigated in vitro. NK cytotoxicity assay was performed while using enriched NK cells as effector cells and Lelystad PRRSV-1-infected PAM as target. NK cytotoxicity against PRRSV-infected PAM decreased, starting from 6 hpi till 12 hpi. UV inactivated PRRSV also suppressed NK activity, but much less than infectious PRRSV, and co-incubation with infected PAM inhibited the degranulation of NK cells. By using supernatant from infected PAM, data showed that the suppressive effect of PRRSV in NK cytotoxicity was not mediated by soluble factors [101]. Successively, Cao et al. still considered the involvement of NK and γδ T cells during a vaccination study with a recombinant MLV vaccine that was incorporated with the porcine IL15 or IL18 gene fused to a signal that can anchor the cytokines to the cell membrane. In this case, immunization enhanced NK and γδ T cells responses and conferred improved protection against heterologous challenge (NADC20) [102].

Even with a limited number of studies, the data indicated that NK and γδ T cells interaction during PRRSV infection is altered with a suppressive effect on NK and the modulation of γδ T cells during the course of the infection. In particular, this is relevant when considering that γδ T cells are an important source of IFNγ during PRRSV infection (Figures 1 and 2).

4. Innate Cellular Immune Responses Triggered by SwIV

4.1. Macrophages and Dendritic Cells

It is worth mentioning some in vitro experiments by several groups that attempted to understand the interaction of these cells with SwIVs. Kim et al. (2009) showed the MΦ culture supernatant from MΦ infected with SwIV H1N2. Significant differences in TNFα concentration between SwIV-infected and uninfected alveolar MΦ were detected at different hpi, with a peak at 36 hpi. These results suggested that TNFα might be an important mediator in the pathophysiology of SwIV infection [103].

Another in vitro study used three-dimensional/four (3D/4) cells, a spontaneously transformed line of swine MΦ (ATCC), infected with a pandemic H1N1 virus [104]. This report demonstrated that A (H1N1)pdm/2009 retains the ability to infect and replicate in swine MΦ, inducing a typical cytopathic effect (16 h pi) and destroying the cell monolayer (32 h pi). This study also examined the pattern of cytokine responses in pH1N1-infected swine MΦ by real time RT-PCR. IL6 and IL8 levels were up regulated at 16 h and the level of IL8 continued to rise up at 36 hpi. The robust induction of antiviral IFNβ and TNF family members, which may be attributable to cell death, was also observed. FasL and TNFα remained undetectable, while the TNF-related apoptosis-inducing ligand (TRAIL) seemed to be the most abundant one before infection. FasL and TNFα were most robustly induced, but TRAIL was only mildly induced in response to infection. The level of IL1β remained unchanged throughout the infection (different from Barbe et al. [105]), indicating that IL6 and IL8, as well as TNFα, were the main pro-inflammatory cytokines that were up-regulated. The authors also observed the induction of RIG-1 and MDA-5, which appeared to be completely suppressed by inhibitors of ERK1/2 or JNK1/2. This indicated that the induction of RIG-1 or MDA-5 depends on the activation of ERK1/2 and JNK1/2 in pig MΦ [104].

For the first time, our group described the interaction between porcine bone marrow-derived DC (poBMDC) (cDC) and SwIV H3N2 in vitro. The infection of poBMDC resulted in a structure resembling IV inside vesicles and also free in the cytoplasm of the cells. Viral progeny was undetectable in the supernatant but limited replication was detected in the first 8 hpi. However, the viral particles from infected-poBMDC were only able to induce a cytopathic effect in susceptible cells when cell-to-cell interaction was favored [106]. Additionally, they observed that similarly to the SwIV H3N2, porcine DC also supported a limited replication of other IVs during the first 8 hpi, without release of infectious progeny [106]. Additionally, these viruses similarly modulated the expression of NFκB, TGFβ and IL10 genes. However, they induced different kinetics and levels of inflammatory cytokines. Infection of poBMDC with SwIV induced a peak of IFNα secretion at 24 hpi, whereas, with the others, the production of IFNα was not detected. SwIV and highly pathogenic avian influenza (HPAI) induced more TNFα when compared to huIV and low pathogenic avian influenza (LPAI). SwIV, LPAI, and HPAI induced an increase of IL12 from 16 to 24 hpi and all of the viruses used induced IL18 secretion in a time-dependent manner [107].

Summerfield's group also used GM-CSF derived DC infected with other avian and porcine IVs. They also generated recombinant reassortants by reverse genetics to elucidate the role of the single gene segments in the activation of cDC. The highest IFN type I responses were achieved by porcine virus reassortants that contained the avian polymerase gene PB2. This finding was not due to the differential tropism, since all of the viruses infected GM-CSF derived DC equally (and also porcine PK-15 epithelial cells) and infectivity was independent of HA expressed by the virus. All of the viruses induced MHCII, but porcine H1N1 expressing the avian viral PB2 more prominently induced nuclear NFkB translocation when compared to its parental strains. Therefore, in the case of porcine DC, PB2 was defined as an important viral element controlling IFN type I. While all the viruses had a comparable ability to infect DC, to initiate replication and to activate the cells in terms of MHCII induction, only those expressing PB2 derived from H5N1 were unable to prevent IFN type I induction; however, no viral progeny was detected [108].

When considering the distinct features of pDC and the crucial role of IFN in fighting virus infections, Bel at al. [109] analyzed the interactions of different influenza A viruses isolated from avian, human and swine with pDC obtained from pigs. Their results demonstrated that porcine pDC could produce high levels of IFNα in response to all of the tested strains, with subtype-specific differences in a virus-dose dependent manner. High levels of IFNα were detected upon live, chemically inactivated, or UV-inactivated virus stimulation. In contrast, heat-inactivated virus failed to induce a response. The observation that chemical and UV-inactivation did not abolish IFNα release indicated that non-infectious particles are also stimulatory for pDC. Additionally, these treatments did not abolish hemagglutination, suggesting that the integrity of HA and its binding function are necessary in inducing IFNα responses in pDC. At low viral doses, H5N1 and H7N1 avian viruses are more efficient in infecting pDC when compared to human H1N1 and at inducing the secretion of IFNα [109].

In vivo infection with SwIV mainly occurs in the respiratory-tract and the lungs of infected pigs, thus innate cells in the lungs are the first ones encountering the virus. One of the main components of the respiratory immune system is the DC/MΦ network that is involved in sensing foreign antigens, controlling inflammation, and initiating the adaptive immune responses. We have adapted a recently proposed nomenclature from Guilliams et al. [110] distinguishing between two levels of identification. The first level focuses on the origin of the cell-type progenitor (adult bone-marrow proDC for conventional DC (cDC), adult blood monocytes for monocyte-derived cells (moCells), or embryonic monocyte-derived precursors that were settled in peripheral tissues for MΦs. The second level focuses on the cell functions (MΦ-like or DC-like). We have recently finely defined the phenotypes and functions of DC/MΦ populations in the different compartments of the swine respiratory tract at a steady state and upon IAV infections in the pig [31]. We have defined six populations within the MΦ-DC network in pig trachea and lungs: 1—Porcine alveolar MΦ (AM) CD163hi/CD11b-likeneg and expressed high levels of MerTK and CD64; 2—AM-like population, the CD163hi 'interstitial' AM, unambiguously localized in the interstitium and representing >50% of the SLAIIhi parenchymal cells; 3—A third MΦ-like cell was described as SLAIIhi lung population: the CD163int cells. According to their MΦ features and their CCR2 and CX3CR1 expressions, they can be considered as moMΦ; 4—inflammatory moDC CD163low; 5-cDC1, FLT3, CD172a− expressing XCR1; cDC2, CD163−/CD172a+/XCR1−/Langerin+. After the infection of pigs with two field isolates, the CD163low/moDC population was the only one that significantly increased in numbers after both swine (sw)H3N2 and swH1N2 infections. Sorted lung CD172a−/cDC1 produced more IL12A mRNA, the Th1 inducer cytokine, than CD163−/cDC1 and CD163low/moDC, both in mock and IAV-infected animals in agreement with their Th1-inducing capacities in allogeneic reactions. Neither IL13 nor IL4 transcripts, which are the Th2-inducing cytokines, were detected. Finally, no differences in IL6 transcription were observed between the three DC subsets, both at steady state and upon infections, which is in agreement with the absence of a specific allogenic Th17-inducing DC subset [31].

Recently, a study highlighted the role of the inflammasome activation within influenza virus infection, in which a 2009 pandemic H1N1 induced less IL1β than swine influenza viruses (SwIVs). Their in vitro studies revealed that the NS1 C terminus of pandemic H1N1, but not that of SwIV was able to significantly inhibit NLRP3 inflammasome-mediated IL1β production, revealing a new mechanism of innate immune evasion achieved by the NS1 protein in pH1N1/09 [111].

In summary, data showed that SwIV interacts with DC in vitro by inducing different kinetics and levels of inflammatory cytokines. Porcine pDC can produce high levels of IFNα, with subtype-specific differences in a virus-dose dependent manner, with PB2 being an important control factor for IFNα secretion in pDC. However, in vivo only CD163low/moDC population significantly increased in numbers after SwIV and lung CD172a−/cDC1 produced more IL12A mRNA than their counterparts, showing a distinctive activation pattern (Figures 2 and 3).

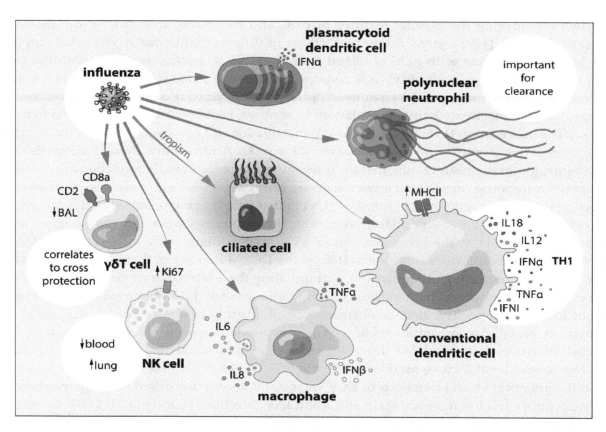

Figure 3. SwIV interaction with cells from the innate immune system and the main effects reported.

4.2. Neutrophils

Neutrophils are important host defense cells against influenza virus during the phase of innate immunity. Although the role of neutrophils against influenza virus infections has been debated, neutrophils have been shown to play a role in the control and clearance of the influenza virus in experimental models [112–115].

The results from the study from Kim et al. demonstrated SwIV nucleic acid that is present in neutrophils by in situ hybridization yet, it was not clear whether the SwIV virus could replicate in the porcine neutrophil although the human influenza virus can replicate in human neutrophils [116]. One important function of neutrophils is phagocytosis. Hence, the SwIV that was detected in the neutrophils may have resulted from uptake (Figure 3). Further study needs to determine whether SwIV can replicate in porcine neutrophils and their role in influenza infection in the pig, as the role of neutrophils in SwIV infection is far from understood (Figures 2 and 3).

4.3. NK and γδ T

Upon binding to the influenza virus, HA, the receptors trigger the NK cells to lyse the infected cell [117]. It has been suggested that invariant NKT (iNKT) cells stimulate the induction of cellular immunity and regulate infection-induced pathology [118]. With the identification of specific NK cell markers in pigs [42], some studies regarding the role of these cells in influenza infected pigs have been addressed. However, there are still few reports on the role of NK cells in swine during influenza virus infection.

Recently, it was demonstrated that NKp46+ lymphocytes accumulate in the vicinity of influenza A-infected cells in the lung of infected pigs. NKp46+NKcells are recruited from the blood to infected parts of the lungs in swine that were inoculated with the 2009 pandemic influenza virus at the same time as a decline in NKp46+ NK cells was demonstrated in the blood of infected pigs. Moreover, influenza virus does not infect the NKp46+ cells in the lungs and they do not undergo apoptosis [119].

Another study investigated the possibility that, besides NKp46+ NK cells, CD3+NKp46+ cells might also be involved in influenza infection. Thus, this lymphocyte population was analyzed in animals that were experimentally infected with the 2009 pandemic H1N1 influenza virus strain. A significant decrease in the total number of CD3+NKp46+ lymphocytes in PBMC could be observed in infected animals 1 dpi when compared with control animals. Furthermore, a significant increase in the frequency of CD3+NKp46+ lymphocytes could be detected in the lungs of infected animals as compared with the control group on day 3 pi. When compared with analyses from day 1 pi, a significant increase in proliferation by Ki67+ cells could be detected within CD3+NKp46+ cells in the lungs on day 3 pi [43]. Although anti-NKp46 mAb has been used to define NK during SwIV studies, the same approach has not been considered during PRRSV infection studies.

Likewise, few studies have been performed on the role of porcine γδ T cells during swine influenza infection. It has been shown that this subset increases in the lung following infection with H1N1 virus [120], in particular, the levels of γδ T cells were significantly higher in BAL and lower in tonsils of infected pigs when compared with control. Conversely, in another previous work, the γδ T cells percentage in the lung remained unchanged during H3N2 and H1N1 infections [121], showing a marked discrepancy in the results.

During a vaccination study, the level of γδ T cells was considered in cross-protection. A reverse genetics-derived H3N2 SwIV with truncated NS1 and wild type viruses were used to evaluate T cell priming and cross-protective efficacy against heterosubtypic H1N1 challenge. In control animals that were challenged with H1N1, there were no changes in the γδ T populations along the experiment, whereas immunization induces antigen-specific γδ T cells, including IFNγ and IL10 recall responses, before and after heterologous challenge. The group with the most robust γδ T cell responses correlated with the greatest cross-protection, suggesting that these cells may have had a protective role during the infection [122].

Finally, in a comparative study with PRRSV infection, using H1N1 SwIV in germ free piglets, the different subpopulation of NK and γδ T cells were evaluated. In the BAL of infected pigs, a decrease in the proportion of γδ T cells or NK cells was shown. The CD2+CD8a− γδ T subset was comparable to control animals, whereas CD2+CD8a+ γδ T increased, and CD2−CD8a− γδ T subset was lower than the control. In the tracheobronchial draining lymph node, there were no differences in the frequencies of NK and γδ T, but the distributions of the CD2+CD8α− subset increased. Similarly, the mesenteric lymph node analysis of γδ T cell subpopulations revealed no significant change in the proportion of any subset [97].

The few studies on the role of NK and γδ T cells during SwIV infections show that they may have a relevant function during infection and clearance, yet their interaction is far from understood (Figures 2 and 3).

5. Innate Immune Responses Triggered by SwIV and PRRSV Co-Infection

While considering PRRSV and influenza virus co-infection, it is important to point out that both of the viruses have a different cell tropism, with macrophages being the main target of PRRSV and respiratory epithelial cells the main target of SwIV. Taking into account these premises, very few studies considered PRRSV-SwIV co-infection at the molecular level in the experimental set up, although both of the viruses are relevant contributors during PRDC and lung infections [1,123,124], and their presence is frequently observed during serological studies under field conditions [4].

Epidemiological studies have been performed to construct statistical models to evaluate a significant association between PRRSV and SwIV or other co-infectious agents, and to assess the effects of changes in age and management system on coinfection status, serological profiles, lung lesions, and histological lesions. One study was performed in piglets with different ages and logistic regression models were used to assess the co-infection. Clinically ill PRRSV-positive pigs were more likely than PRRSV-negative pigs to be co-infected with SwIV and to have lung scores that were in the 11 to 50% range. Nine and 16-week old pigs were 15.57 and 5.75 times as likely to be co-infected with

SwIV, respectively [125]. Similarly, a statistically important association between pre-weaning infection with SwIV and PRRSV and post-weaning mortality was detected, with the season and number of days on feed also being associated [126]. US seroprevalence of PRRSV and SwIV co-infection in finisher herds was also estimated by the USDA NAHMS swine 2000 national study, with 4.9% herds serologically positive and 5.9% finishers (regardless the vaccination status) [127].

Early studies during the 1990s were mainly related to clinical and histopathological findings, where the inflammation of the bronchiolar wall was more pronounced in PRRSV/SwIV infected pigs than PRRSV, bronchiolar and lung lymph nodes were larger in the co-infection than in SwIV alone, but, at the end the PRRSV infection did not aggravate the acute stage of SwIV [128], or SwIV was only slightly affected by prior PRRSV [129].

Only in the last five years, Meurens' group has been the one primarily investigating the interaction between SwIV and PRRSV in an experimental in vitro system. The first study was performed in porcine alveolar macrophages (PAM) and precision cut lung slices (PCLS) from eight-week-old pigs. They used the PRRSV-2 VR-2385 and SwIV Canadian strain H1N1 applied simultaneously or 3 h apart on PAM and PCLS for 18 h. Interference that was caused by the first virus on replication of the second was observed and a synergic effect between PRRSV and SwIV was observed for some transcripts, such as TLR3, RIG1, and IFNβ in PCLS. PRRSV infection 3 h prior SwIV reduced the response to SwIV, while the SwIV infection prior to PRRSV infection had limited impact [130]. The second recent study was performed in a trachea epithelial cell line expressing CD163 (NPTr-CD163), which is the main receptor for PRRSV. The cell line was receptive to both viruses and was used to assess the interference between the two. SwIV and PRRSV interacted differently with the modified cell line, but they were interfering each other in terms of replication when infected in the same cell with consequence on the antiviral response (LGP2, MDA5, TLR8, IFNα, IFNβ, IFNλ1, MX2, OAS, PKR) [131].

More studies are required to precisely define the interaction of both viruses on the immune system and the consequences for disease and vaccination.

6. Conclusions

Given the importance of the innate immune system during the first critical hours and days of exposure to a new pathogen, it is surprising to realize how scattered the information is when speaking about two of the main players in PRDC. PRRSV interaction with MΦ and DC has been studied in some detail, but there are controversial data between different groups. For SwIV, the picture seems more in agreement, but the whole picture of fine-tuning mechanisms of virus interaction with the host innate immune is still far from complete. The modulation of NK, PMN, or γδ T cells, in general, has not received as much attention as their APC counterparts and there are numerous gaps in the knowledge regarding the role of these cells in both virus infections and their interaction between them. Finally, studies on the co-infection of PRRSV-SwIV have received little attention within the scientific community, and even epidemiological studies have shown significant association between PRRSV and SwIV. Studies in these directions will pave the way to understand PRDC in better detail and possible design strategies to combat this disease.

Acknowledgments: The authors thank Rada Ellegård for Figures 1–3 and Kyle Miskell for editing English language.

References

1. Opriessnig, T.; Gimenez-Lirola, L.G.; Halbur, P.G. Polymicrobial respiratory disease in pigs. *Anim. Health Res. Rev.* **2011**, *12*, 133–148. [CrossRef] [PubMed]

2. Susan, L.; Brockmeier, P.G.H.; Thacker, E.L. Porcine Respiratory Disease Complex. In *Polymicrobial Diseases*; Brogden, K.A., Guthmiller, J.M., Eds.; ASM Press: Washington, DC, USA, 2002. [CrossRef]

3. Thacker, E.L. Immunology of the porcine respiratory disease complex. *Vet. Clin. N. Am. Food Anim. Pract.* **2001**, *17*, 551–565. [CrossRef]

4. Fraile, L.; Alegre, A.; Lopez-Jimenez, R.; Nofrarias, M.; Segales, J. Risk factors associated with pleuritis and cranio-ventral pulmonary consolidation in slaughter-aged pigs. *Vet. J.* **2010**, *184*, 326–333. [CrossRef] [PubMed]

5. Sassu, E.L.; Bosse, J.T.; Tobias, T.J.; Gottschalk, M.; Langford, P.R.; Hennig-Pauka, I. Update on Actinobacillus pleuropneumoniae-knowledge, gaps and challenges. *Transbound. Emerg. Dis.* **2018**, *65* (Suppl. 1), 72–90. [CrossRef] [PubMed]

6. Zimmerman, J.J. *Diseases of Swine*, 10th ed.; Locke, A., Karriker, J.Z., Alejandro, R., Kent, S., Gregory, S., Eds.; Wiley—Blackwell: Chichester, West Sussex, UK, 2012.

7. Qin, S.; Ruan, W.; Yue, H.; Tang, C.; Zhou, K.; Zhang, B. Viral communities associated with porcine respiratory disease complex in intensive commercial farms in Sichuan province, China. *Sci. Rep.* **2018**, *8*, 13341. [CrossRef] [PubMed]

8. Yassin, A.F.; Hupfer, H.; Siering, C.; Schumann, P. Comparative chemotaxonomic and phylogenetic studies on the genus Arcanobacterium Collins et al. 1982 emend. Lehnen et al. 2006: Proposal for Trueperella gen. nov. and emended description of the genus Arcanobacterium. *Int. J. Syst. Evol. Microbiol.* **2011**, *61*, 1265–1274. [CrossRef] [PubMed]

9. Butler, J.E.; Lager, K.M.; Golde, W.; Faaberg, K.S.; Sinkora, M.; Loving, C.; Zhang, Y.I. Porcine reproductive and respiratory syndrome (PRRS): An immune dysregulatory pandemic. *Immunol. Res.* **2014**, *59*, 81–108. [CrossRef] [PubMed]

10. Lunney, J.K.; Fang, Y.; Ladinig, A.; Chen, N.; Li, Y.; Rowland, B.; Renukaradhya, G.J. Porcine Reproductive and Respiratory Syndrome Virus (PRRSV): Pathogenesis and Interaction with the Immune System. *Annu. Rev. Anim. Biosci.* **2016**, *4*, 129–154. [CrossRef] [PubMed]

11. Kappes, M.A.; Faaberg, K.S. PRRSV structure, replication and recombination: Origin of phenotype and genotype diversity. *Virology* **2015**, *479–480*, 475–486. [CrossRef] [PubMed]

12. Kuhn, J.H.; Lauck, M.; Bailey, A.L.; Shchetinin, A.M.; Vishnevskaya, T.V.; Bao, Y.; Ng, T.F.; LeBreton, M.; Schneider, B.S.; Gillis, A.; et al. Reorganization and expansion of the nidoviral family Arteriviridae. *Arch. Virol.* **2016**, *161*, 755–768. [CrossRef] [PubMed]

13. Duan, X.; Nauwynck, H.J.; Pensaert, M.B. Effects of origin and state of differentiation and activation of monocytes/macrophages on their susceptibility to porcine reproductive and respiratory syndrome virus (PRRSV). *Arch. Virol.* **1997**, *142*, 2483–2497. [CrossRef] [PubMed]

14. Bordet, E.; Maisonnasse, P.; Renson, P.; Bouguyon, E.; Crisci, E.; Tiret, M.; Descamps, D.; Bernelin-Cottet, C.; Urien, C.; Lefevre, F.; et al. Porcine Alveolar Macrophage-like cells are pro-inflammatory Pulmonary Intravascular Macrophages that produce large titers of Porcine Reproductive and Respiratory Syndrome Virus. *Sci. Rep.* **2018**, *8*, 10172. [CrossRef] [PubMed]

15. Zhang, Q.; Yoo, D. PRRS virus receptors and their role for pathogenesis. *Vet. Microbiol.* **2015**, *177*, 229–241. [CrossRef] [PubMed]

16. Burkard, C.; Lillico, S.G.; Reid, E.; Jackson, B.; Mileham, A.J.; Ait-Ali, T.; Whitelaw, C.B.; Archibald, A.L. Precision engineering for PRRSV resistance in pigs: Macrophages from genome edited pigs lacking CD163 SRCR5 domain are fully resistant to both PRRSV genotypes while maintaining biological function. *PLoS Pathog.* **2017**, *13*, e1006206. [CrossRef] [PubMed]

17. Whitworth, K.M.; Rowland, R.R.; Ewen, C.L.; Trible, B.R.; Kerrigan, M.A.; Cino-Ozuna, A.G.; Samuel, M.S.; Lightner, J.E.; McLaren, D.G.; Mileham, A.J.; et al. Gene-edited pigs are protected from porcine reproductive and respiratory syndrome virus. *Nat. Biotechnol.* **2016**, *34*, 20–22. [CrossRef] [PubMed]

18. Krammer, F.; Smith, G.J.D.; Fouchier, R.A.M.; Peiris, M.; Kedzierska, K.; Doherty, P.C.; Palese, P.; Shaw, M.L.; Treanor, J.; Webster, R.G.; et al. Influenza. *Nat. Rev. Dis. Primers* **2018**, *4*, 4. [CrossRef] [PubMed]

19. Tong, S.; Zhu, X.; Li, Y.; Shi, M.; Zhang, J.; Bourgeois, M.; Yang, H.; Chen, X.; Recuenco, S.; Gomez, J.; et al. New world bats harbor diverse influenza A viruses. *PLoS Pathog.* **2013**, *9*, e1003657. [CrossRef] [PubMed]

20. Medina, R.A.; Garcia-Sastre, A. Influenza A viruses: New research developments. *Nat. Rev. Microbiol.* **2011**, *9*, 590–603. [CrossRef] [PubMed]

21. Webster, R.G.; Bean, W.J.; Gorman, O.T.; Chambers, T.M.; Kawaoka, Y. Evolution and ecology of influenza A viruses. *Microbiol. Rev.* **1992**, *56*, 152–179. [PubMed]

22. Vincent, A.; Awada, L.; Brown, I.; Chen, H.; Claes, F.; Dauphin, G.; Donis, R.; Culhane, M.; Hamilton, K.; Lewis, N.; et al. Review of influenza A virus in swine worldwide: A call for increased surveillance and research. *Zoonoses Public Health* **2014**, *61*, 4–17. [CrossRef] [PubMed]

23. Bourret, V. Avian influenza viruses in pigs: An overview. *Vet. J.* **2018**, *239*, 7–14. [CrossRef] [PubMed]

24. Solorzano, A.; Foni, E.; Cordoba, L.; Baratelli, M.; Razzuoli, E.; Bilato, D.; Martin del Burgo, M.A.; Perlin, D.S.; Martinez, J.; Martinez-Orellana, P.; et al. Cross-Species Infectivity of H3N8 Influenza Virus in an Experimental Infection in Swine. *J. Virol.* **2015**, *89*, 11190–11202. [CrossRef] [PubMed]

25. Kahn, R.E.; Ma, W.; Richt, J.A. Swine and influenza: A challenge to one health research. *Curr. Top. Microbiol. Immunol.* **2014**, *385*, 205–218. [CrossRef] [PubMed]

26. Crisci, E.; Mussa, T.; Fraile, L.; Montoya, M. Review: Influenza virus in pigs. *Mol. Immunol.* **2013**, *55*, 200–211. [CrossRef] [PubMed]

27. Mair, K.H.; Sedlak, C.; Kaser, T.; Pasternak, A.; Levast, B.; Gerner, W.; Saalmuller, A.; Summerfield, A.; Gerdts, V.; Wilson, H.L.; et al. The porcine innate immune system: An update. *Dev. Comp. Immunol.* **2014**, *45*, 321–343. [CrossRef] [PubMed]

28. Summerfield, A.; McCullough, K.C. The porcine dendritic cell family. *Dev. Comp. Immunol.* **2009**, *33*, 299–309. [CrossRef] [PubMed]

29. Carrasco, C.P.; Rigden, R.C.; Schaffner, R.; Gerber, H.; Neuhaus, V.; Inumaru, S.; Takamatsu, H.; Bertoni, G.; McCullough, K.C.; Summerfield, A. Porcine dendritic cells generated in vitro: Morphological, phenotypic and functional properties. *Immunology* **2001**, *104*, 175–184. [CrossRef] [PubMed]

30. Edwards, J.C.; Everett, H.E.; Pedrera, M.; Mokhtar, H.; Marchi, E.; Soldevila, F.; Kaveh, D.A.; Hogarth, P.J.; Johns, H.L.; Nunez-Garcia, J.; et al. CD1(−) and CD1(+) porcine blood dendritic cells are enriched for the orthologues of the two major mammalian conventional subsets. *Sci. Rep.* **2017**, *7*, 40942. [CrossRef] [PubMed]

31. Maisonnasse, P.; Bouguyon, E.; Piton, G.; Ezquerra, A.; Urien, C.; Deloizy, C.; Bourge, M.; Leplat, J.J.; Simon, G.; Chevalier, C.; et al. The respiratory DC/macrophage network at steady-state and upon influenza infection in the swine biomedical model. *Mucosal Immunol.* **2016**, *9*, 835–849. [CrossRef] [PubMed]

32. Ezquerra, A.; Revilla, C.; Alvarez, B.; Perez, C.; Alonso, F.; Dominguez, J. Porcine myelomonocytic markers and cell populations. *Dev. Comp. Immunol.* **2009**, *33*, 284–298. [CrossRef] [PubMed]

33. Arora, S.; Dev, K.; Agarwal, B.; Das, P.; Syed, M.A. Macrophages: Their role, activation and polarization in pulmonary diseases. *Immunobiology* **2018**, *223*, 383–396. [CrossRef] [PubMed]

34. Sang, Y.; Rowland, R.R.; Blecha, F. Interaction between innate immunity and porcine reproductive and respiratory syndrome virus. *Anim. Health Res. Rev.* **2011**, *12*, 149–167. [CrossRef] [PubMed]

35. Sica, A.; Mantovani, A. Macrophage plasticity and polarization: In vivo veritas. *J. Clin. Investig.* **2012**, *122*, 787–795. [CrossRef] [PubMed]

36. Liegeois, M.; Legrand, C.; Desmet, C.J.; Marichal, T.; Bureau, F. The interstitial macrophage: A long-neglected piece in the puzzle of lung immunity. *Cell. Immunol.* **2018**, *330*, 91–96. [CrossRef] [PubMed]

37. Thanawongnuwech, R.; Halbur, P.G.; Thacker, E.L. The role of pulmonary intravascular macrophages in porcine reproductive and respiratory syndrome virus infection. *Anim. Health Res. Rev.* **2000**, *1*, 95–102. [CrossRef] [PubMed]

38. Brea, D.; Meurens, F.; Dubois, A.V.; Gaillard, J.; Chevaleyre, C.; Jourdan, M.L.; Winter, N.; Arbeille, B.; Si-Tahar, M.; Gauthier, F.; et al. The pig as a model for investigating the role of neutrophil serine proteases in human inflammatory lung diseases. *Biochem. J.* **2012**, *447*, 363–370. [CrossRef] [PubMed]

39. Denyer, M.S.; Wileman, T.E.; Stirling, C.M.; Zuber, B.; Takamatsu, H.H. Perforin expression can define CD8 positive lymphocyte subsets in pigs allowing phenotypic and functional analysis of natural killer, cytotoxic T, natural killer T and MHC un-restricted cytotoxic T-cells. *Vet. Immunol. Immunopathol.* **2006**, *110*, 279–292. [CrossRef] [PubMed]

40. Takamatsu, H.H.; Denyer, M.S.; Stirling, C.; Cox, S.; Aggarwal, N.; Dash, P.; Wileman, T.E.; Barnett, P.V. Porcine gammadelta T cells: Possible roles on the innate and adaptive immune responses following virus infection. *Vet. Immunol. Immunopathol.* **2006**, *112*, 49–61. [CrossRef] [PubMed]

41. Gerner, W.; Kaser, T.; Saalmuller, A. Porcine T lymphocytes and NK cells—An update. *Dev. Comp. Immunol.* **2009**, *33*, 310–320. [CrossRef] [PubMed]

42. Mair, K.H.; Essler, S.E.; Patzl, M.; Storset, A.K.; Saalmuller, A.; Gerner, W. NKp46 expression discriminates porcine NK cells with different functional properties. *Eur. J. Immunol.* **2012**, *42*, 1261–1271. [CrossRef] [PubMed]

43. Mair, K.H.; Stadler, M.; Talker, S.C.; Forberg, H.; Storset, A.K.; Mullebner, A.; Duvigneau, J.C.; Hammer, S.E.; Saalmuller, A.; Gerner, W. Porcine CD3(+)NKp46(+) Lymphocytes Have NK-Cell Characteristics and Are Present in Increased Frequencies in the Lungs of Influenza-Infected Animals. *Front. Immunol.* **2016**, *7*, 263. [CrossRef] [PubMed]

44. Stepanova, K.; Sinkora, M. The expression of CD25, CD11b, SWC1, SWC7, MHC-II, and family of CD45 molecules can be used to characterize different stages of gammadelta T lymphocytes in pigs. *Dev. Comp. Immunol.* **2012**, *36*, 728–740. [CrossRef] [PubMed]

45. Stepanova, K.; Sinkora, M. Porcine gammadelta T lymphocytes can be categorized into two functionally and developmentally distinct subsets according to expression of CD2 and level of TCR. *J. Immunol.* **2013**, *190*, 2111–2120. [CrossRef] [PubMed]

46. Holtkamp, D.J.; Kliebenstein, J.B.; Neumann, E.J. Assessment of the economic impact of porcine reproductive and respiratory syndrome virus on United States pork producers. *J. Swine Health Prod.* **2013**, *21*, 72–84.

47. Loving, C.L.; Osorio, F.A.; Murtaugh, M.P.; Zuckermann, F.A. Innate and adaptive immunity against Porcine Reproductive and Respiratory Syndrome Virus. *Vet. Immunol. Immunopathol.* **2015**, *167*, 1–14. [CrossRef] [PubMed]

48. Bordet, E.; Blanc, F.; Tiret, M.; Crisci, E.; Bouguyon, E.; Renson, P.; Maisonnasse, P.; Bourge, M.; Leplat, J.J.; Giuffra, E.; et al. Porcine Reproductive and Respiratory Syndrome Virus Type 1.3 Lena Triggers Conventional Dendritic Cells 1 Activation and T Helper 1 Immune Response Without Infecting Dendritic Cells. *Front. Immunol.* **2018**, *9*, 2299. [CrossRef] [PubMed]

49. Darwich, L.; Diaz, I.; Mateu, E. Certainties, doubts and hypotheses in porcine reproductive and respiratory syndrome virus immunobiology. *Virus Res.* **2010**, *154*, 123–132. [CrossRef] [PubMed]

50. Wang, L.; Hu, S.; Liu, Q.; Li, Y.; Xu, L.; Zhang, Z.; Cai, X.; He, X. Porcine alveolar macrophage polarization is involved in inhibition of porcine reproductive and respiratory syndrome virus (PRRSV) replication. *J. Vet. Med. Sci.* **2017**, *79*, 1906–1915. [CrossRef] [PubMed]

51. Jiang, Z.; Zhou, X.; Michal, J.J.; Wu, X.L.; Zhang, L.; Zhang, M.; Ding, B.; Liu, B.; Manoranjan, V.S.; Neill, J.D.; et al. Reactomes of porcine alveolar macrophages infected with porcine reproductive and respiratory syndrome virus. *PLoS ONE* **2013**, *8*, e59229. [CrossRef] [PubMed]

52. Zeng, N.; Wang, C.; Liu, S.; Miao, Q.; Zhou, L.; Ge, X.; Han, J.; Guo, X.; Yang, H. Transcriptome Analysis Reveals Dynamic Gene Expression Profiles in Porcine Alveolar Macrophages in Response to the Chinese Highly Pathogenic Porcine Reproductive and Respiratory Syndrome Virus. *BioMed Res. Int.* **2018**, *2018*, 1538127. [CrossRef] [PubMed]

53. Wang, L.; Zhou, L.; Hu, D.; Ge, X.; Guo, X.; Yang, H. Porcine reproductive and respiratory syndrome virus suppresses post-transcriptionally the protein expression of IFN-beta by upregulating cellular microRNAs in porcine alveolar macrophages in vitro. *Exp. Ther. Med.* **2018**, *15*, 115–126. [CrossRef] [PubMed]

54. Zhang, J.; Sun, P.; Gan, L.; Bai, W.; Wang, Z.; Li, D.; Cao, Y.; Fu, Y.; Li, P.; Bai, X.; et al. Genome-wide analysis of long noncoding RNA profiling in PRRSV-infected PAM cells by RNA sequencing. *Sci. Rep.* **2017**, *7*, 4952. [CrossRef] [PubMed]

55. Wang, C.; Shi, X.; Zhang, X.; Wang, A.; Wang, L.; Chen, J.; Deng, R.; Zhang, G. The Endoribonuclease Activity Essential for the Nonstructural Protein 11 of Porcine Reproductive and Respiratory Syndrome Virus to Inhibit NLRP3 Inflammasome-Mediated IL-1beta Induction. *DNA Cell Biol.* **2015**, *34*, 728–735. [CrossRef] [PubMed]

56. Bi, J.; Song, S.; Fang, L.; Wang, D.; Jing, H.; Gao, L.; Cai, Y.; Luo, R.; Chen, H.; Xiao, S. Porcine reproductive and respiratory syndrome virus induces IL-1beta production depending on TLR4/MyD88 pathway and NLRP3 inflammasome in primary porcine alveolar macrophages. *Mediat. Inflamm.* **2014**, *2014*, 403515. [CrossRef] [PubMed]

57. Liang, W.; Ji, L.; Zhang, Y.; Zhen, Y.; Zhang, Q.; Xu, X.; Liu, B. Transcriptome Differences in Porcine Alveolar Macrophages from Tongcheng and Large White Pigs in Response to Highly Pathogenic Porcine Reproductive and Respiratory Syndrome Virus (PRRSV) Infection. *Int. J. Mol. Sci.* **2017**, *18*, 1475. [CrossRef] [PubMed]

58. Charerntantanakul, W.; Platt, R.; Roth, J.A. Effects of porcine reproductive and respiratory syndrome virus-infected antigen-presenting cells on T cell activation and antiviral cytokine production. *Viral Immunol.* **2006**, *19*, 646–661. [CrossRef] [PubMed]

59. Flores-Mendoza, L.; Silva-Campa, E.; Resendiz, M.; Osorio, F.A.; Hernandez, J. Porcine reproductive and respiratory syndrome virus infects mature porcine dendritic cells and up-regulates interleukin-10 production. *Clin. Vaccine Immunol.* **2008**, *15*, 720–725. [CrossRef] [PubMed]

60. Loving, C.L.; Brockmeier, S.L.; Sacco, R.E. Differential type I interferon activation and susceptibility of dendritic cell populations to porcine arterivirus. *Immunology* **2007**, *120*, 217–229. [CrossRef] [PubMed]

61. Pineyro, P.E.; Subramaniam, S.; Kenney, S.P.; Heffron, C.L.; Gimenez-Lirola, L.G.; Meng, X.J. Modulation of Proinflammatory Cytokines in Monocyte-Derived Dendritic Cells by Porcine Reproductive and Respiratory Syndrome Virus Through Interaction with the Porcine Intercellular-Adhesion-Molecule-3-Grabbing Nonintegrin. *Viral Immunol.* **2016**, *29*, 546–556. [CrossRef] [PubMed]

62. Rodriguez-Gomez, I.M.; Kaser, T.; Gomez-Laguna, J.; Lamp, B.; Sinn, L.; Rumenapf, T.; Carrasco, L.; Saalmuller, A.; Gerner, W. PRRSV-infected monocyte-derived dendritic cells express high levels of SLA-DR and CD80/86 but do not stimulate PRRSV-naive regulatory T cells to proliferate. *Vet. Res.* **2015**, *46*, 54. [CrossRef] [PubMed]

63. Silva-Campa, E.; Cordoba, L.; Fraile, L.; Flores-Mendoza, L.; Montoya, M.; Hernandez, J. European genotype of porcine reproductive and respiratory syndrome (PRRSV) infects monocyte-derived dendritic cells but does not induce Treg cells. *Virology* **2010**, *396*, 264–271. [CrossRef] [PubMed]

64. Singleton, H.; Graham, S.P.; Bodman-Smith, K.B.; Frossard, J.P.; Steinbach, F. Establishing Porcine Monocyte-Derived Macrophage and Dendritic Cell Systems for Studying the Interaction with PRRSV-1. *Front. Microbiol.* **2016**, *7*, 832. [CrossRef] [PubMed]

65. Liu, J.; Wei, S.; Liu, L.; Shan, F.; Zhao, Y.; Shen, G. The role of porcine reproductive and respiratory syndrome virus infection in immune phenotype and Th1/Th2 balance of dendritic cells. *Dev. Comp. Immunol.* **2016**, *65*, 245–252. [CrossRef] [PubMed]

66. Proll, M.J.; Neuhoff, C.; Schellander, K.; Uddin, M.J.; Cinar, M.U.; Sahadevan, S.; Qu, X.; Islam, M.A.; Poirier, M.; Muller, M.A.; et al. Transcriptome profile of lung dendritic cells after in vitro porcine reproductive and respiratory syndrome virus (PRRSV) infection. *PLoS ONE* **2017**, *12*, e0187735. [CrossRef] [PubMed]

67. Resendiz, M.; Valenzuela, O.; Hernandez, J. Response of the cDC1 and cDC2 subtypes of tracheal dendritic cells to porcine reproductive and respiratory syndrome virus. *Vet. Microbiol.* **2018**, *223*, 27–33. [CrossRef] [PubMed]

68. Wang, X.; Eaton, M.; Mayer, M.; Li, H.; He, D.; Nelson, E.; Christopher-Hennings, J. Porcine reproductive and respiratory syndrome virus productively infects monocyte-derived dendritic cells and compromises their antigen-presenting ability. *Arch. Virol.* **2007**, *152*, 289–303. [CrossRef] [PubMed]

69. Park, J.Y.; Kim, H.S.; Seo, S.H. Characterization of interaction between porcine reproductive and respiratory syndrome virus and porcine dendritic cells. *J. Microbiol. Biotechnol.* **2008**, *18*, 1709–1716. [PubMed]

70. Chen, X.; Bai, J.; Liu, X.; Song, Z.; Zhang, Q.; Wang, X.; Jiang, P. Nsp1alpha of Porcine Reproductive and Respiratory Syndrome Virus Strain BB0907 Impairs the Function of Monocyte-Derived Dendritic Cells via the Release of Soluble CD83. *J. Virol.* **2018**, *92*, e00366-18. [CrossRef] [PubMed]

71. Chen, X.; Zhang, Q.; Bai, J.; Zhao, Y.; Wang, X.; Wang, H.; Jiang, P. The Nucleocapsid Protein and Nonstructural Protein 10 of Highly Pathogenic Porcine Reproductive and Respiratory Syndrome Virus Enhance CD83 Production via NF-kappaB and Sp1 Signaling Pathways. *J. Virol.* **2017**, *91*, e00986-17. [CrossRef] [PubMed]

72. Zhang, H.; Guo, X.; Nelson, E.; Christopher-Hennings, J.; Wang, X. Porcine reproductive and respiratory syndrome virus activates the transcription of interferon alpha/beta (IFN-alpha/beta) in monocyte-derived dendritic cells (Mo-DC). *Vet. Microbiol.* **2012**, *159*, 494–498. [CrossRef] [PubMed]

73. Silva-Campa, E.; Flores-Mendoza, L.; Resendiz, M.; Pinelli-Saavedra, A.; Mata-Haro, V.; Mwangi, W.; Hernandez, J. Induction of T helper 3 regulatory cells by dendritic cells infected with porcine reproductive and respiratory syndrome virus. *Virology* **2009**, *387*, 373–379. [CrossRef] [PubMed]

74. Gimeno, M.; Darwich, L.; Diaz, I.; de la Torre, E.; Pujols, J.; Martin, M.; Inumaru, S.; Cano, E.; Domingo, M.; Montoya, M.; et al. Cytokine profiles and phenotype regulation of antigen presenting cells by genotype-I porcine reproductive and respiratory syndrome virus isolates. *Vet. Res.* **2011**, *42*, 9. [CrossRef] [PubMed]

75. Weesendorp, E.; Stockhofe-Zurwieden, N.; Popma-De Graaf, D.J.; Fijten, H.; Rebel, J.M. Phenotypic modulation and cytokine profiles of antigen presenting cells by European subtype 1 and 3 porcine reproductive and respiratory syndrome virus strains in vitro and in vivo. *Vet. Microbiol.* **2013**, *167*, 638–650. [CrossRef] [PubMed]

76. Li, Y.L.; Darwich, L.; Mateu, E. Characterization of the attachment and infection by Porcine reproductive and respiratory syndrome virus 1 isolates in bone marrow-derived dendritic cells. *Vet. Microbiol.* **2018**, *223*, 181–188. [CrossRef] [PubMed]

77. Doeschl-Wilson, A.; Wilson, A.; Nielsen, J.; Nauwynck, H.; Archibald, A.; Ait-Ali, T. Combining laboratory and mathematical models to infer mechanisms underlying kinetic changes in macrophage susceptibility to an RNA virus. *BMC Syst. Biol.* **2016**, *10*, 101. [CrossRef] [PubMed]

78. Frydas, I.S.; Verbeeck, M.; Cao, J.; Nauwynck, H.J. Replication characteristics of porcine reproductive and respiratory syndrome virus (PRRSV) European subtype 1 (Lelystad) and subtype 3 (Lena) strains in nasal mucosa and cells of the monocytic lineage: Indications for the use of new receptors of PRRSV (Lena). *Vet. Res.* **2013**, *44*, 73. [CrossRef] [PubMed]

79. Colonna, M.; Trinchieri, G.; Liu, Y.J. Plasmacytoid dendritic cells in immunity. *Nat. Immunol.* **2004**, *5*, 1219–1226. [CrossRef] [PubMed]

80. Calzada-Nova, G.; Schnitzlein, W.; Husmann, R.; Zuckermann, F.A. Characterization of the cytokine and maturation responses of pure populations of porcine plasmacytoid dendritic cells to porcine viruses and toll-like receptor agonists. *Vet. Immunol. Immunopathol.* **2010**, *135*, 20–33. [CrossRef] [PubMed]

81. Calzada-Nova, G.; Schnitzlein, W.M.; Husmann, R.J.; Zuckermann, F.A. North American porcine reproductive and respiratory syndrome viruses inhibit type I interferon production by plasmacytoid dendritic cells. *J. Virol.* **2011**, *85*, 2703–2713. [CrossRef] [PubMed]

82. Baumann, A.; Mateu, E.; Murtaugh, M.P.; Summerfield, A. Impact of genotype 1 and 2 of porcine reproductive and respiratory syndrome viruses on interferon-alpha responses by plasmacytoid dendritic cells. *Vet. Res.* **2013**, *44*, 33. [CrossRef] [PubMed]

83. Garcia-Nicolas, O.; Auray, G.; Sautter, C.A.; Rappe, J.C.; McCullough, K.C.; Ruggli, N.; Summerfield, A. Sensing of Porcine Reproductive and Respiratory Syndrome Virus-Infected Macrophages by Plasmacytoid Dendritic Cells. *Front. Microbiol.* **2016**, *7*, 771. [CrossRef] [PubMed]

84. Abella, G.; Pena, R.N.; Nogareda, C.; Armengol, R.; Vidal, A.; Moradell, L.; Tarancon, V.; Novell, E.; Estany, J.; Fraile, L. A WUR SNP is associated with European Porcine Reproductive and Respiratory Virus Syndrome resistance and growth performance in pigs. *Res. Vet. Sci.* **2016**, *104*, 117–122. [CrossRef] [PubMed]

85. Dekkers, J.; Rowland, R.R.R.; Lunney, J.K.; Plastow, G. Host genetics of response to porcine reproductive and respiratory syndrome in nursery pigs. *Vet. Microbiol.* **2017**, *209*, 107–113. [CrossRef] [PubMed]

86. Koltes, J.E.; Fritz-Waters, E.; Eisley, C.J.; Choi, I.; Bao, H.; Kommadath, A.; Serao, N.V.; Boddicker, N.J.; Abrams, S.M.; Schroyen, M.; et al. Identification of a putative quantitative trait nucleotide in guanylate binding protein 5 for host response to PRRS virus infection. *BMC Genomics* **2015**, *16*, 412. [CrossRef] [PubMed]

87. Reiner, G. Genetic resistance—An alternative for controlling PRRS? *Porcine Health Manag.* **2016**, *2*, 27. [CrossRef] [PubMed]

88. Han, D.; Hu, Y.; Li, L.; Tian, H.; Chen, Z.; Wang, L.; Ma, H.; Yang, H.; Teng, K. Highly pathogenic porcine reproductive and respiratory syndrome virus infection results in acute lung injury of the infected pigs. *Vet. Microbiol.* **2014**, *169*, 135–146. [CrossRef] [PubMed]

89. Girard, M.; Cleroux, P.; Tremblay, P.; Dea, S.; St-Pierre, Y. Increased proteolytic activity and matrix metalloprotease expression in lungs during infection by porcine reproductive and respiratory syndrome virus. *J. Gen. Virol.* **2001**, *82*, 1253–1261. [CrossRef] [PubMed]

90. Wan, B.; Qiao, S.; Li, P.; Jin, Q.; Liu, Y.; Bao, D.; Liu, M.; Wang, Y.; Zhang, G. Impairment of the antibody-dependent phagocytic function of PMNs through regulation of the FcgammaRs expression after porcine reproductive and respiratory syndrome virus infection. *PLoS ONE* **2013**, *8*, e66965. [CrossRef] [PubMed]

91. Liu, J.; Hou, M.; Yan, M.; Lu, X.; Gu, W.; Zhang, S.; Gao, J.; Liu, B.; Wu, X.; Liu, G. ICAM-1-dependent and ICAM-1-independent neutrophil lung infiltration by porcine reproductive and respiratory syndrome virus infection. *Am. J. Physiol. Lung Cell. Mol. Physiol.* **2015**, *309*, L226–L236. [CrossRef] [PubMed]

92. Liu, Y.; Du, Y.; Wang, H.; Du, L.; Feng, W.H. Porcine reproductive and respiratory syndrome virus (PRRSV) up-regulates IL-8 expression through TAK-1/JNK/AP-1 pathways. *Virology* **2017**, *506*, 64–72. [CrossRef] [PubMed]

93. Lopez Fuertes, L.; Domenech, N.; Alvarez, B.; Ezquerra, A.; Dominguez, J.; Castro, J.M.; Alonso, F. Analysis of cellular immune response in pigs recovered from porcine respiratory and reproductive syndrome infection. *Virus Res.* **1999**, *64*, 33–42. [CrossRef]

94. Samsom, J.N.; de Bruin, T.G.; Voermans, J.J.; Meulenberg, J.J.; Pol, J.M.; Bianchi, A.T. Changes of leukocyte phenotype and function in the broncho-alveolar lavage fluid of pigs infected with porcine reproductive and respiratory syndrome virus: A role for CD8(+) cells. *J. Gen. Virol.* **2000**, *81*, 497–505. [CrossRef] [PubMed]

95. Weesendorp, E.; Rebel, J.M.; Popma-De Graaf, D.J.; Fijten, H.P.; Stockhofe-Zurwieden, N. Lung pathogenicity of European genotype 3 strain porcine reproductive and respiratory syndrome virus (PRRSV) differs from that of subtype 1 strains. *Vet. Microbiol.* **2014**, *174*, 127–138. [CrossRef] [PubMed]

96. Lamontagne, L.; Page, C.; Larochelle, R.; Magar, R. Porcine reproductive and respiratory syndrome virus persistence in blood, spleen, lymph nodes, and tonsils of experimentally infected pigs depends on the level of CD8high T cells. *Viral Immunol.* **2003**, *16*, 395–406. [CrossRef] [PubMed]

97. Sinkora, M.; Butler, J.E.; Lager, K.M.; Potockova, H.; Sinkorova, J. The comparative profile of lymphoid cells and the T and B cell spectratype of germ-free piglets infected with viruses SIV, PRRSV or PCV2. *Vet. Res.* **2014**, *45*, 91. [CrossRef] [PubMed]

98. Olin, M.R.; Batista, L.; Xiao, Z.; Dee, S.A.; Murtaugh, M.P.; Pijoan, C.C.; Molitor, T.W. Gammadelta lymphocyte response to porcine reproductive and respiratory syndrome virus. *Viral Immunol.* **2005**, *18*, 490–499. [CrossRef] [PubMed]

99. Xiao, Z.; Batista, L.; Dee, S.; Halbur, P.; Murtaugh, M.P. The level of virus-specific T-cell and macrophage recruitment in porcine reproductive and respiratory syndrome virus infection in pigs is independent of virus load. *J. Virol.* **2004**, *78*, 5923–5933. [CrossRef] [PubMed]

100. Dwivedi, V.; Manickam, C.; Binjawadagi, B.; Linhares, D.; Murtaugh, M.P.; Renukaradhya, G.J. Evaluation of immune responses to porcine reproductive and respiratory syndrome virus in pigs during early stage of infection under farm conditions. *Virol. J.* **2012**, *9*, 45. [CrossRef] [PubMed]

101. Cao, J.; Grauwet, K.; Vermeulen, B.; Devriendt, B.; Jiang, P.; Favoreel, H.; Nauwynck, H. Suppression of NK cell-mediated cytotoxicity against PRRSV-infected porcine alveolar macrophages in vitro. *Vet. Microbiol.* **2013**, *164*, 261–269. [CrossRef] [PubMed]

102. Cao, Q.M.; Ni, Y.Y.; Cao, D.; Tian, D.; Yugo, D.M.; Heffron, C.L.; Overend, C.; Subramaniam, S.; Rogers, A.J.; Catanzaro, N.; et al. Recombinant Porcine Reproductive and Respiratory Syndrome Virus Expressing Membrane-Bound Interleukin-15 as an Immunomodulatory Adjuvant Enhances NK and gammadelta T Cell Responses and Confers Heterologous Protection. *J. Virol.* **2018**, *92*. [CrossRef] [PubMed]

103. Kim, B.; Ahn, K.K.; Ha, Y.; Lee, Y.H.; Kim, D.; Lim, J.H.; Kim, S.H.; Kim, M.Y.; Cho, K.D.; Lee, B.H.; et al. Association of tumor necrosis factor-alpha with fever and pulmonary lesion score in pigs experimentally infected with swine influenza virus subtype H1N2. *J. Vet. Med. Sci.* **2009**, *71*, 611–616. [CrossRef] [PubMed]

104. Gao, W.; Sun, W.; Qu, B.; Cardona, C.J.; Powell, K.; Wegner, M.; Shi, Y.; Xing, Z. Distinct regulation of host responses by ERK and JNK MAP kinases in swine macrophages infected with pandemic (H1N1) 2009 influenza virus. *PLoS ONE* **2012**, *7*, e30328. [CrossRef] [PubMed]

105. Barbe, F.; Atanasova, K.; Van Reeth, K. Cytokines and acute phase proteins associated with acute swine influenza infection in pigs. *Vet. J.* **2011**, *187*, 48–53. [CrossRef] [PubMed]

106. Mussa, T.; Rodriguez-Carino, C.; Pujol, M.; Cordoba, L.; Busquets, N.; Crisci, E.; Dominguez, J.; Fraile, L.; Montoya, M. Interaction of porcine conventional dendritic cells with swine influenza virus. *Virology* **2011**, *420*, 125–134. [CrossRef] [PubMed]

107. Mussa, T.; Ballester, M.; Silva-Campa, E.; Baratelli, M.; Busquets, N.; Lecours, M.P.; Dominguez, J.; Amadori, M.; Fraile, L.; Hernandez, J.; et al. Swine, human or avian influenza viruses differentially activates porcine dendritic cells cytokine profile. *Vet. Immunol. Immunopathol.* **2013**, *154*, 25–35. [CrossRef] [PubMed]

108. Ocana-Macchi, M.; Ricklin, M.E.; Python, S.; Monika, G.A.; Stech, J.; Stech, O.; Summerfield, A. Avian influenza A virus PB2 promotes interferon type I inducing properties of a swine strain in porcine dendritic cells. *Virology* **2012**, *427*, 1–9. [CrossRef] [PubMed]

109. Bel, M.; Ocana-Macchi, M.; Liniger, M.; McCullough, K.C.; Matrosovich, M.; Summerfield, A. Efficient sensing of avian influenza viruses by porcine plasmacytoid dendritic cells. *Viruses* **2011**, *3*, 312–330. [CrossRef] [PubMed]

110. Guilliams, M.; Ginhoux, F.; Jakubzick, C.; Naik, S.H.; Onai, N.; Schraml, B.U.; Segura, E.; Tussiwand, R.; Yona, S. Dendritic cells, monocytes and macrophages: A unified nomenclature based on ontogeny. *Nat. Rev. Immunol.* **2014**, *14*, 571–578. [CrossRef] [PubMed]

111. Park, H.S.; Liu, G.; Thulasi Raman, S.N.; Landreth, S.L.; Liu, Q.; Zhou, Y. NS1 Protein of 2009 Pandemic Influenza A Virus Inhibits Porcine NLRP3 Inflammasome-Mediated Interleukin-1 Beta Production by Suppressing ASC Ubiquitination. *J. Virol.* **2018**, *92*, e00022-18. [CrossRef] [PubMed]

112. Fujisawa, H. Neutrophils play an essential role in cooperation with antibody in both protection against and recovery from pulmonary infection with influenza virus in mice. *J. Virol.* **2008**, *82*, 2772–2783. [CrossRef] [PubMed]

113. Salvatore, M.; Garcia-Sastre, A.; Ruchala, P.; Lehrer, R.I.; Chang, T.; Klotman, M.E. alpha-Defensin inhibits influenza virus replication by cell-mediated mechanism(s). *J. Infect. Dis.* **2007**, *196*, 835–843. [CrossRef] [PubMed]

114. Tate, M.D.; Ioannidis, L.J.; Croker, B.; Brown, L.E.; Brooks, A.G.; Reading, P.C. The role of neutrophils during mild and severe influenza virus infections of mice. *PLoS ONE* **2011**, *6*, e17618. [CrossRef] [PubMed]

115. Tripathi, S.; White, M.R.; Hartshorn, K.L. The amazing innate immune response to influenza A virus infection. *Innate Immun.* **2015**, *21*, 73–98. [CrossRef] [PubMed]

116. Zhao, Y.; Lu, M.; Lau, L.T.; Lu, J.; Gao, Z.; Liu, J.; Yu, A.C.; Cao, Q.; Ye, J.; McNutt, M.A.; et al. Neutrophils may be a vehicle for viral replication and dissemination in human H5N1 avian influenza. *Clin. Infect. Dis.* **2008**, *47*, 1575–1578. [CrossRef] [PubMed]

117. Mandelboim, O.; Lieberman, N.; Lev, M.; Paul, L.; Arnon, T.I.; Bushkin, Y.; Davis, D.M.; Strominger, J.L.; Yewdell, J.W.; Porgador, A. Recognition of haemagglutinins on virus-infected cells by NKp46 activates lysis by human NK cells. *Nature* **2001**, *409*, 1055–1060. [CrossRef] [PubMed]

118. Paget, C.; Ivanov, S.; Fontaine, J.; Blanc, F.; Pichavant, M.; Renneson, J.; Bialecki, E.; Pothlichet, J.; Vendeville, C.; Barba-Spaeth, G.; et al. Potential role of invariant NKT cells in the control of pulmonary inflammation and CD8+ T cell response during acute influenza A virus H3N2 pneumonia. *J. Immunol.* **2011**, *186*, 5590–5602. [CrossRef] [PubMed]

119. Forberg, H.; Hauge, A.G.; Valheim, M.; Garcon, F.; Nunez, A.; Gerner, W.; Mair, K.H.; Graham, S.P.; Brookes, S.M.; Storset, A.K. Early responses of natural killer cells in pigs experimentally infected with 2009 pandemic H1N1 influenza A virus. *PLoS ONE* **2014**, *9*, e100619. [CrossRef] [PubMed]

120. Khatri, M.; Dwivedi, V.; Krakowka, S.; Manickam, C.; Ali, A.; Wang, L.; Qin, Z.; Renukaradhya, G.J.; Lee, C.W. Swine influenza H1N1 virus induces acute inflammatory immune responses in pig lungs: A potential animal model for human H1N1 influenza virus. *J. Virol.* **2010**, *84*, 11210–11218. [CrossRef] [PubMed]

121. Heinen, P.P.; de Boer-Luijtze, E.A.; Bianchi, A.T. Respiratory and systemic humoral and cellular immune responses of pigs to a heterosubtypic influenza A virus infection. *J. Gen. Virol.* **2001**, *82*, 2697–2707. [CrossRef] [PubMed]

122. Kappes, M.A.; Sandbulte, M.R.; Platt, R.; Wang, C.; Lager, K.M.; Henningson, J.N.; Lorusso, A.; Vincent, A.L.; Loving, C.L.; Roth, J.A.; et al. Vaccination with NS1-truncated H3N2 swine influenza virus primes T cells and confers cross-protection against an H1N1 heterosubtypic challenge in pigs. *Vaccine* **2012**, *30*, 280–288. [CrossRef] [PubMed]

123. Choi, Y.K.; Goyal, S.M.; Joo, H.S. Retrospective analysis of etiologic agents associated with respiratory diseases in pigs. *Can. Vet. J.* **2003**, *44*, 735–737. [PubMed]

124. Fablet, C.; Marois-Crehan, C.; Simon, G.; Grasland, B.; Jestin, A.; Kobisch, M.; Madec, F.; Rose, N. Infectious agents associated with respiratory diseases in 125 farrow-to-finish pig herds: A cross-sectional study. *Vet. Microbiol.* **2012**, *157*, 152–163. [CrossRef] [PubMed]

125. A Dorr, P.M.; Gebreyes, W.A.; Almond, G.W. Porcine reproductive and respiratory syndrome virus: Age and management system disease modeling for pathogenic co-infection. *J. Swine Health Prod.* **2007**, *15*, 258–264.

126. Alvarez, J.; Sarradell, J.; Kerkaert, B.; Bandyopadhyay, D.; Torremorell, M.; Morrison, R.; Perez, A. Association of the presence of influenza A virus and porcine reproductive and respiratory syndrome virus in sow farms with post-weaning mortality. *Prev. Vet. Med.* **2015**, *121*, 240–245. [CrossRef] [PubMed]

127. Bush, E.J.; Thacker, E.L.; Swenson, S.L. *National Seroprevalence of PRRS, Mycoplasma and Swine Influenza Virus*; American Association Of Swine Veterinarians: Iowa, IA, USA, 2003.

128. Pol, J.M.; van Leengoed, L.A.; Stockhofe, N.; Kok, G.; Wensvoort, G. Dual infections of PRRSV/influenza or PRRSV/Actinobacillus pleuropneumoniae in the respiratory tract. *Vet. Microbiol.* **1997**, *55*, 259–264. [CrossRef]

129. Van Reeth, K.; Nauwynck, H.; Pensaert, M. Dual infections of feeder pigs with porcine reproductive and respiratory syndrome virus followed by porcine respiratory coronavirus or swine influenza virus: A clinical and virological study. *Vet. Microbiol.* **1996**, *48*, 325–335. [CrossRef]

130. Dobrescu, I.; Levast, B.; Lai, K.; Delgado-Ortega, M.; Walker, S.; Banman, S.; Townsend, H.; Simon, G.; Zhou, Y.; Gerdts, V.; et al. In vitro and ex vivo analyses of co-infections with swine influenza and porcine reproductive and respiratory syndrome viruses. *Vet. Microbiol.* **2014**, *169*, 18–32. [CrossRef] [PubMed]

131. Provost, C.; Hamonic, G.; Gagnon, C.A.; Meurens, F. Dual infections of CD163 expressing NPTr epithelial cells with influenza A virus and PRRSV. *Vet. Microbiol.* **2017**, *207*, 143–148. [CrossRef] [PubMed]

2

A Serological Survey on Swine Brucellosis using Standard Procedures, Dot Blot, and Western Blot in Finisher Pigs in Central-North Italy

Fabrizio Bertelloni [†,*] , Mario Forzan [†] , Barbara Turchi, Simona Sagona, Maurizio Mazzei, Antonio Felicioli, Filippo Fratini and Domenico Cerri

Department of Veterinary Science, University of Pisa, Viale delle Piagge 2, 56124 Pisa, Italy; mario.forzan@unipi.it (M.F.); barbara.turchi@unipi.it (B.T.); simonasagona@tiscali.it (S.S.); maurizio.mazzei@unipi.it (M.M.); antonio.felicioli@unipi.it (A.F.); filippo.fratini@unipi.it (F.F.); domenico.cerri@unipi.it (D.C.)
* Correspondence: fabriziobertelloni@gmail.com
† These authors contributed equally to the study.

Abstract: In recent years, *Brucella suis* has been sporadically reported in Italy in domestic and wild swine. Since standard serological tests can determine false positive results, the development of alternative tests with improved sensitivity and specificity is rather essential. We analyzed 1212 sera collected at slaughterhouse from healthy pigs belonging to 62 farms of North-Central Italy. Sera were tested by Rose Bengal Test, Complement Fixation Test, and subsequently by a Dot Blot (DB) and Western Blot assays (WB). Only one serum resulted positive to all tests, indicating that swine brucellosis has a very limited spread. DB and WB could represent a support to the available serological tests; however, further studies to validate these tests are needed. In the presence of reemerging diseases, a prompt and continuous monitoring design is necessary to acquire epidemiological information for the subsequent application of specific health emergency plans.

Keywords: swine; brucellosis; serology; Dot Blot; Western Blot

1. Introduction

Swine brucellosis is primarily caused by *Brucella suis* (*B. suis*) [1]. *B. suis* can be divided into five biovars of which 1, 2, and 3 are the most relevant for pigs and are globally distributed [2,3]. Brucellosis caused by *Brucella suis* biovar 2 (*B. suis* bv. 2) is emerging in Europe, and although this biovar is not pathogenic for humans, it could be a cause of reproductive failure in pigs, which results in important economic losses for the swine industry [2,4–7].

Wild boars and hares represent reservoir hosts for *B. suis* bv. 2; these animals are the main sources of infection for domestic pigs, contributing to the spreading of the disease [2,8]. Moreover, wild boars and hares imported for hunting purposes could represent sources of introduction of the pathogen in infection-free areas [8,9]. Recently, *B. suis* bv. 2 was reported for the first time in wild boars [9,10] and later it was reported in swine in different Italian regions [11,12].

Serology plays an important role in brucellosis surveillance and eradication [13]. Nowadays, according to World Organization for Animal Health (OIE) [14], several validated serological tests are available for brucellosis diagnosis in swine: Rose Bengal Test (RBT), Fluorescence Polarisation Assay (FPA), Complement Fixation Test (CFT), and Indirect/Competitive Enzyme-Linked Immunosorbent Assay (I/C ELISA). All these serological tests are routinely used and are based on the detection of antibodies against the smooth lipopolysaccharides (sLPS) of smooth strains. Although these serological tests are globally validated, each of them shows limitations, especially for the screening of individual animals, in particular in swine serum samples [14].

Particularly, it is well documented that antibodies against *Yersinia enterocolitica* O:9 cross-react with *Brucella* sLPS antigens [15]. *Y. enterocolitica* O:9 is particularly widespread in swine populations [16] and represents a frequent cause of false positive serological reactions (FPSR) [13,14]. For these reasons, several authors developed different immunoblotting methods in order to improve sensitivity and specificity of the serological diagnosis [17–19].

The aim of this survey was to evaluate the diffusion of *Brucella* spp. in domestic pigs of North-Central Italy by a serological investigation of samples collected at the slaughterhouse from healthy animals employing standard methods and immune assays.

2. Materials and Methods

From September to December 2015, 1212 swine blood samples were collected at slaughterhouses from healthy animals belonging to 62 different farms located in five different Italian regions: 33 in Lombardy (660 sera), 15 in Tuscany (274 sera), 7 in Emilia Romagna (138 sera), 5 in Veneto (100 sera), and 2 in Piedmont (40 sera) (Table S1). When it was feasible, from each farm, sera from 20 pigs were collected. Blood samples were quickly transported in refrigerated condition; obtained sera were stored at $-20\,°C$ until processed.

All collected sera were screened for anti-brucella antibody by Rose Bengal Test [14]. The sera from farms in which at least one positive sample was present were also analyzed by Complement Fixation Test [14] and by Dot Blot assay (DB). Antigens prepared from a smooth strain of *B. abortus* W99 were produced by "Istituto Zooprofilattico della Lombardia e dell'Emilia Romagna Bruno Ubertini, Brescia" and by "Istituto Zooprofilattico Sperimentale dell'Abruzzo e del Molise G. Caporale, Teramo" for CFTs and for RBTs, respectively.

Antigen employed in DB was Brucellergene OCB (Rhône-Mérieux, Lyon, France), produced from *Brucella melitensis* rough strain B115. DB was performed according to Iovinella et al. [20], with modifications. The antigen (2 µL) was adsorbed on a 0.45 µm size nitrocellulose membrane (Thermo Fisher Scientific, Waltham, MA, USA) and incubated overnight in 3% semi-skimmed milk, 0.05% Tween 20, 100 mM phosphate buffer saline, pH 7.5. The membrane was exposed to serum samples at different concentrations (1:50, 1:100, 1:200), with different incubation times (15, 30, and 45 min) and with or without heat treatment at $58\,°C \pm 2\,°C$ for 60 min. Afterwards, the membrane was incubated for 1 h at Room Temperature (RT) with a horseradish peroxidase (HRP)-conjugated polyclonal Rabbit anti-Pig IgG-(H+L) antibody (Bethyl Laboratories, Montgomery, TX, USA) diluted 1:10000. The reaction was detected by Immun-Star™ WesternC™ Kit (Biorad Laboratories, Richmond, CA, USA) using a Nikon D5100 camera [21]. Sera scored positive by DB were subsequently analyzed by Western Blot assay (WB) according to Iovinella et al. [20]. The Brucellergene total protein content was measured by Qubit 2.0 Fluorometer (Invitrogen, Waltham, MA, USA). Ten micrograms of Brucellergene total protein were loaded into 12% T and 7.5% T, 2.6% C separating polyacrylamide gels (1.5 mm thick); a 10–250 kDa pre-stained protein Sharpmass™ V plus protein MW marker (Euroclone, Milan, Italy) was used. Sodium Dodecyl Sulphate - PolyAcrylamide Gel Electrophoresis (SDS-PAGE) was performed at 20 mA/ gel at 15 °C using SE 260 mini vertical electrophoresis (GE Healthcare, Little Chalfont Buckinghamshire, UK). Gels were stained in Coomassie brilliant G colloidal solution, scanned by an Epson Perfection V750 Pro, and elaborated by Image J software (National Institutes of Health, Maryland, USA) [22]. Proteins were transferred on the nitrocellulose membrane by ECL TE 70 PWR Semi-dry transfer unit (GE Healthcare) at 75 mA for 4 h and 30 min. The membrane was processed as described for DB; serum concentration, incubation time and heat treatment were chosen on the basis of DB results (1:200, 30 min, and heat treatment at $58\,°C \pm 2\,°C$ for 60 min, respectively). In order to avoid false positive serological reactions (FPSRs) due to *Y. enterocolitica* O:9, a hyperimmune anti-Yersinia rabbit serum was also tested both by DB and by WB using Goat anti-Rabbit IgG (H+L)-HRP conjugate (Biorad laboratories) as secondary antibody.

All employed antigens were provided by "Istituto Zooprofilattico Sperimentale dell'Abruzzo e del Molise G. Caporale, Teramo".

3. Results

Among 1212 serum samples, only one serum resulted positive to RBT and CFT (titer 1:4 corresponding to 20 International Complement Fixation Test Units for milliliter—ICFTU/mL) and was confirmed by Dot Blot assay. A second serum that was negative to RBT resulted positive to CFT (titer 1:4 corresponding to 20 ICFTU), but it scored negative when tested by Dot Blot. Both these sera obviously belonged to the same farm, located in South Tuscany (Siena province). The best DB experimental conditions were: serum dilution 1:200 at 30 min of incubation (Figure S1, Table S2). Heat treatment of sera was useful for the interpretation of the negative samples. The positive serum was also confirmed by WB (Figures S2 and S3); this test highlighted a band of 53.5 kDa corresponding to the one with the same molecular weight and the same relative mobility (Rm) observed by SDS-PAGE. Hyperimmune anti-Yersinia rabbit serum resulted negative in both assays (Figure S4, Table S3).

4. Discussion

Brucella suis biovar 2 has been recently introduced in Italy [9–12]. This bacterium is generally considered a pathogen only for swine that represent, along with wild boars and hares, the most important host for this biovar [2]. However, human infection caused by *B. suis* biovar 2 has been described in France in immuno-compromised hunters [23]. Furthermore, rare cases of asymptomatic infection have been reported in Europe in ruminants after exposure to infected wild boars [24,25]. For these reasons, a constant serological monitoring of wild and domestic swine populations could be essential in order to acquire as much epidemiological information as possible.

In Italy, pig farms are mainly located in the central and northern parts of the country [26]; consequently, the improvement of swine health monitoring in this area is advisable. To the best of our knowledge, there is only one report on the seroprevalence of *Brucella* spp. in breeding pigs in Central-North Italy [11].

Our survey aimed to increase the epidemiological information concerning swine brucellosis in this geographical area. Based on our results, swine brucellosis seems to have a very limited spread. In fact, only one sample resulted positive. One serum resulted positive to CFT but not to RBT and DB. CFT is more specific than RBT, but it is not capable of eliminating the FPSR problem, and can be recommended only as a complementary test, especially in swine, as suggested by WHO [14]. To consolidate the obtained serological results and to exclude possible cross-reactions with other bacteria, two different kinds of antigens were employed: one based on LPS (RBT and CFT) and the other one of protein nature (DB and WB). In our study, therefore, only the serum that resulted positive to all tests employed was considered as positive.

The positive serum came from a free ranged farm of "cinta senese" pigs, in South Tuscany (Siena province), a region characterized by the presence of many wild boars [27] and close to the area where *B. suis* bv. 2 was reported in pigs for the first time [11]. A retrospective investigation highlighted that the positive herd was a free ranged farm of "cinta senese" pigs, where animals could frequently come into contact with wild boars.

Although serological tests cannot discriminate among *Brucella* species, it seems plausible to assume that *B. suis* bv. 2 could be involved in this case, considering also that Tuscany is free from bovine and ovine brucellosis.

Brucellergene was previously employed in swine for in vitro serological test, such as ELISA [13], and for in vivo skin test [7], showing significant performance, especially in term of specificity and in the ability to distinguish FPSR. Moreover, Brucellergene is safe to handle, standardized, and, in some countries, commercially available. For these reasons, it was chosen as an antigen for confirmatory tests. Our results confirm its validity and ease of use in swine brucellosis serological diagnosis.

WB assay resulted useful to confirm and support traditional serology, as also reported previously by other authors [17–19]. However, WB execution requires specialized and trained personnel, it is time consuming, and previous work has showed that its sensitivity is low [28]. In this perspective, DB, although its sensibility is probably low, is less time consuming, easier to perform, and applicable to a higher number of samples in comparison to WB. In our study, WB confirmed the results obtained by DB. However, before this method could be applied to support conventional serological tests, such as RBT and CFT, it would be necessary to perform more accurate investigations to precisely evaluate and define its specificity and sensitivity.

5. Conclusions

Despite the recent reports, swine brucellosis seems to have a limited diffusion in the investigated area. However, considering the possible hazard for farmed animals, especially swine, and the possible risk for humans, a continuous monitoring plan is advisable. In light of the considerable number of animals to test, slaughterhouses represent the best places for sampling. Serology is a useful and valid tool to obtain epidemiological data, but the development of methods with increased performance characteristics is required. DB and WB could represent possible candidates for this purpose, but, on the other hand, it is necessary to perform additional studies to fully validate those experimental approaches in order to evaluate their performances and usefulness.

Supplementary Materials:
Table S1: Farms included in this study; Figure S1: SDS-PAGE of Brucellergene antigen; Figure S2: Dot Blot at different experimental condition: a = serum without heat treatment; b = serum after heat treatment; 1:100 and 1:200 = sera dilution in PBS; 45′, 30′, and 15′ = sera incubation times in minutes; + serum and − serum = positive and negative sera, respectively; Table S2: Optical density measured from Dot Blot assay from different experimental conditions; Figure S3: Dot Blot of different sera: P+ = positive serum; P+/− = serum positive to CFT and negative to RBT; P− = negative serum; R Yersinia + = rabbit serum positive to *Yersinia enterocolitica* O:9; R Yersinia − = SPF rabbit serum; Table S3: Optical density measured from Dot Blot assay of different serum samples; Figure S4: Western Blot analysis: proteins of Brucellergene were separated by SDS-PAGE and blotted on nitrocellulose membrane using a semidry system. +: positive serum; −: negative serum.

Author Contributions: D.C., A.F., and F.F. planned and supervised the study; D.C. and A.F. supported and financed the project the work; F.B. and F.F. collected the samples; F.B., M.F., and S.S. carried out laboratory experiments; F.B., B.T., and M.M. wrote and edited the manuscript. All authors reviewed and approved the final version of the article.

Acknowledgments: The authors wish to thank the Istituto Zooprofilattico Sperimentale dell'Abruzzo e del Molise G. Caporale, Teramo, Italy, which provided the antigens employed in all serological tests.

References

1. Olsen, S.C.; Garin-Bastuji, B.; Blasco, J.M.; Nicola, A.M.; Samartino, L. Brucellosis. In *Stevenson, Diseases of Swine*, 10th ed.; Zimmerman, J.J., Karriker, L.A., Ramirez, A., Schwartz, G.W., Eds.; John Wiley & Sons, Inc.: Hoboken, NJ, USA, 2012; pp. 697–708.
2. Godfroid, J.; Scholz, H.C.; Barbier, T.; Nicolas, C.; Wattiau, P.; Fretin, D.; Whatmore, A.M.; Cloeckaert, A.; Blasco, J.M.; Moriyon, I.; et al. Brucellosis at the animal/ecosystem/human interface at the beginning of the 21st century. *Prev. Vet. Med.* **2011**, *102*, 118–131. [CrossRef] [PubMed]
3. Duvnjak, S.; Račić, I.; Špičić, S.; Zdelar-Tuk, M.; Reil, I.; Cvetnić, Ž. Characterisation of *Brucella suis* isolates from Southeast Europe by multi-locus variable-number tandem repeat analysis. *Vet. Microbiol.* **2015**, *180*, 146–150. [CrossRef] [PubMed]
4. Cvetnić, Z.; Spicić, S.; Toncić, J.; Majnarić, D.; Benić, M.; Albert, D.; Thiébaud, M.; Garin-Bastuji, B. *Brucella suis* infection in domestic pigs and wild boar in Croatia. *Rev. Sci. Tech.* **2009**, *28*, 1057–1067. [CrossRef] [PubMed]
5. Ferreira, A.C.; Almendra, C.; Cardoso, R.; Pereira, M.S.; Beja-Pereira, A.; Luikart, G.; de Sá, M.I.C. Development and evaluation of a selective medium for *Brucella suis*. *Res. Vet. Sci.* **2012**, *93*, 565–567. [CrossRef] [PubMed]

6. Szulowski, K.; Iwaniak, W.; Weiner, M.; Zlotnicka, J. Characteristics of *Brucella* strains isolated from animals in Poland. *Pol. J. Vet. Sci.* **2013**, *16*, 757–758. [CrossRef] [PubMed]

7. Dieste-Pérez, L.; Blasco, J.M.; De Miguel, M.J.; Marín, C.M.; Barberán, M.; Conde-Álvarez, R.; Moriyón, I.; Muñoz, P.M. Performance of skin tests with allergens from *B. melitensis* B115 and rough *B. abortus* mutants for diagnosing swine brucellosis. *Vet. Microbiol.* **2014**, *168*, 161–168. [CrossRef]

8. Kreizinger, Z.; Foster, J.T.; Rónai, Z.; Sulyok, K.M.; Wehmann, E.; Jánosi, S.; Gyuranecz, M. Genetic relatedness of *Brucella suis* biovar 2 isolates from hares, wild boars and domestic pigs. *Vet. Microbiol.* **2014**, *172*, 492–498. [CrossRef] [PubMed]

9. De Massis, F.; di Provvido, A.; di Sabatino, D.; di Francesco, D.; Zilli, K.; Ancora, M.; Tittarelli, M. Isolation of *Brucella suis* biovar 2 from a wild boar in the Abruzzo Region of Italy. *Vet. Ital.* **2012**, *48*, 397–404. [PubMed]

10. Bergagna, S.; Zoppi, S.; Ferroglio, E.; Gobetto, M.; Dondo, A.; Di Giannatale, E.; Gennero, M.S.; Grattarola, C. Epidemiologic survey for *Brucella suis* biovar 2 in a wild boar (*Sus scrofa*) population in northwest Italy. *J. Wildl. Dis.* **2009**, *45*, 1178–1181. [CrossRef] [PubMed]

11. Barlozzari, G.; Franco, A.; Macrì, G.; Lorenzetti, S.; Maggiori, F.; Dottarelli, S.; Maurelli, M.; Di Giannatale, E.; Tittarelli, M.; Battisti, A.; Gamberale, F. First report of *Brucella suis* biovar 2 in a semi free-range pig farm, Italy. *Vet. Ital.* **2015**, *51*, 151–154. [CrossRef] [PubMed]

12. Pilo, C.; Tedde, M.T.; Orrù, G.; Addis, G.; Liciardi, M. *Brucella suis* infection in domestic pigs in Sardinia (Italy). *Epidemiol. Infect.* **2015**, *143*, 2170–2177. [CrossRef] [PubMed]

13. McGiven, J.A.; Nicola, A.; Commander, N.J.; Duncombe, L.; Taylor, A.V.; Villari, S.; Dainty, A.; Thirlwall, R.; Bouzelmat, N.; Perrett, L.L.; et al. An evaluation of the capability of existing and novel serodiagnostic methods for porcine brucellosis to reduce false positive serological reactions. *Vet. Microbiol.* **2012**, *160*, 378–386. [CrossRef] [PubMed]

14. World Organization for Animal Health. Manual of Diagnostic Tests and Vaccines for Terrestrial Animals. In *Brucella abortus, B. melitensis and B. suis Office International Des Epizooties*; OIE: Paris, France, 2017.

15. Jungersen, G.; Sørensen, V.; Giese, S.B.; Stack, J.A.; Riber, U. Differentiation between serological responses to *Brucella suis* and *Yersinia enterocolitica* serotype O:9 after natural or experimental infection in pigs. *Epidemiol. Infect.* **2006**, *134*, 347–357. [CrossRef] [PubMed]

16. EFSA (European Food Safety Authority) and ECDC (European Centre for Disease Prevention and Control). The European Union summary report on trends and sources of zoonoses, zoonotic agents and food-borne outbreaks in 2015. *EFSA J.* **2016**, *14*, 231. [CrossRef]

17. Spencer, S.A.; Broughton, E.S.; Hamid, S.; Young, D.B. Immunoblot studies in the differential diagnosis of porcine brucellosis: An immunodominant 62 kDa protein is related to the mycobacterial 65 kDa heat shock protein (HSP-65). *Vet. Microbiol.* **1994**, *39*, 47–60. [CrossRef]

18. Corrente, M.; Desario, C.; Greco, G.; Buonavoglia, D.; Pratelli, A.; Madio, A.; Scaltrito, D.; Consenti, B.; Buonavoglia, C. Development of a western blotting assay to discriminate *Brucella* spp. and *Yersinia enterocolitica* O:9 infections in sheep. *New Microbiol.* **2004**, *27*, 155–161. [PubMed]

19. Wareth, G.; Melzer, F.; Weise, C.; Neubauer, H.; Roesler, U.; Murugaiyan, J. Proteomics-based identification of immunodominant proteins of Brucellae using sera from infected hosts points towards enhanced pathogen survival during the infection. *Biochem. Biophys. Res. Commun.* **2015**, *456*, 202–206. [CrossRef] [PubMed]

20. Iovinella, I.; Dani, F.R.; Niccolini, A.; Sagona, S.; Michelucci, E.; Gazzano, A.; Turillazzi, S.; Felicioli, A.; Pelosi, P. Differential expression of odorant-binding proteins in the mandibular glands of the honey bee according to caste and age. *J. Proteome Res.* **2011**, *10*, 3439–3449. [CrossRef] [PubMed]

21. Khoury, M.K.; Parker, I.; Aswad, D.W. Acquisition of chemiluminescent signals from immunoblots with a digital single-lens reflex camera. *Anal. Biochem.* **2010**, *397*, 129–131. [CrossRef] [PubMed]

22. Abramoff, M.D.; Magalhaes, P.J.; Ram, S.J. Image Processing with Image. *J. Biophoton. Int.* **2004**, *11*, 36–42.

23. Pappas, G. The changing *Brucella* ecology: Novel reservoirs, new threats. *Int. J. Antimicrob. Agents* **2010**, *36*, S8–S11. [CrossRef] [PubMed]

24. Fretin, D.; Mori, M.; Czaplicki, G.; Quinet, C.; Maquet, B.; Godfroid, J.; Saegerman, C. Unexpected *Brucella suis* biovar 2 infection in a dairy cow, Belgium. *Emerg. Infect. Dis.* **2013**, *19*, 2053–2054. [CrossRef] [PubMed]

25. Szulowski, K.; Iwaniak, W.; Weiner, M.; Złotnicka, J. *Brucella suis* biovar 2 isolations from cattle in Poland. *Ann. Agric. Environ. Med.* **2013**, *20*, 672–675. [PubMed]

26. ISTAT. 6° Censimento Generale dell'Agricoltura. Available online: https://www.istat.it/it/archivio/66591 (accessed on 13 July 2012).

27. Carnevali, L.; Pedrotti, L.; Riga, F.; Toso, S. Banca Dati Ungulati: Status, distribuzione, consistenza, gestione e prelievo venatorio delle popolazioni di Ungulati in Italia. Rapporto 2001–2005. *Biol. Cons. Fauna* **2009**, *117*, 1–168, [Italian-English text].

28. Kittelberger, R.; Hilbink, F.; Hansen, M.F.; Penrose, M.; de Lisle, G.W.; Letesson, J.J.; Garin-Bastuji, B.; Searson, J.; Fossati, C.A.; Cloeckaert, A.; et al. Serological crossreactivity between *Brucella abortus* and *Yersinia enterocolitica* O:9 I immunoblot analysis of the antibody response to *Brucella* protein antigens in bovine brucellosis. *Vet. Microbiol.* **1995**, *47*, 257–270. [CrossRef]

Evaluation of the Efficiency of Active and Passive Surveillance in the Detection of African Swine Fever in Wild Boar

Vincenzo Gervasi [1], **Andrea Marcon** [1]🆔, **Silvia Bellini** [2] and **Vittorio Guberti** [2,*]

[1] Wildlife Department, Istituto Superiore per la Protezione e la Ricerca Ambientale, 40064 Ozzano Emilia (BO), Italy; vincent.gervasi@gmail.com (V.G.); amarcon.work@gmail.com (A.M.)

[2] Istituto Zooprofilattico della Lombardia ed Emilia-Romagna, 25124 Brescia, Italy; silvia.bellini@izsler.it

* Correspondence: vittorio.guberti@isprambiente.it

Abstract: African swine fever (ASF) is one of the most severe diseases of pigs and has a drastic impact on pig industry. Wild boar populations play the role of ASF genotype II virus epidemiological reservoir. Disease surveillance in wild boar is carried out either by testing all the wild boar found sick or dead for virus detection (passive surveillance) or by testing for virus (and antibodies) all hunted wild boar (active surveillance). When virus prevalence and wild boar density are low as it happens close to eradication, the question on which kind of surveillance is more efficient in detecting the virus is still open. We built a simulation model to mimic the evolution of the host-parasite interaction in the European wild boar and to assess the efficiency of different surveillance strategies. We constructed a deterministic SIR model, which estimated the probability to detect the virus during the 8 years following its introduction, using both passive and active surveillance. Overall, passive surveillance provided a much larger number of ASF detections than active surveillance during the first year. During subsequent years, both active and passive surveillance exhibited a decrease in their probability to detect ASF. Such decrease, though, was more pronounced for passive surveillance. Under the assumption of 50% of carcasses detection, active surveillance became the best detection method when the endemic disease prevalence was lower than 1.5%, when hunting rate was >60% and when population density was lower than 0.1 individuals/km^2. In such a situation, though, the absolute probability to detect the disease was very low with both methods, and finding almost every carcass is the only way to ensure virus detection. The sensitivity analysis shows that carcass search effort is the sole parameter that increases proportionally the chance of ASF virus detection. Therefore, an effort should be made to promote active search of dead wild boar also in endemic areas, since reporting wild boar carcasses is crucial to understand the epidemiological situation in any of the different phases of ASF infection at any wild boar density.

Keywords: African swine fever; wild boar; surveillance; early detection; endemic; SIR model

---

1. Introduction

African swine fever (ASF) is one of the most severe diseases of pigs and has a drastic impact on pig industry [1]. The disease is caused by the ASF virus (ASFV), which belongs to the family *Asfarviridae* and affects both domestic pigs and wild boar with a high case fatality rate. No effective vaccine or treatment exists to aid in the control of the disease. The disease is present in Africa, Europe and Asia.

In Europe, there are currently two main clusters of ASFV infection. One of them is in Sardinia where the disease was introduced in 1978 and it is caused by strains of ASFV belonging to genotype I. The second cluster is occurring in a large part of North Eastern Europe and it is caused by strains of

ASFV belonging to genotype II. The latter is a highly virulent strain inducing an acute form of ASF that results in a mortality rate of 94.5–100% in both wild boar and domestic pigs [2]. In the European Union (EU), ASF was detected for the first time in Lithuania in January 2014 and since then, the disease has spread to Estonia, Latvia, Poland, Czech Republic, Hungary, Romania, Bulgaria, Belgium, Slovakia. In most of the affected areas, wild boar populations play the role of ASF virus epidemiological reservoir, maintaining indefinitely the virus in the environment, independently from any other susceptible species or vector [3]. In virgin wild boar populations, ASF is introduced either by human related activities, such as transfer of infected food or illegal trade (e.g., Czech Republic and Belgium) or through a geographical continuity of the infected wild boar or domestic pig populations (e.g., Hungary, Slovakia) [4], although in the specific cases it was not possible to trace back the specific cause of virus introduction. In wild boar, following its introduction, the virus shows an epidemic wave that tends to spread toward free areas while it remains endemic in the previously affected ones, despite the low wild boar local density resulting from virus lethality and/or control measures (hunting/culling) [4]; this pattern was observed in most of the European countries affected so far, such as Poland, Lithuania, Estonia and Latvia [4]; the virus persists in the environment since it remains viable in wild boar carcasses. The epidemiological pattern is further complicated by the presence of infected domestic pigs and the long distance transport of the virus [4]. The transportation of infected pigs and pork meat or other contaminated material is considered as the most important factor contributing to the spread of the ASF virus over long distances [4].

In the EU, ASF surveillance in wild boar addresses both early detection in free areas and the follow up of the implemented control measures in endemic areas. Passive surveillance is carried out by testing all the wild boar found sick or dead for virus detection. Active surveillance is performed by testing all hunted wild boar for virus (and antibodies) [5]. Information collected by the European Food Safety Authority (EFSA) from the Baltic countries and Poland indicates that passive surveillance provides the higher probability of early detecting ASF, although the probability has not been quantified. Indeed, most of the primary cases in wild boar were found by passive surveillance [4]. Previous studies and the examples provided by the spread of the ASF virus in the Eastern European countries have shown that the disease can persist with a very low prevalence, even when wild boar density is kept low through intensive hunting [4]. However, since the infection became endemic in many infected wild boar populations, the question on which kind of surveillance (passive or active) is more efficient in detecting the virus at low prevalence and low wild boar density is still open, in particular considering that most of the countries are eradicating ASF in wild boar through a progressive population management aimed at reducing at a very low density the infected populations; in these epidemiological situations there is a window of uncertainty where ASF virus, if still present, is hardly detected, thus making any further policy management more complicated, including a possible exit strategy addressed at re-gaining the ASF free status.

The efficiency of ASF surveillance in wild boar is determined by a combination of epidemiological parameters, by field management practices, and by the time since virus introduction. Prevalence, lethality, and recovery rates are the epidemiological parameters determining the number of affected animals to be targeted by surveillance, whereas hunting effort and carcass search patterns are the field activities which allow the collection of samples for the diagnosis of ASF in wild boar.

The aim of this study was to compare the potential efficiency of active and passive surveillance in detecting ASF genotype II in wild boar populations and in particular:

a.   first virus detection in a naive wild boar population (early detection);
b.   monitoring the epidemic period following the virus invasion of the previously ASF free wild boar population;
c.   monitoring the trend of the infection during the years following the introduction of the virus;

For such purpose, we built a simulation model, developed to broadly mimic the epidemiological evolution of the host-parasite interaction in the European wild boar infected populations. We analysed the results of such model to highlight the field conditions in which each detection method is more likely to provide a significant probability of early detecting the disease and monitoring it through time.

2. Materials and Methods

To assess the efficiency of different surveillance strategies in ASF endemic areas, we constructed a deterministic SIR model with a one-day step, which estimated the probability to detect the virus during the 8 years following its introduction, using both passive and active surveillance. The simulation assumed a homogeneous mixing. The model comprised eight compartments: S = susceptible; I = infected; R = recovered (immune); SH = susceptible hunted; IH = infected hunted; RH = recovered hunted; D = dead due to ASF, C = dead and recovered as carcass. We parameterized the system using an infection-induced mortality model, following Keeling and Rohani [6]. The transition of individuals from one compartment to the other is illustrated in the diagram in Figure 1, and analytically defined by the following system of differential equations:

$$\begin{cases} \frac{dS}{dt} = \mu(S+R) - \beta SI - \varepsilon S \\ \frac{dI}{dt} = \beta SI - \frac{(\varepsilon+\theta)}{(1-\rho)}I \\ \frac{dR}{dt} = \theta I - \varepsilon R \\ \frac{dSH}{dt} = \varepsilon S \\ \frac{dIH}{dt} = \varepsilon I \\ \frac{dRH}{dt} = \varepsilon R \\ \frac{dD}{dt} = \gamma I - \phi D \\ \frac{dC}{dt} = \phi D \end{cases}$$

In which μ is the parameter controlling the recruitment of new individuals into the susceptible compartment, β is the disease transmission rate, ε represents hunting rate, θ is the daily recovery probability (i.e., the daily probability to survive the disease and become immune), ϕ is the carcass recovery rate, ρ is the overall probability to die from ASF, and γ is the disease lethality.

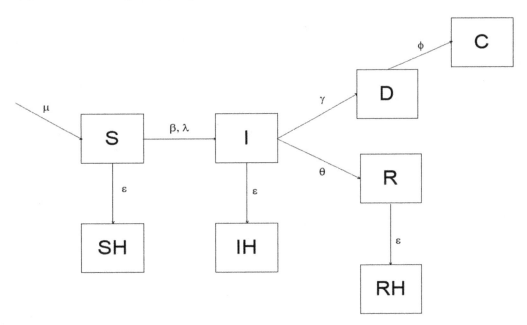

Figure 1. Conceptual diagram illustrating the structure of the compartmental model of the African Swine Fever (ASF) dynamics in a simulated wild boar population. The model comprised eight compartments: S = susceptible; I = infected; R = recovered; SH = susceptible hunted; IH = infected hunted; RH = recovered hunted; D = dead due to ASF; C = carcass recovered. The parameters controlling the transitions were: μ = recruitment; β = transmission rate; λ = force of the infection; ε = hunting rate; θ = recovery rate; γ = lethality; ϕ = carcass detection rate.

We initially focused on the first year after the disease outbreak and divided it into an early detection phase corresponding to the 100 days following recruitment, and an epidemic phase, comprising the remaining 265 days of the year. In order to have a better control on the disease prevalence during the epidemic phase, the model was forced to obtain a 10% disease prevalence at its onset and a 2% endemic prevalence (Figure 2).

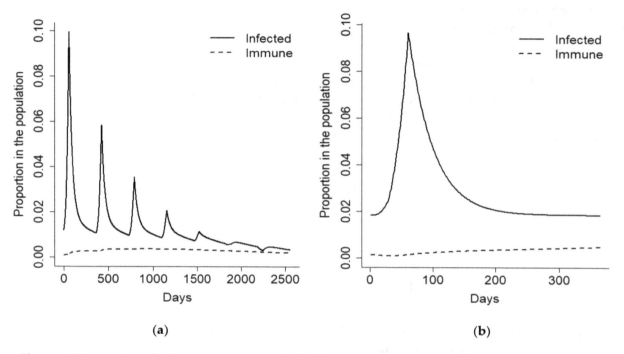

(a)   (b)

Figure 2. Proportion of infected and immune individuals in a simulated wild boar population affected by an African Swine Fever (ASF) epidemic during an 8-year period, as resulting from a compartmental model of the disease. The plot is illustrated for the whole 8-year period (**a**) and for just the first year (**b**).

We set the yearly hunting rate to 40% of the post-reproductive population and used two different values (10% and 50%) for the proportion of carcasses recovered during the passive surveillance of ASF. We simulated three scenarios, corresponding to three wild boar populations of different size, namely 100, 400 and 1000 individuals, all living at an initial density of 1 wild boar/km^2. The complete list of parameter values for the model is provided in Table 1.

Table 1. Description, symbology and values of the main parameters used to build an epidemiological model of the African Swine Fever (ASF) in a simulated wild boar population.

Parameter	Symbol	Description	Rates
Lethality	γ	% of infected wild boar that die due to ASF	95% after five days from the infection = 0.19 day^{-1}
Recovery rate	θ	% of infected individuals who survive and develop immunity	5% after 15 days from the infection = 0.0033 day^{-1}
Hunting rate	ε	% of hunted wild boars in 365 days	40% of the post reproductive population in one year = 0.0011 day^{-1}
Recruitment	μ	% of new-borns who enter the population	100% increase in a 30-days period = 0.033 day^{-1}
Carcass recovery rate	ϕ	% of dead wild boars found and recovered	10% and 50%

The processes of hunting and carcass recovery were simulated accounting for their stochastic nature. For each day, we generated the number of hunted ASF positive individuals (compartment IH) from a Poisson distribution with mean equal to the number of infected individuals in that day, and probability corresponding to the daily hunting rate ε. We followed the same procedure to generate the number of immune hunted individuals which survived the infection and developed antibodies (compartment RH) and the number of carcasses recovered in any given day of the study period (compartment C). For this last randomization, we defined as available carcasses only those belonging to the individuals dead due to ASF during the last 30 days. We ran the stochastic process over 1000 iterations.

After running the model, which provided us with the absolute number of individuals in each compartment during each day of the simulated study period, we reported the total number of ASF infected carcasses recovered, and the number of antigen and antibodies positive wild boars shot during hunting. We did so for each simulated population size, and separately for the early detection (days 1–100) and epidemic periods (days 101–365). Additionally, we estimated the proportion of iterations in which the disease was detected by each of the two surveillance methods, the average day of first detection of the disease and the average time interval between two successive ASF detections.

After exploring the main model dynamics during the first year of the epidemic, we focused on assessing the relative performance of active and passive surveillance during subsequent years, and accounting for a wider range of epidemiologic and management scenarios. We re-ran the model over 1000 iterations and for a period of 8 years. This time, though, we randomly extracted the values for the main model parameters from a set of uniform distributions. We simulated the disease prevalence during the endemic phase in a range between 1 and 4%, hunting rate between 20 and 70%, carcass recovery rate between 10 and 90%, and the initial population size between 100 and 1000 individuals. After running all model iterations, we estimated the average number of runs in which the disease was detected by either active or passive surveillance each year. In addition, we pooled all model iterations in which active surveillance exhibited a higher probability to detect the disease than passive surveillance. By plotting the range of parameter values of this set of iterations, we obtained an overview of the epidemiologic and management conditions in which active surveillance was more likely to detect ASF than passive surveillance.

Finally, in order to highlight how parameter values influenced the final model output, we performed a sensitivity analysis according to Keeling and Gilligan [7]. We increased by 10% each parameter value in the model and compared the equivalent changes in the day of first ASF detection, with respect to the baseline values for both passive and active surveillance. Sensitivity values >0 and <1 indicated a less than proportional increase in the likelihood of disease detection; a sensitivity value equal to 1 indicated a true proportional increase in the likelihood of detection; sensitivity values <0 indicated that any increase in the parameter value produced a decrease in the disease detection probability.

3. Results

During the first year, including the early detection and epidemic periods, passive surveillance was always the most effective method to detect the disease, but the relative efficacy of the two methods was strongly influenced by population size. For a population of 100 wild boars, passive surveillance exhibited a 100% probability to early detect the disease whereas hunting revealed the disease only in 43% of cases (Figure 3).

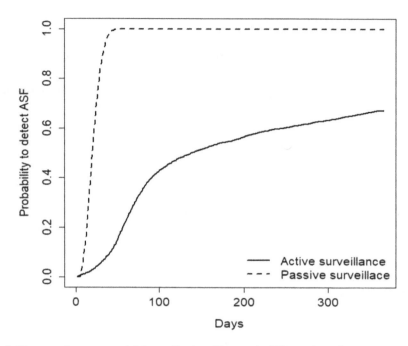

Figure 3. Probability to detect an African Swine Fever (ASF) outbreak with passive and active surveillance in a simulated wild boar population of 100 individuals, as resulting from a compartmental model of the disease. The plot refers to the first year after the initial disease outbreak.

Such difference between the two strategies became less pronounced when population size increased (Table 2). Depending on population size, the day of first ASF detection when using carcass finding as detection method ranged between 1–12 days, about half of the time necessary to detect the disease when using hunting. The average number of days between two successive ASF detections was several times shorter for passive than for active surveillance (Table 2).

Table 2. Relative performance of passive and active surveillance in the early detection of African Swine Fever (ASF) in wild boars, as resulting from a compartmental model. The results refer to the first year after the first disease outbreak.

Wild Boar Pop. Size	Early Detection (Days 1–100)						Epidemic Phase (Days 101–365)					
	Probability to Detect the Disease		Day of First Detection		Days between Detections		Probability to Detect the Disease		Day of First Detection		Days between Detections	
	Passive ($\phi^a = 0.1$)	Active	Passive ($\phi^a = 0.1$)	Active	Passive ($\phi^a = 0.1$)	Active	Passive ($\phi = 0.1$)	Active	Passive ($\phi = 0.1$)	Active	Passive ($\phi = 0.1$)	Active
100	100%	43%	41	78	12	90	100%	62%	49	178	43	242
400	100%	87%	24	57	4	61	100%	100%	34	76	10	149
1000	100%	99%	15	35	1	24	100%	100%	31	54	3	58

[a] Probability to detect a carcass of a wild boar dead for ASF.

Overall, passive surveillance provided a much higher number of ASF detections than active surveillance during the first year following the virus invasion (Table 3). On average, the number of ASF positive carcasses found was about 10 times higher than the number of antigen or antibodies positive wild boars shot. Such difference increased to 20–40 folds when simulating a 50% carcass recovery rate (Table 3), mimicking the so-called active search of carcasses. Compared to the shooting of an infected wild boar, antibodies detection always had a negligible probability to detect the infection (Table 3).

Table 3. Average number of African Swine Fever (ASF) detections obtained through active and passive surveillance, as resulting from a compartmental model of the disease dynamics in a wild boar population. The results refer to the first year after the first disease outbreak.

	Early Detection (Days 1–100)				Epidemic Phase (Days 101–365)			
	Passive Surveillance		Active Surveillance		Passive Surveillance		Active Surveillance	
Wild Boar Population Size	N. Carcasses ($\phi = 0.1$)	N. Carcasses ($\phi = 0.5$)	N. Shot Wild Boar ASFV Positive	N. Shot Wild Boar Ab Positive	N. Carcasses ($\phi = 0.1$)	N. Carcasses ($\phi = 0.5$)	N. Shot Wild Boar ASFV Positive	N. Shot Wild Boar Ab Positive
100	6.9	27.5	0.7	0.01	4.4	16.2	0.4	0.08
400	28.5	112.1	2.8	0.07	17.2	64.2	1.7	0.3
1000	71.1	279.9	6.8	0.2	43.3	160.9	4.4	0.8

During subsequent years, both active and passive surveillance exhibited a decrease in their probability to detect ASF (Figure 4a). Such decrease, though, was more pronounced for passive surveillance, so that in the last year the two methods exhibited similar performances, corresponding to about 20% success rate in detecting the disease (Figure 4a). Active surveillance performance exhibited a linear relationship with population density, whereas passive surveillance provided high detection probabilities when population density was higher than 0.1 individuals/km^2, but rapidly decreased its detection probability for lower density values (Figure 4b).

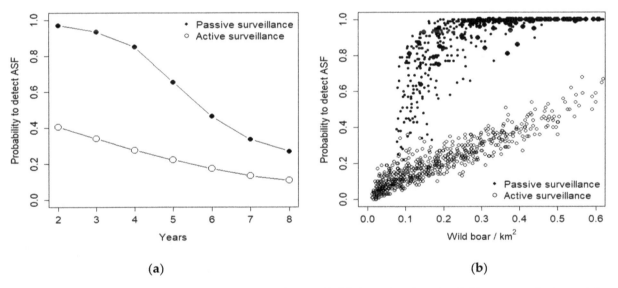

(a)

(b)

Figure 4. Probability to detect African Swine Fever (ASF) in a simulated wild boar population with passive and active surveillance, as resulting from a compartmental model of the disease. The plot provides the temporal trend in virus detection probability (**a**) and its relationship with population density (**b**).

Under the hypotheses of 50% carcass detection, active surveillance was the best detection method when the endemic disease prevalence was lower than 1.5%, when hunting rate was >60%, and when population density was lower than 0.1 individuals/km^2 (Figure 5). In such a situation, though, the absolute probability to detect the disease is very low with both methods (Figure 4b), and finding almost every carcass is the only way to ensure virus detection. Additionally, the sensitivity analysis shows that carcass search effort is the sole parameter that increases proportionally the chance of ASF virus detection.

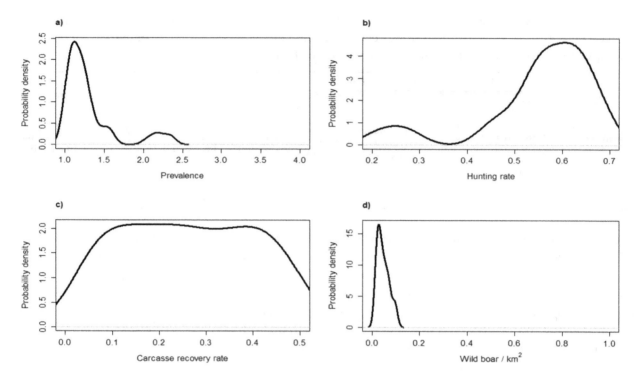

Figure 5. Frequency distribution of four parameter values (endemic prevalence (**a**), hunting rate (**b**), carcass recovery rate (**c**), population density (**d**)) corresponding to the simulated scenarios in which active surveillance was more effective than passive surveillance in revealing an African Swine Fever (ASF) outbreak.

Sensitivity values of all parameters are shown in Table 4. In the case of passive surveillance, increased lethality and force of the infection (the rate at which susceptible individuals acquire the disease, λ [8]) reduced the time of detection in a less than a proportional manner. A 10% increase of the above-mentioned parameters reduced detection times of 2.4 and 2.2%, respectively. Intuitively, the increased proportion of carcasses found in the forest proportionally decreased the time necessary to detect the virus. An increase in the hunting effort mathematically decreased the probability to detect the virus through passive surveillance (−0.6%). The 10% increased hunting effort increased the efficiency of active surveillance in a non-proportional way, allowing a 3% reduction in the time necessary to reveal the disease. Also, the increased 10% in the force of the infection (λ) non-proportionally increased the performance of active surveillance, providing an 8.6% reduced time to detect it through both antigens and antibodies.

Table 4. Results of a sensitivity analysis performed on a compartmental model of African Swine Fever (ASF) in wild boars, following the method of Keeling and Gilligan [7]. Sensitivity values refer to the variation in the time necessary to first detect the disease, corresponding to a 10% variation in each parameter value.

Parameter	Passive	Active (ASFV Positive)	Active (Ab Positive)
Force of infection (λ)	0.22	0.86	0.86
Lethality (γ)	0.24	−0.06	−0.04
Hunting effort (ε)	−0.06	0.30	0.30
Recovery rate (θ)	0.00	0.00	0.40
% found carcasses (ϕ)	1.00	0.00	0.00

4. Discussion

Passive surveillance is the most effective way of detecting the presence of ASF in wild boar and to follow the epidemic phase in a wild boar infected population. Hence, surveillance aimed at early detection and to follow the first epidemic phase should not be based on sampling of hunted animals.

Among the parameters that drive surveillance activities, only hunting and carcass finding can be modified by management authorities. Any reasonable increasing of hunting, though, will not achieve the same probability to detect the virus than the one exhibited by passive surveillance. Our results showed than only by hunting more than 60% of the wild boar post-reproductive population, active surveillance would achieve the same probability to detect the virus than the one exhibited by passive surveillance. Such hunting effort is not considered achievable in short term and could be even counter effective, as it would likely increase animal movement due to disturbance [9]. When the infection was simulated in a small population, only passive surveillance had a 100% detection probability, whereas active surveillance exhibited a much lower detection capacity. In practice, at hunting ground level, if passive surveillance is not fully implemented, hunters might be unaware to hunt in an infected area, even when the infection is already/still present. In larger populations, the epidemiological patterns are easier to be monitored because of the increased chance that at least one ASF infected carcass will be found, or an infected individual will be shot. Still, the highest probability to detect the infection was associated to passive surveillance.

In both cases, simulations showed that disease detection during the endemic phase is unlikely and rather problematic, regardless of the method used. The pattern highlighted was consistent with the epidemiological findings in the field, where the virus seems to have locally disappeared, but it is again newly detected after several months [4]. Only in relatively large endemic areas a steady detection of the virus is likely to be observed in both dead and hunted animals, even if most of the virus detections are still from dead animals. At low wild boar density, the virus detection (both passive and active) is mainly driven by stochasticity. In such a scenario, only a progressive increase in carcass detection rate, inversely correlated with wild boar density, ensures the efficiency of surveillance. Variability of seasonal hunting, depopulation attempts, rewards for reporting dead wild boar, have the potential to modify the patterns highlighted by the model, thus also modifying the efficiency of both passive and active surveillance. It is worth to underline that the sensitivity analysis identifies the search of dead wild boar as the sole parameter having a linear connection between field effort and surveillance efficiency.

The use of serology, according to the model outcome, is of poor value (if any) in the first phases of the infection. Active surveillance aimed at detecting Abs positive animals, though, could be useful or even preferable at a later stage of the endemic phase; however, since Abs can be detected even in the absence of virus circulation, the use of serological surveillance has to be further fine-tuned considering all the epidemiological factors determining the possible surveillance outcomes.

Therefore, to enhance surveillance efficiency in each of the epidemiological phases characterizing ASF in wild boar, an effort should be made to promote reporting of dead wild boar, by maintaining or increasing awareness amongst the persons that in any way could report wild boar carcasses to the competent authorities; this is particularly important in those areas where ASF eradication is almost achieved and where surveillance has the main task to demonstrate the absence of the virus.

5. Conclusions

At very low wild boar density (i.e., 100/1000 km^2), the virus is hardly detected through the usual surveillance strategies (both passive and active); in such epidemiological scenario, the available resources should be addressed at increasing passive surveillance with the aim of understanding where the virus is still present and removing infected carcasses. A low wild boar density, in fact, carcasses are the main responsible for maintaining the chain of infection in the wild.

Author Contributions: Conceptualization, V.G. and S.B.; methodology, V.G., V.G. and A.M.; formal analysis, V.G. and V.G.; writing—original draft preparation, all authors; writing—review and editing, all authors; project administration, V.G.; funding acquisition, V.G. All authors have read and agreed to the published version of the manuscript.

References

1.   Pitts, N.; Whitnall, T. Impact of African swine fever on global markets. *Agric. Commod.* **2019**, *9*, 52–54.

2.   Gallardo, C.; Fernández-Pinero, J.; Pelayo, V.; Gazaev, I.; Markowska-Daniel, I.; Pridotkas, G.; Nieto, R.; Fernández-Pacheco, P.; Bokhan, S.; Nevolko, O.; et al. Genetic variation among African swine fever genotype II viruses, Eastern and Central Europe. *Emerg. Infect. Dis.* **2014**, *20*, 1544–1547. [CrossRef] [PubMed]

3.   Chenais, E.; Sternberg-Lewerin, S.; Boqvist, S.; Liu, L.; LeBlanc, N.; Aliro, T.; Masembe, C.; Ståhl, K. African swine fever outbreak on a medium-sized farm in Uganda: Biosecurity breaches and within-farm virus contamination. *Trop. Anim. Health Prod.* **2017**, *49*, 337–346. [CrossRef] [PubMed]

4.   EFSA; Boklund, A.; Cay, B.; Depner, K.; Földi, Z.; Guberti, V.; Masiulis, M.; Miteva, A.; More, S.; Olsevskis, E.; et al. Epidemiological analyses of African swine fever in the European Union (November 2017 until November 2018). *EFSA J.* **2018**, *16*, 5494.

5.   Chenais, E.; Depner, K.; Guberti, V.; Dietze, K.; Viltrop, A.; Ståhl, K. Epidemiological considerations on African swine fever in Europe 2014–2018. *Porc. Heal. Manag.* **2019**, *5*, 1–10. [CrossRef] [PubMed]

6.   Keeling, M.J.; Rohani, P. *Modeling Infectious Diseases*; Princeton University Press: Princeton, NJ, USA, 2008.

7.   Keeling, M.J.; Gilligan, C.A. Bubonic plague: A metapopulation model of a zoonosis. *Proc. R. Soc. B Biol. Sci.* **2000**, *267*, 2219–2230. [CrossRef] [PubMed]

8.   Diekmann, O.; Heesterbeek, J.A.P. *Mathematical epidemiology of infectious diseases: Model building, analysis and interpretation*; Jon Wiley & Sons: New York, NY, USA, 2000.

9.   Keuling, O.; Stier, N.; Roth, M. How does hunting influence activity and spatial usage in wild boar Sus scrofa L.? *Eur. J. Wildl. Res.* **2008**, *54*, 729–737. [CrossRef]

4

Development of a High-Throughput Serum Neutralization Test using Recombinant Pestiviruses Possessing a Small Reporter Tag

Madoka Tetsuo [1], Keita Matsuno [1,2], Tomokazu Tamura [3,4], Takasuke Fukuhara [3], Taksoo Kim [1], Masatoshi Okamatsu [1], Norbert Tautz [5], Yoshiharu Matsuura [3] and Yoshihiro Sakoda [1,2,*]

[1] Laboratory of Microbiology, Division of Disease Control, Faculty of Veterinary Medicine, Hokkaido University, Sapporo, Hokkaido 060-0818, Japan; doma2_1996@eis.hokudai.ac.jp (M.T.); matsuno@vetmed.hokudai.ac.jp (K.M.); tatatataksoo-u2@eis.hokudai.ac.jp (T.K.); okamatsu@vetmed.hokudai.ac.jp (M.O.)

[2] Global Station for Zoonosis Control, Global Institute for Collaborative Research and Education (GI-CoRE), Hokkaido University, Sapporo 001-0020, Japan

[3] Department of Molecular Virology, Research Institute for Microbial Diseases, Osaka University, Osaka 565-0871, Japan; ttamura@princeton.edu (T.T.); fukut@biken.osaka-u.ac.jp (T.F.); matsuura@biken.osaka-u.ac.jp (Y.M.)

[4] Department of Molecular Biology, Princeton University, Washington Road, Princeton, NJ 08540, USA

[5] Institute of Virology and Cell Biology, University of Lübeck, D-23562 Lübeck, Germany; norbert.tautz@vuz.uni-luebeck.de

* Correspondence: sakoda@vetmed.hokudai.ac.jp

Abstract: A serum neutralization test (SNT) is an essential method for the serological diagnosis of pestivirus infections, including classical swine fever, because of the cross reactivity of antibodies against pestiviruses and the non-quantitative properties of antibodies in an enzyme-linked immunosorbent assay. In conventional SNTs, an immunoperoxidase assay or observation of cytopathic effect after incubation for 3 to 7 days is needed to determine the SNT titer, which requires labor-intensive or time-consuming procedures. Therefore, a new SNT, based on the luciferase system and using classical swine fever virus, bovine viral diarrhea virus, and border disease virus possessing the 11-amino-acid subunit derived from NanoLuc luciferase was developed and evaluated; this approach enabled the rapid and easy determination of the SNT titer using a luminometer. In the new method, SNT titers can be determined tentatively at 2 days post-infection (dpi) and are comparable to those obtained by conventional SNTs at 3 or 4 dpi. In conclusion, the luciferase-based SNT can replace conventional SNTs as a high-throughput antibody test for pestivirus infections.

Keywords: border disease; bovine viral diarrhea; classical swine fever; pestivirus; serum neutralization test; reporter virus

1. Introduction

Pestiviruses are enveloped positive-strand RNA viruses that belong to the genus *Pestivirus*, within the family *Flaviviridae*. Pestiviruses can infect farmed pigs and ruminants with significant economic impact and have also been detected in wild boar, wild ruminants, rodents, bats, and aquatic mammals [1,2]. Pestiviruses possess a single-stranded positive-sense RNA of approximately 12.3 kb in length, with one large open reading frame (ORF) flanked by 5′ and 3′ untranslated regions. The ORF encodes a single polyprotein cleaved by cellular and viral proteases co- and post-translationally into four structural proteins (C, E^{rns}, E1, and E2) and eight non-structural proteins (N^{pro}, p7, NS2, NS3, NS4A, NS4B, NS5A, and NS5B) [1]. The genus *Pestivirus* currently comprises 11 species, *Pestivirus A* to

Pestivirus K, with bovine viral diarrhea virus (BVDV), classical swine fever virus (CSFV), and border disease virus (BDV) classified into *Pestivirus A* (BVDV-1), *Pestivirus B* (BVDV-2), *Pestivirus C* (CSFV), and *Pestivirus D* (BDV), respectively [3]. Originally, the taxonomic classification of pestiviruses was based on the host species from which they were isolated (e.g., CSFV from pigs and BVDV from cattle), but it is now well known that many pestiviruses are capable of interspecies transmission (e.g., BVDV infections in pigs and BDV infections in cattle) [4,5].

Classical swine fever (CSF) is one of the most important diseases of domestic pigs and wild boar. Because of its tremendous impact on animal health and the pig industry, CSF is notifiable to the World Organization for Animal Health (OIE) [6–8]. The diagnosis of CSF consists of (1) clinical observation, (2) gross pathological findings, (3) antigen detection, and (4) antibody detection [9,10]. Diagnosis during the early stages of a CSF outbreak usually relies on 1 and 2 (i.e., clinical and pathological diagnoses), however, these features may vary and can sometimes be atypical [7,11,12]. Thus, for the confirmation of CSFV infection, antigen and antibody detection following the early clinical and pathological diagnoses is necessary. In the diagnostic laboratory, antigen detection by virus isolation and reverse transcriptase-polymerase chain reaction (RT-PCR) is highly recommended to confirm clinical cases. The detection of virus-specific antibodies is particularly useful for herds suspected of having been infected at least 21 days previously with CSFV [8]. Anti-CSFV antibody detection methods, such as enzyme-linked immunosorbent assay (ELISA), are valuable tools for surveillance that requires high-throughput, although this approach can be hampered by antibodies that cross-react with CSFV antigens, which can occasionally be raised in animals infected with other pestiviruses [13]. Some ELISAs are relatively CSFV-specific, but the definitive method of choice for differentiation is the comparative serum neutralization test (SNT), which compares the neutralizing titer of antibodies against different pestivirus isolates [8,14].

In September 2018, the first CSF outbreak in Japan for 26 years was reported [15,16]. Despite countermeasures being taken, including the culling of infected herds and movement restrictions, the infection has continued to spread in 10 prefectures, resulting in 57 outbreaks and a total of 165,186 pigs culled as of 2 March 2020 [17]. In addition, 1944 cases of CSFV infection in wild boar have been reported as of 21 February 2020 [17]. To control CSF in wild boar, a vaccination program using the bait dosed with vaccine containing a live attenuated C strain [18] was initiated in March 2019, in addition to efforts to reduce the wild boar population by trapping or hunting, based on previous experiences in Europe [19,20]. Furthermore, in addition to the improvements in biosecurity, a vaccination program using an injectable vaccine containing a live attenuated GPE⁻ strain [21] was also started in October 2019, to help minimize the CSF outbreak in domestic pigs. The vaccination of domestic pigs is only permitted in high-risk prefectures where CSFV infection in wild boar has been confirmed. Currently, large-scale serological monitoring is being conducted using ELISA, to evaluate the effects of the vaccination program and monitor the CSF-free status in non-vaccinated areas. In addition, BVDV and BDV infections in domestic pigs have also previously been reported in Japan [22,23]. Hence, the necessity for a comparative SNT is now increasing, both to discriminate CSFV-specific antibodies from those against BVDV or BDV and to understand quantitative aspects of antibody levels following the vaccination of wild boar and domestic pigs.

Despite the intense demands for the use of an SNT to test the sera of domestic pigs and wild boar, conventional SNTs based on an immunoperoxidase assay or cytopathic effect (CPE) observation are time- and labor-intensive when testing a large number of samples [8,24]. Thus, in this study, a new, high-throughput SNT method using recombinant viruses carrying a reporter gene was developed. Since the first recombinant pestivirus carrying a marker gene was constructed [25], various reporter genes have been applied for pestivirus research [26–28]. Recently, to reduce the risk of undesirable effects following the insertion of a large foreign gene into a viral genome, NanoLuc binary technology (NanoBiT) [29] was employed for the construction of recombinant CSFV and BVDV-1 carrying a small reporter gene [30,31]. NanoBiT is a split reporter protein consisting of two subunits: a high-affinity NanoBiT (HiBiT) consisting of just 11 amino acids and a large NanoBiT (LgBiT). Neither subunit has enzymatic activity individually but regains this activity when the subunits associate to form a heterodimer, either in cells or in vitro [32]. The detection of HiBiT-fusion viral protein is simple and scalable in comparison with the currently used methods.

In the present study, a recombinant BDV carrying the HiBiT gene was newly constructed and applied for SNT, together with previously established recombinant CSFV and BVDV-1 possessing HiBiT [30,31], to reduce the time and effort required to detect specific neutralizing antibodies. This new SNT method using these recombinant viruses showed the same sensitivity and specificity as conventional SNTs. The HiBiT recombinant-virus-based SNT will provide a more simple and rapid procedure for the serological diagnosis of pestivirus infections.

2. Results

2.1. Rescue of Border Disease Virus (BDV) Possessing a Small Reporter High-Affinity NanoBiT (HiBiT) Tag, vBDV FNK/HiBiT

In our previous studies, recombinant *Flaviviridae* viruses possessing a small reporter HiBiT tag were developed as tools to understand the viral life cycle and pathogenesis and to provide a robust platform for the development of novel antivirals [30,31]. For those studies, two recombinant pestiviruses, vCSFV GPE⁻/HiBiT and vBVDV-1 NCP7/HiBiT, were established from the recombinant full-length cDNA of CSFV GPE⁻ and BVDV-1 NCP7 strains, respectively. To establish a novel SNT using pestiviruses possessing a small reporter tag, the recombinant full-length cDNA of the BDV FNK2012-1 strain, BDV subgenotype-1 (BDV-1) isolated from domestic pigs in Japan [22] was newly established and a BDV recombinant was generated by inserting HiBiT between C and E^{rns} (vBDV FNK/HiBiT, Figure 1A), since the N-termini of E^{rns} of CSFV and BVDV tolerate the exogenous tag [27,30,31]. To compare the growth of recombinant vBDV FNK/HiBiT with the wild-type BDV, swine kidney line-L (SK-L) cells were inoculated with 200 50% tissue-culture infective doses ($TCID_{50}$) of either virus. The growth of the recombinant BDV was relatively lower at the early period, but finally identical to that of the wild-type BDV (Figure 1B). Next, the genetic stability of the newly constructed recombinant BDV was evaluated by passaging it at five times in SK-L cells. The infectious titer through the passages was sufficient (Figure 1C); however, the luciferase activities of vBDV FNK/HiBiT P3, P4 and P5 were significantly lower than that of original virus, vBDV FNK/HiBiT P0 (Figure 1D), suggesting low stability of this marker virus. For this reason, the serial passage of vBDV FNK/HiBiT for the SNT was kept to a minimum.

2.2. Characterization of Reporter Pestiviruses with HiBiT Tags

To check the increasing luciferase activity associated with virus growth, the luciferase activity in the infected cells and culture supernatant was measured during the time course of infection with vCSFV GPE⁻/HiBiT, vBVDV-1 NCP7/HiBiT, and vBDV FNK/HiBiT, respectively (Figure 2). Luciferase activity became detectable at 2 days post-infection (dpi) in the cells and the culture supernatant. For all infection experiments, the luminescence value in the cell lysate was higher than that of the respective culture supernatant. The luciferase activity in cells inoculated with vCSFV GPE⁻/HiBiT was the highest, followed by vBVDV-1 NCP7/HiBiT, while the lowest activity was measured for the cells inoculated with vBDV FNK/HiBiT. Taking these findings together, it was evident that the growth of each recombinant virus could be monitored based on luciferase activity in the cell lysate. The growth of vCSFV GPE⁻/HiBiT could also be monitored in culture supernatant.

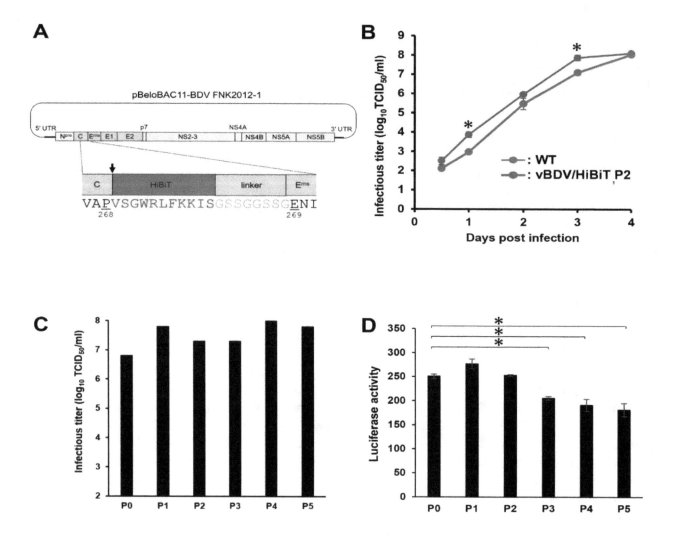

Figure 1. Construction and characterization of recombinant border disease virus (BDV) carrying high-affinity NanoBiT (HiBiT). (**A**) Schematic diagram of the BDV cDNA clone encoding the HiBiT luciferase gene. Amino acid sequence of HiBiT (red) and linker (green) was inserted upstream of E^{rns} of BDV FNK2012-1 strain (indicated by arrow). (**B**) Swine kidney line-L (SK-L) cells were infected with 200 50% tissue-culture infective doses ($TCID_{50}$) of BDV FNK-WT (WT) and the recombinant vBDV FNK/HiBiT P2 (vBDV/HiBiT P2). Infectious titers in the culture supernatant were determined at the indicated time points. Data are presented as mean ± standard error (SE) ($n = 3$). Asterisks indicate significant differences (*, $p < 0.05$) versus the result of the vBDV/HiBiT P2. (**C**) SK-L cells were infected with 200 $TCID_{50}$ of vBDV FNK/HiBiT, then the recombinant BDV was passaged five times. Undiluted culture supernatant (100 μL) at 3 days post-infection (dpi) was used for the next passage in naïve cells, and infectious titers in the culture supernatant were determined at 4 dpi after each passage. (**D**) SK-L cells were infected with 200 $TCID_{50}$ of vBDV FNK/HiBiT, then the recombinant BDV was passaged five times. Luciferase activity in the cells was determined at 4 dpi after each passage. Data are presented as mean ± standard error (SE) ($n = 3$). Asterisks indicate significant differences (*, $p < 0.05$) versus the result of the vBDV FNK/HiBiT P0.

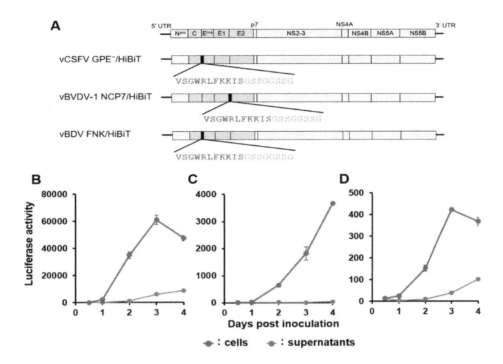

Figure 2. Construction and luciferase activity of the recombinant pestiviruses carrying HiBiT. Schematic preparation of the reporter pestiviruses (**A**). Coding regions of the recombinant viruses are displayed as boxes divided by each protein gene; structural protein (blue) and non-structural protein (grey). Amino acid sequence of HiBiT (red) and linker (green) was inserted upstream of E^{rns} of classical swine fever virus (CSFV) and BDV or upstream of E2 of BVDV-1. The luciferase activities following the infection of recombinant vCSFV GPE⁻/HiBiT in swine kidney line-L (SK-L) cells (**B**), vBVDV-1 NCP7/HiBiT in Madin–Darby bovine kidney (MDBK) cells (**C**), and vBDV FNK/HiBiT in SK-L cells (**D**) at 200 $TCID_{50}$ were determined in the cell lysate or the culture supernatant, respectively. Data are presented as mean ± standard error (SE) ($n = 3$).

To confirm whether the antigenicity of the recombinant viruses was affected by the insertion of HiBiT, both recombinants and parental viruses were tested using reference antisera in a conventional SNT based on the immunoperoxidase assay (Table 1). Convalescent sera derived from pigs experimentally infected with CSFV GPE⁻, BVDV-1 Nose, BVDV-2 KZ91, or BDV FNK2012-1 strains were used as reference antisera. These four pestiviruses are generally used as reference virus strains of pestiviruses for SNTs performed in Japan. In addition, the reference virus strain BVDV-1 Nose-WT was also tested, because the antiserum against BVDV-1 NCP7 was not available for this study. In the SNT using CSFV, the serum against CSFV showed the highest SNT titer, 1024, for both recombinant and wild-type viruses, while the other sera showed titers of <2. In the SNT using BVDV-1, however, the sera against BVDV-1 as well as BVDV-2 showed the highest SNT titer, 32, for the recombinant vBVDV-1 NCP7/HiBiT and the original vBVDV-1 NCP7-WT, while the other sera showed lower titers of <2. In terms of the neutralizing activities of antisera against BVDV-1 Nose and BVDV-2 KZ91-NCP to BVDV-1 Nose-WT, the serum against BVDV-1 Nose showed the highest SNT titer, 64, and the others against BVDV-2 KZ91-NCP showed lower titers of 8. In the SNT using BDV, serum against BDV showed the highest SNT titer, 128, for the recombinant and the wild-type viruses, and the other sera showed lower titers, of between 2 to 8. Each type of serum showed the highest SNT titer when the homologous virus was used, regardless of whether it was the wild-type virus or the recombinant virus, and there were few differences in SNT titer between the recombinant and wild-type viruses. Thus, the antigenicity of the recombinants was not altered by the insertion of HiBiT, although the BVDV-1 NCP7 strain with and without HiBiT showed different antigenicity compared with that of the BVDV-1 Nose strain. Hence, these recombinants carrying HiBiT were employed for the development of a new SNT.

Table 1. Comparative serum neutralization tests (SNTs) of pestiviruses based on the conventional immunoperoxidase assay.

Marker Virus	SNT Titer* of Antiserum against			
	CSFV GPE⁻	BVDV-1 Nose	BVDV-2 KZ91-NCP	BDV FNK2012-1
vCSFV GPE⁻/HiBiT	1024	<2	<2	<2
vCSFV GPE⁻-WT	1024	<2	<2	<2
vBVDV-1 NCP7/HiBiT	<2	32	32	<2
vBVDV-1 NCP7-WT	<2	32	32	<2
BVDV-1 Nose-WT	<2	64	8	<2
vBDV FNK/HiBiT	8	2	4	128
BDV FNK-WT	8	4	8	128

* SNT titers were determined at 4 days post-infection (dpi).

2.3. Development of the Serum Neutralization Test (SNT) Based on the Luciferase Assay

The luciferase activity became detectable on 2 dpi for all viruses tested (Figure 2), therefore the new luciferase-based SNTs were first tested on 2, 3, and 4 dpi to determine the most appropriate incubation time for measuring luciferase activity (Supplementary Materials Figures S1–S3). Luciferase activity was monitored using the culture medium (for CSFV) or cell lysate (for BVDV-1 and BDV), because only CSFV luciferase activity in the culture medium was sufficient for the test. Luciferase activity increased depending on the serum dilution and the time following inoculation with the virus. At some of the low serum dilutions, luciferase activity was initially not detectable (e.g., vBDV FNK/HiBiT with the reference anti-BDV serum diluted 8 times, shown in Figure S3D), but became detectable by 4 dpi. On the other hand, at levels of serum dilution where the virus could be completely neutralized, the luciferase activity did not increase during the study period. Next, the SNT titers of the luciferase-based SNT were determined for each dpi and compared with the titers of the conventional SNT, determined on 4 dpi (Table 2). Following the luciferase-based assay from 2 to 4 dpi, each serum sample showed the highest SNT titer and 50% effective concentration (EC_{50}) against the homologous strain and could be differentiated from the heterologous strains, with the exception of vBVDV-1 NCP7/HiBiT, which showed cross reactivity with the serum against BVDV-2. These findings were observed in both the luciferase-based and conventional SNT, with SNT titers based on luciferase activity decreasing in a time-dependent manner and finally becoming comparable with SNT titers from the conventional SNT at 3 or 4 dpi.

Table 2. Comparative SNTs of pestiviruses when using the new luciferase-based assay and the conventional immunoperoxidase assay.

Marker Virus	SNT Method (dpi)		SNT Titer and EC_{50}* of Antiserum against							
			CSFV GPE⁻		BVDV-1 Nose		BVDV-2 KZ91-NCP		BDV FNK2012-1	
vCSFV GPE⁻/HiBIT	Luciferase-based	(2)	1024	11.3	2	6.73	2	7.04	4	5.19
		(3)	1024	11.1	<2	2.46	<2	4.59	<2	3.65
		(4)	1024	10.8	<2	1.65	<2	3.75	<2	1.86
	Immunoperoxidase	(4)	1024		<2		<2		<2	
vBVDV-1 NCP7/HiBiT	Luciferase-based	(2)	2	4.98	128	8.47	128	9.57	<2	2.77
		(3)	<2	3.97	32	8.17	32	7.97	<2	2.01
		(4)	<2	2.93	32	7.91	64	9.52	<2	N/A
	Immunoperoxidase	(4)	<2		32		32		<2	
vBDV FNK/HiBiT	Luciferase-based	(2)	64	7.36	8	4.92	64	7.20	2048	10.83
		(3)	8	4.77	2	2.22	2	3.34	256	9.01
		(4)	2	1.01	<2	N/A	<2	1.22	128	7.11
	Immunoperoxidase	(4)	8		2		4		128	

* The EC_{50} number of the Luciferase-based SNT method was indicated by an index with a base of 2. N/A: not available.

3. Discussion

ELISAs involve simple, rapid procedures and are therefore widely used for the serological diagnosis of pestivirus infections, including CSF. Because of the cross reactivity of antibodies against pestiviruses, the definitive method of choice for differentiation of pestiviruses is the comparative SNT, which compares neutralizing titers of antibodies to different pestivirus isolates [8]. However, the conventional SNT requires a high-containment laboratory able to handle infectious viruses and involves labor-and time-intensive procedures. Therefore, recombinant pestiviruses were employed to establish a novel SNT based on the luciferase system, which allows virus growth to be easily and rapidly monitored and enables SNT titers for pestiviruses to be determined.

Four pestiviruses, including CSFV, BVDV-1, BVDV-2, and BDV, are usually used as reference viruses for SNTs. The CSFV GPE$^-$ strain, which shows a CPE in CPK-NS cells [24], the BVDV-1 Nose and BVDV-2 KZ91-CP strains, which show a CPE regardless of the cell line used, and the BDV FNK2012-1 strain, which does not show a CPE, are usually selected for conventional comparative SNTs in Japan. In SNTs using reference viruses which do not show a CPE, the immunoperoxidase assay is performed to determine the SNT titers following incubation for 3 to 4 days, which is indicated in the OIE manual to be the "gold standard" [8], even though it is time-consuming. In the present study, SNT titers determined by a luciferase-based SNT using recombinant pestiviruses were comparable with those determined using conventional SNTs, although some differences in SNT titers were observed; this might reflect the experimental conditions, such as the type of cells or viruses used. The luciferase assay used to determine SNT titers is less time-consuming and more straightforward than the immunoperoxidase assay when dealing with a large number of samples, although the recombinant pestiviruses can only be handled by a limited number of laboratories. In addition, the SNT titers can be determined within 3 or 4 days of inoculation, which is the same as the conventional SNT based on the immunoperoxidase assay and earlier than the conventional SNT based on CPE observation. Additionally, the SNT titers can be tentatively determined earlier, at 2 dpi, although they are slightly higher than those at 4 dpi, suggesting that earlier confirmation of pestivirus infection may be possible using the present method of SNT.

In Japan, CSFV infection has spread among domestic pigs and wild boar since the first outbreak at a domestic pig farm in September 2018. Control of CSFV infection in wild boar should be prioritized for preventing the spread of CSF, because direct or indirect contact with wild boar infected with CSFV can be a primary route for the introduction of the virus to pig farms [33,34]. To prevent the spread of this infection in wild boar, an oral vaccination program targeting wild boar commenced in the spring of 2019. So far, the efficacy of vaccination in wild boar has been evaluated by ELISA only, while the cross-reaction to antibodies against other ruminant pestiviruses and non-specific reactions to the low-quality sera derived from wild boar have not been investigated. Hence, SNTs should be performed at reference laboratories to confirm the ELISA results and possibly also provide information about the spread of CSFV in the field. In addition to the vaccination of wild boar, a vaccination program for domestic pigs was re-started in October 2019. The vaccine being used in the present program is the same as that used in the previous program conducted in Japan between 1969 and 2006, in which domestic piglets aged from 30 to 40 days were vaccinated once [35]. Thus, in this program, in which it is recommended that all pigs in the at-risk area are vaccinated regardless of their age, the vaccine performance should be revisited according to the neutralizing antibody titer derived from acquired and/or maternal immunity. Hence, the SNT titer after the vaccination of domestic pigs, in addition to wild boar, should be investigated using this luciferase-based SNT.

The N-termini of E^{rns} of both CSFV and BVDV are capable of expressing an exogenous tag [27,30,31]. Based on these findings, we generated a BDV recombinant by inserting HiBiT between C and E^{rns} (vBDV FNK/HiBiT) (Figure 1A). However, the luciferase activity of vBDV FNK/HiBiT was lower than those of the others (Figure 2). In addition, the luciferase activities of serially passaged recombinant virus were significantly lower than that of original virus (Figure 1D); suggesting low genetic stability of the vBDV FNK/HiBiT. The luciferase activity of recombinant virus carrying HiBiT should be related to the expression level of HiBiT fused with a viral protein; therefore, HiBiT inserted into recombinant BDV might not be appropriately expressed, resulting in its lower luciferase activity. The vBDV FNK/HiBiT was designed following vCSFV GPE⁻/HiBiT to express HiBiT and the linker fused with the N-terminus of Eʳⁿˢ and presumably cleaved upstream of HiBiT by a signal peptidase. However, the signal sequence at the C-terminus of the C is not conserved among the pestiviruses (Figure 3); therefore, HiBiT inserted downstream of the signal sequence might disturb the post-translational cleavage of the BDV protein. Indeed, the growth of vBVDV-1 NCP7/HiBiT and vBDV FNK/HiBiT needs to be monitored by measuring luciferase activity in the cells, whereas vCSFV GPE⁻/HiBiT is able to be monitored by measuring luciferase activity in the culture supernatant (Figure 2). Measuring luciferase activity in the culture supernatant enables the assessment of viral growth at several time points after infection of a single cell culture. Thus, recombinant viruses need to be detectable in culture supernatants for an assay to be efficient. On the other hand, we evaluated vBVDV-1 NCP7/HiBiT, which has been previously reported [30,31], but the significant cross reactivity of vBVDV-1 NCP7-WT with the serum against BVDV-2 was confirmed. In addition, the subgenotypes of BDV are more diverse, and selection of a reference strain for the SNT seems to be more complicated, although only BDV subgenotype 1 (BDV-1) has previously been isolated in Japan [22]. Hence, appropriate reference viruses should be selected based on the local prevalence of pestiviruses, and genetically stable recombinant viruses, which express the HiBiT fused with a viral protein efficiently, should be generated for the luciferase-based SNT. These localized recombinant reporter pestiviruses would be useful for luciferase-based SNTs for the surveillance not only of CSFV but also, in certain areas, of BVDV and BDV.

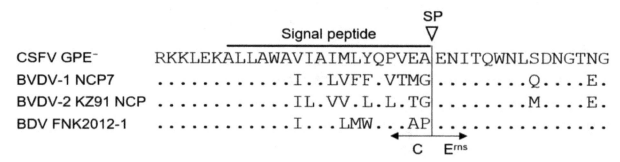

Figure 3. Amino acid sequences of pestiviruses around the cleavage site between C and Eʳⁿˢ. The sequences were compared using GENETIX network ver. 12.0.1 (GENETYX Corp., Japan). The region of the signal peptide sequence and the site of cleavage by signal peptidase is indicated on top of the alignment (SP). The line and arrow indicate part of the C and Eʳⁿˢ proteins, respectively, at the bottom of the alignment.

Altogether, the present luciferase-based SNT enables SNT titers to be determined simply and rapidly, replacing conventional SNTs. Therefore, this luciferase-based SNT could be a powerful tool for high-throughput serological testing, providing useful information for the investigation and control of pestiviruses, including CSFV in the field.

4. Materials and Methods

4.1. Cells and Viruses

The SK-L and MDBK cells were propagated in Eagle's Minimum Essential Medium (Nissui Pharmaceutical, Tokyo, Japan) supplemented with 0.3 mg/mL L-glutamine (Nacalai tesque, Kyoto, Japan), 100 U/mg penicillin G (Meiji Seika Pharma, Tokyo, Japan), 8 µg/mL gentamycin (TAKATA Pharmaceutical, Saitama, Japan), sodium bicarbonate (Nacalai tesque), 0.1 mg/mL streptomycin (Meiji Seika Pharma), 0.295% tryptose phosphate broth (Becton, Dickinson and Company, Franklin Lakes, NJ, USA), 10 mM N,N-bis-(2-hydroxyethyl)-2-aminoethanesulfonic acid (BES; MilliporeSigma, St. Louis,

MO, USA), and 10% horse serum (Thermo Fisher Scientific, Waltham, MA, USA). Both types of cells were incubated at 37 °C in the presence of 5% CO_2.

Three recombinant pestiviruses encoding the HiBiT luciferase gene were used for the new luciferase-based SNT; vCSFV GPE$^-$/HiBiT was derived from recombinant full-length cDNA of the CSFV GPE$^-$ strain, which expressed HiBiT luciferase fused with the N-terminus of viral E^{rns} [31]. vBVDV-1 NCP7/HiBiT was derived from recombinant full-length cDNA of the BVDV-1 NCP7 strain, which expressed HiBiT luciferase fused with the N-terminus of viral E2 [30,36]. vBDV FNK/HiBiT was derived from recombinant full-length cDNA of the BDV-1 FNK2012-1 strain [22], which expressed HiBiT luciferase fused with the N-terminus of viral E^{rns}. This full-length cDNA of the BDV FNK2012-1 strain and vBDV FNK/HiBiT was newly developed for this study. Details of the construction of the recombinant full-length cDNA clone of BDV are given below.

In addition, the wild-type viruses in the conventional SNT were selected as follows: vGPE$^-$, which was derived from recombinant full-length cDNA of the CSFV GPE$^-$ strain [37], described as vCSFV GPE$^-$-WT, BVDV-1 Nose strain [38] described as BVDV-Nose-WT, vNCP7 which was derived from the recombinant full-length cDNA of the BVDV-1 NCP7 strain [36] described as vBVDV-1 NCP7-WT, and BDV FNK2012-1 strain [22] described as BDV FNK-WT. The BDV FNK2012-1 strain was isolated from domestic pigs and propagated in SK-L cells.

4.2. Reference Antisera

Four reference porcine sera were used for the SNTs. Each serum sample was obtained from a pig in the convalescent phase following infection with CSFV GPE$^-$ strain, BVDV-1 Nose strain, BVDV-2 KZ91-NCP strain, or BDV FNK2012-1 strain. CSFV GPE$^-$ strain was intramuscularly inoculated in 6-week-old pigs, and serum against CSFV was collected at 6 months post-inoculation. BDV FNK2012-1 strain was intramuscularly inoculated in four-week-old pigs, followed by intramuscular inoculation with adjuvant; serum against BDV was collected at 42 dpi. Porcine sera against BVDV-1 Nose strain and BVDV-2 KZ91-CP strain were previously established [14]. All sera were inactivated by heating at 56 °C for 30 min before SNTs were performed.

4.3. Construction of BDV FNK2012-1 Full-Length cDNA

The cDNA clone of BDV FNK2012-1 was constructed according to a previously reported methodology [39]. Viral RNA was extracted from the supernatant of virus-infected cells using TRIzol LS Reagent (Thermo Fisher Scientific), 1-bromo-3-chloropropane (MilliporeSigma), and RNeasy Mini Kit (Qiagen, Hilden, Germany), according to the manufacturer's instructions. The extracted RNA was reverse transcribed (RT) with RT primer (Table S1) using SuperScript III Reverse Transcriptase (Thermo Fisher Scientific), and subsequently 2 μL of cDNA was subjected to polymerase chain reaction (PCR) with gene-specific primers (Table S1) using Q5 Hot Start High-Fidelity DNA Polymerase (New England Biolabs, Ipswich, MA, USA). The linearized fragment of pBeloBAC11 (New England Biolabs) was also amplified with the primers indicated in Table S1, using Q5 Hot Start High-Fidelity DNA Polymerase. Then, the bacterial artificial chromosome (BAC) containing full-length cDNA corresponding to FNK2012-1 was obtained using an In-Fusion HD Cloning Kit (TaKaRa Bio, Shiga, Japan). The nucleotide sequences of the purified PCR products of the cDNA clones used in the present study were confirmed using an ABI 3500 Genetic Analyzer (Thermo Fisher Scientific).

4.4. Construction of HiBiT Recombinant Full-Length cDNA of BDV

The BDV cDNA clone encoding the HiBiT luciferase gene (Figure 1) was constructed following the method described in a previous report for CSFV and BVDV-1 [30,31], using a KOD-plus-mutagenesis kit (TOYOBO, Osaka, Japan) and the respective oligonucleotide primers. Briefly, the BAC carrying the BDV cDNA clone was used as a template for inverse PCR following DpnI digestion, with primers including the HiBiT sequence (Table S1), and then the product was self-ligated, according to the manufacturer's protocol.

4.5. In Vitro Transcription and RNA Transfection

The recombinant clones of BVDV-1 and BDV were used as templates for full genome PCR to add the T7 promoter sequence with the respective primers (Table S1), using AccuPrime *Taq* DNA Polymerase, High Fidelity (Thermo Fisher Scientific), and then the products were purified using a FastGene Gel/PCR Extraction Kit (NIPPON Genetics, Tokyo, Japan), according to the manufacturer's protocol. The recombinant full-length cDNA clone of CSFV was linearized at the SrfI site located at the end of the viral genomic cDNA sequence, followed by purification by phenol-chloroform extraction and ethanol precipitation. The purified PCR products of the BVDV-1 and BDV clones and the linearized product of the CSFV clones were used as templates for run-off transcription using a MEGAscript T7 kit (Thermo Fisher Scientific). After DNase I digestion and purification in S-400 HR Sephadex columns (GE Healthcare, Chicago, IL, USA), RNA was transfected to SK-L cells for CSFV and BDV or MDBK cells for BVDV-1 by electroporation using a Gene Pulser Xcell (Bio-Rad, Hercules, CA, USA), set at 200 V and 500 μF for SK-L cells or 180 V and 950 μF for MDBK cells, followed by incubation at 37 °C for 3 days. Virus recovery was confirmed by an immunostaining assay using anti-CSFV NS3 antibodies, as described below. The entire genomes of rescued viruses were verified by sequencing with an ABI 3500 Genetic Analyzer. The rescued viruses were stored at −80 °C for the SNTs.

4.6. Immunoperoxidase Assay to Detect Pestivirus Antigens

The immunoperoxidase assay was performed as previously described [40]. Briefly, cells inoculated with viruses were washed with PBS and heat-fixed at 80 °C for 1 h. The cells were then incubated at room temperature for 1 h in the presence of the primary monoclonal antibody for NS3, 46/1. The cells were washed with PBS and then incubated at 37 °C for 1 h in the presence of goat anti-mouse IgG (H+L) horseradish peroxidase conjugate (Bio-Rad). The cells were washed again and then stained with 3-amino-9-ethyl carbazole (MilliporeSigma).

4.7. Virus Titration

SK-L cells were infected with 10-fold serially diluted CSFV or BDV, and MDBK cells were infected with 10-fold serially diluted BVDV-1, in 96-well plates and incubated at 37 °C for 4 days. Then, the plates were immunostained, as described above. Virus titers were calculated and expressed as $TCID_{50}$ per mL [41].

4.8. Luciferase Assay

The luciferase activity of culture supernatants or cell lysates was measured using a Nano-Glo HiBiT lytic detection system (Promega, Madison, WI, USA), according to the manufacturer's protocol. To measure luciferase activity in the cell culture supernatant, 20 μL of culture medium was mixed with an equal volume of Nano-Glo HiBiT lytic buffer. To measure luciferase activity in cell lysate, all culture medium was removed, and the cells were lysed using 20 μL of Nano-Glo HiBiT lytic buffer for 20 min at room temperature. Luciferase activity was measured in a 96-well LumiNunc™ plate (Thermo Fisher Scientific) using a POWERSCAN 4 (DS Pharma Biomedical, Osaka, Japan).

4.9. Serum Neutralization Tests (SNTs)

Most of the SNTs were performed according to previously described protocols [8,14]. Equal volumes (25 μL) of serially diluted serum and 200 $TCID_{50}$ of CSFV, BVDV-1, or BDV were mixed and incubated at 37 °C for 1 h. This mixture plus SK-L or MDBK cell suspension was incubated in 96-well plates at 37 °C and 5% CO_2. Viral antigens were detected at 4 dpi using the conventional SNT by immunostaining assay, as described above.

For the new luciferase-based SNT, viral antigens were detected from the culture medium (for CSFV) or cell lysate (for BVDV-1 and BDV) on each day by the luciferase assay, as described above. The cut-off value for the luciferase activity to signal complete neutralization (i.e., no virus growth) for the new SNT was calculated based on that of mock-infected 96-well plates. The average number of mock-infected 96-well plates plus five times the standard deviation of this population (i.e., luciferase activity = 70) was set as the cut-off value.

The neutralizing antibody titer of each test was expressed as the reciprocal of the highest serum dilution which showed complete neutralization of the virus.

4.10. The 50% Effective Concentration (EC$_{50}$) of Each Serum against Marker Virus

For the calculation of EC$_{50}$, the diagram of obtained luciferase activity was figured out as a sigmoid curve using ImageJ (version 1.52t) [42] Then, the EC$_{50}$ was calculated based on the maximum and minimum value of each test.

4.11. Ethics Statement

The animal experiments were authorized by the Institutional Animal Care and Use Committee of the Faculty of Veterinary Medicine, Hokkaido University (approval number 18-0038), and performed according to the guidelines of this committee.

Supplementary Materials:
Figure S1: Serum neutralization test (SNT) using recombinant CSFV carrying HiBiT and anti-pestivirus serum; Figure S2: SNT using recombinant BVDV-1 carrying HiBiT and anti-pestivirus serum; Figure S3: SNT using recombinant BDV carrying HiBiT and anti-pestivirus serum, Table S1: Primers for the construction of HiBiT recombinant full-length cDNA of BDV and the virus rescue for BVDV-1 and BDV.

Author Contributions: Conceptualization, K.M. and Y.S.; methodology, T.T., T.F., N.T., and Y.S.; validation, K.M. and M.O.; formal analysis, M.T.; investigation, M.T. and T.K.; resources, Y.M. and Y.S.; data curation, M.T.; writing—original draft preparation, M.T.; writing—review and editing, K.M. and Y.S.; supervision, Y.S.; funding acquisition, K.M., M.O., and Y.S. All authors have read and agree to the published version of the manuscript.

Acknowledgments: Our great appreciation is extended to T. B. Rasmussen and C. Johnston, National Veterinary Institute, Technical University of Denmark, for the revision of constructing the BAC clone.

References

1. Tautz, N.; Tews, B.A.; Meyers, G. *The Molecular Biology of Pestiviruses*; Academic Press: Cambridge, MA, USA, 2015; Volume 93, ISBN 9780128021798.
2. Wu, Z.; Liu, B.; Du, J.; Zhang, J.; Lu, L.; Zhu, G.; Han, Y.; Su, H.; Yang, L.; Zhang, S.; et al. Discovery of diverse rodent and bat pestiviruses with distinct genomic and phylogenetic characteristics in several Chinese provinces. *Front. Microbiol.* **2018**, *9*, 2562.
3. Smith, D.B.; Meyers, G.; Bukh, J.; Gould, E.A.; Monath, T.; Muerhoff, A.S.; Pletnev, A.; Rico-Hesse, R.; Stapleton, J.T.; Simmonds, P.; et al. Proposed revision to the taxonomy of the genus Pestivirus, family Flaviviridae. *J. Gen. Virol.* **2017**, *98*, 2106–2112.
4. Tao, J.; Liao, J.; Wang, Y.; Zhang, X.; Wang, J.; Zhu, G. Bovine Viral Diarrhea Virus (BVDV) infections in pigs. *Vet. Microbiol.* **2013**, *165*, 185–189. [CrossRef]
5. Braun, U.; Hilbe, M.; Peterhans, E.; Schweizer, M. Border disease in cattle. *Vet. J.* **2019**, *246*, 12–20. [CrossRef]
6. Moennig, V.; Becher, P. Pestivirus control programs: How far have we come and where are we going? *Anim. Heal. Res. Rev.* **2015**, *16*, 83–87.
7. Blome, S.; Staubach, C.; Henke, J.; Carlson, J.; Beer, M. Classical swine fever—An updated review. *Viruses* **2017**, *9*, 86. [CrossRef] [PubMed]
8. World Organisation for Animal Health. Classical swine fever. Manual of Diagnostic Tests and Vaccines for Terrestrial Animals. 2019. Available online: https://www.oie.int/standard-setting/terrestrial-manual/access-online/ (accessed on 3 March 2020).
9. Greiser-Wilke, I.; Blome, S.; Moennig, V. Diagnostic methods for detection of classical swine fever virus-status quo and new developments. *Vaccine* **2007** *25*, 5524–5530. [CrossRef] [PubMed]

10. Postel, A.; Austermann-Busch, S.; Petrov, A.; Moennig, V.; Becher, P. Epidemiology, diagnosis and control of classical swine fever: Recent developments and future challenges. *Transbound. Emerg. Dis.* **2018**, *65*, 248–261. [CrossRef] [PubMed]

11. Floegel-Niesmann, G.; Bunzenthal, C.; Fischer, S.; Moennig, V. Virulence of recent and former classical swine fever virus isolates evaluated by their clinical and pathological signs. *J. Vet. Med. Ser. B* **2003**, *50*, 214–220. [CrossRef]

12. Moennig, V.; Floegel-Niesmann, G.; Greiser-Wilke, I. Clinical signs and epidemiology of classical swine fever: A review of new knowledge. *Vet. J.* **2003**, *165*, 11–20. [CrossRef]

13. Terpstra, C.; Bloemraad, M.; Gielkens, A.L.J. The neutralizing peroxidase-linked assay for detection of antibody against swine fever virus. *Vet. Microbiol.* **1984**, *9*, 113–120. [CrossRef]

14. Sakoda, Y.; Wakamoto., H.; Tamura, T.; Nomura., T.; Naito., M.; Aoki., H.; Morita., H.; Kida, H.; Fukusho, A. Development and evaluation of indirect enzyme-linked immunosorbent assay for a screening test to detect antibodies against classical swine fever virus. *Jpn. J. Vet. Res.* **2012**, *60*, 85–94. [PubMed]

15. Kameyama, K.; Nishi, T.; Yamada, M.; Masujin, K.; Morioka, K.; Kokuho, T.; Fukai, K. Experimental infection of pigs with a classical swine fever virus isolated in Japan for the first time in 26 years. *J. Vet. Med. Sci.* **2019**, *81*, 1277–1284. [CrossRef] [PubMed]

16. Postel, A.; Nishi, T.; Kameyama, K.; Meyer, D.; Suckstorff, O.; Fukai, K.; Becher, P. Reemergence of classical swine fever, Japan, 2018. *Emerg. Infect. Dis.* **2019**, *25*, 1228–1231. [CrossRef] [PubMed]

17. Ministry of Agriculture, Forestry and Fisheries, Japan. Update of Classical Swine Fever in Japan. Available online: https://www.maff.go.jp/j/syouan/douei/csf/domestic.html (accessed on 3 March 2020).

18. Brauer, A.; Lange, E.; Kaden, V. Oral immunisation of wild boar against classical swine fever: Uptake studies of new baits and investigations on the stability of lyophilised C-strain vaccine. *Eur. J. Wildl. Res.* **2006**, *52*, 271–276. [CrossRef]

19. Rossi, S.; Staubach, C.; Blome, S.; Guberti, V.; Thulke, H.H.; Vos, A.; Koenen, F.; Le Potier, M.F. Controlling of CSFV in European wild boar using oral vaccination: A review. *Front. Microbiol.* **2015**, *6*, 1141. [CrossRef]

20. Moennig, V. The control of classical swine fever in wild boar. *Front. Microbiol.* **2015**, *6*, 1211. [CrossRef]

21. Shimizu, Y.; Furuuchi, S.; Kumagai, T.; Sasahara, J. A mutant of hog cholera virus inducing interference in swine testicle cell cultures. *Am. J. Vet. Res.* **1970**, *31*, 1787–1794.

22. Nagai, M.; Aoki, H.; Sakoda, Y.; Kozasa, T.; Tominaga-Teshima, K.; Mine, J.; Abe, Y.; Tamura, T.; Kobayashi, T.; Nishine, K.; et al. Molecular, biological, and antigenic characterization of a border disease virus isolated from a pig during classical swine fever surveillance in Japan. *J. Vet. Diagn. Investig.* **2014**, *26*, 547–552. [CrossRef]

23. Takaku, H.; Igarashi, Y.; Kiyohara, H.; Ohyama, K.; Kurosawa, A.; Saitoh, M.; Miyane, K.; Hiramatsu, M. Detection of antibodies against Bovine viral diarrhea virus from field pigs. *J. Jpn. Vet. Med. Assoc.* **2007**, *60*, 125–130. [CrossRef]

24. Sakoda, Y.; Hikawa, M.; Tamura, T.; Fukusho, A. Establishment of a serum-free culture cell line, CPK-NS, which is useful for assays of classical swine fever virus. *J. Virol. Methods* **1998**, *75*, 59–68. [CrossRef]

25. Moser, C.; Tratschin, J.D.; Hofmann, M.A. A recombinant classical swine fever virus stably expresses a marker gene. *J. Virol.* **1998**, *72*, 5318–5322. [CrossRef] [PubMed]

26. Fan, Z.C.; Bird, R.C. An improved reverse genetics system for generation of bovine viral diarrhea virus as a BAC cDNA. *J. Virol. Methods* **2008**, *149*, 309–315. [CrossRef]

27. Wegelt, A.; Reimann, I.; Granzow, H.; Beer, M. Characterization and purification of recombinant bovine viral diarrhea virus particles with epitopetagged envelope proteins. *J. Gen. Virol.* **2011**, *92*, 1352–1357. [CrossRef] [PubMed]

28. Shen, L.; Li, Y.; Chen, J.; Li, C.; Huang, J.; Luo, Y.; Sun, Y.; Li, S.; Qiu, H. Generation of a recombinant classical swine fever virus stably expressing the firefly luciferase gene for quantitative antiviral assay. *Antivir. Res.* **2014**, *109*, 15–21. [CrossRef] [PubMed]

29. Dixon, A.S.; Schwinn, M.K.; Hall, M.P.; Zimmerman, K.; Otto, P.; Lubben, T.H.; Butler, B.L.; Binkowski, B.F.; MacHleidt, T.; Kirkland, T.A.; et al. NanoLuc complementation reporter optimized for accurate measurement of protein interactions in cells. *ACS Chem. Biol.* **2016** *11*, 400–408. [CrossRef]

30. Tamura, T.; Fukuhara, T.; Uchida, T.; Ono, C.; Mori, H.; Sato, A.; Fauzyah, Y.; Okamoto, T.; Kurosu, T.; Setoh, Y.X.; et al. Characterization of recombinant,Flaviviridae viruses possessing a small reporter tag. *J. Virol.* **2018**, *92*, e01582-17. [CrossRef]

31. Tamura, T.; Igarashi, M.; Enkhbold, B.; Suzuki, T.; Okamatsu, M.; Ono, C.; Mori, H.; Izumi, T.; Sato, A.; Fauzyah, Y.; et al. In vivo dynamics of reporter Flaviviridae viruses. *J. Virol.* **2019**, *93*, e01191-19. [CrossRef]

32. Schwinn, M.K.; Machleidt, T.; Zimmerman, K.; Eggers, C.T.; Dixon, A.S.; Hurst, R.; Hall, M.P.; Encell, L.P.; Binkowski, B.F.; Wood, K.V. CRISPR-mediated tagging of endogenous proteins with a Luminescent Peptide. *ACS Chem. Biol.* **2018**, *13*, 467–474. [CrossRef]

33. Hayama, Y.; Shimizu, Y.; Murato, Y.; Sawai, K.; Yamamoto, T. Estimation of infection risk on pig farms in infected wild boar areas—Epidemiological analysis for the reemergence of classical swine fever in Japan in 2018. *Prev. Vet. Med.* **2020**, *175*, 104873. [CrossRef]

34. Ito, S.; Jurado, C.; Bosch, J.; Ito, M.; Sánchez-vizcaíno, J.M.; Isoda, N.; Sakoda, Y. Role of Wild Boar in the spread of classical swine fever in Japan. *Pathogens* **2019**, *8*, 206. [CrossRef] [PubMed]

35. Shimizu, Y. Eradication of classical swine fever in Japan. *Bull. NARO Natl. Inst. Anim. Heal.* **2013**, *119*, 1–9.

36. Meyers, G.; Tautz, N.; Becher, P.; Thiel, H.J.; Kümmerer, B.M. Recovery of cytopathogenic and noncytopathogenic bovine viral diarrhea viruses from cDNA constructs. *J. Virol.* **1996**, *70*, 8606–8613. [CrossRef] [PubMed]

37. Tamura, T.; Sakoda, Y.; Yoshino, F.; Nomura, T.; Yamamoto, N.; Sato, Y.; Okamatsu, M.; Ruggli, N.; Kida, H. Selection of classical swine fever virus with enhanced pathogenicity reveals synergistic virulence determinants in E2 and NS4B. *J. Virol.* **2012**, *86*, 8602–8613. [CrossRef] [PubMed]

38. Nagai, M.; Sakoda, Y.; Mori, M.; Hayashi, M.; Kida, H.; Akashi, H. Insertion of cellular sequence and RNA recombination in the structural protein coding region of cytopathogenic bovine viral diarrhoea virus. *J. Gen. Virol.* **2003**, *84*, 447–452. [CrossRef]

39. Fahnøe, U.; Pedersen, A.G.; Risager, P.C.; Nielsen, J.; Belsham, G.J.; Höper, D.; Beer, M.; Rasmussen, T.B. Rescue of the highly virulent classical swine fever virus strain "Koslov" from cloned cDNA and first insights into genome variations relevant for virulence. *Virology* **2014**, *468*, 379–387. [CrossRef]

40. Kameyama, K.; Sakoda, Y.; Tamai, K.; Nagai, M.; Akashi, H.; Kida, H. Genetic recombination at different points in the Npro-coding region of bovine viral diarrhea viruses and the potentials to change their antigenicities and pathogenicities. *Virus Res.* **2006**, *116*, 78–84. [CrossRef]

41. Reed, L.J.; Muench, H. A simple method of estimating fifty percent endpoints. *Am. J. Epidemiol.* **1938**, *27*, 435–469. [CrossRef]

42. Schneider, C.A.; Rasband, W.S.; Eliceiri, K.W. NIH Image to ImageJ: 25 years of image analysis. *Nat. Methods* **2012**, *9*, 671–675. [CrossRef]

Rapid Spread of Classical Swine Fever Virus among South Korean Wild Boars in Areas Near the Border with North Korea

SeEun Choe [1,†], **Ra Mi Cha** [1,†], **Dae-Sung Yu** [2], **Ki-Sun Kim** [1], **Sok Song** [1], **Sung-Hyun Choi** [3], **Byung-Il Jung** [3], **Seong-In Lim** [1], **Bang-Hun Hyun** [1], **Bong-Kyun Park** [1,4] and **Dong-Jun An** [1,*]

[1] Virus Disease Division, Animal and Plant Quarantine Agency, Gimchen, Gyeongbuk-do 39660, Korea; ivvi59@korea.kr (S.C.); rami.cha01@korea.kr (R.M.C.); kisunkim@korea.kr (K.-S.K.); ssoboro@naver.com (S.S.); saint78@korea.kr (S.-I.L.); hyunbh@korea.kr (B.-H.H.); parkx026@korea.kr (B.-K.P.)
[2] Division of Veterinary Epidemiological, Animal and Plant Quarantine Agency, Gimchen, Gyeongbuk-do 39660, Korea; shanuar@korea.kr
[3] Korea Pork Producers Association, Seocho-gu, Seoul 06643, Korea; heechan9@hanmail.net (S.-H.C.); exksa001@daum.net (B.-I.J.)
[4] College of Veterinary Medicine, Seoul University, Gwanak-ro, Gwanak-gu, Seoul 08826, Korea
[*] Correspondence: andj67@korea.kr
[†] These authors made an equal contribution.

Abstract: There has been a rapid increase in the number of classical swine fever (CSF) sero-positive wild boars captured near the demilitarized zone (DMZ), located the border with North Korea. In 2015–2016, few CSFV-positive antibody boars were detected; however, the number has increased steeply since 2017. Most occurred in the northern region of Gyeonggi before spreading slowly to Gangwon (west to east) in 2018–2019. Multi-distance spatial cluster analysis provided an indirect estimate of the time taken for CSFV to spread among wild boars: 46.7, 2.6, and 2.49 days/km. The average CSF serum neutralization antibody titer was 4–10 (log $_2$), and CSFV Ab B-ELISA PI values ranged from 65.5 to 111.5, regardless of the age and sex of wild boars. Full genome analysis revealed that 16 CSFV strains isolated from wild boars between 2017 and 2019 were identical to the YC16CS strain (sub-genotype 2.1d) isolated from an outbreak in breeding pigs near the border with North Korea in 2016. The rapid increase in CSF in wild boars may be due to a continuously circulating infection within hub area and increased population density. The distribution pattern of CSFV in Korean wild boars moves from west to southeast, affected by external factors, including small-scale hunting, geographical features and highways.

Keywords: CSFV; wild boar; antibody; transmission; E2

1. Introduction

Classical swine fever virus (CSFV) is a single-stranded RNA virus belonging to the genus pestivirus (family, Flaviviridae). Classical swine fever (CSF) is one of the most important viral diseases affecting domestic pigs and wild boars [1]. Wild boars are as susceptible to CSFV as domestic pigs; therefore, eradication of CSF from wild boars is of epidemiologic value because it can prevent spread among domestic animals [2]. In Germany, 59% of CSF cases in domestic pigs from 1993 to 1998 were transmitted by direct or indirect contact with wild boars [3]. Over the last decades, several European Union (EU) member states (including Germany, France, and Slovakia) were confronted with outbreaks among wild boar; these outbreaks had a clear tendency to establish endemicity [4,5]. Following EU legislation, surveillance was implemented to ensure that CSFV is not circulating and spreading within wild-boar populations. At the beginning of a CSF outbreak, the antibody prevalence within a population is far below 5%, and it can be several months until the threshold of 5% is reached [5,6]. A previous study suggests that a higher incidence of CSF among wild boars in a particular region is closely related to the population density [7]. A high density of wild boars, particularly young wild boars, drives CSF outbreaks [7]. Recently, CSF have been reported in Gifu Prefecture, affecting domestic pigs and wild boars since September 2019 in Japan [8,9]. The current circulating CSFV in Japan was identified moderate pathogenicity and most closely matched in nucleotide identity, with CSFVs recently isolated in China and Mongolia [8]. A space–time permutation analysis in Japan showed virus transmission spread (10.3 and 4.9 days/km) among wild boars in two significant clusters [9]. After overlaying of a map of habitat quality, approximately 82% and 75% of CSF notifications in two clusters were found in the areas with potential contact between pigs and wild boars [9]. Monitoring of CSF in 5620 Korean wild boars captured between 2010 and 2014 identified only seven animals with CSFV and 23 animals with CSFV antibodies [10]. CSFV (YC16CS strain) isolated from an outbreak in breeding pigs in the north of Gyeonggi in 2016 shows a high genetic similarity and the same sub-genotype (2.1d) as the CSFV (CW17WB) strain isolated from wild boars in 2017 [11]. The risk of CSFV transmission from wild boars to breeding pigs is clear [11]. Therefore, we attempted to identify the reasons underlying the rapid spread of CSF infection among wild boars to guide development of prevention measures.

2. Results

2.1. CSF Antibody Prevalence According to Province

Korean wild boars captured between 2016 and 2019 comprised 40.2% females, 48.2% males, and 11.6% unknown. Of these, 4.7% (132/2799) of females, 3.6% (123/3362) of males, and 2.3% (19/809) of unknown animals were positive for CSFV antibodies (Table 1). With respect to age, 34.2% (2387/6970) of captured boars were under 1 year old, and 39.7% (2771/6970) were 1–2 years old (Table 1). In addition, 2.1% (51/2387) of boars under 1 year old, 4.9% (136/2771) aged 1–2 years old, 6.1% (36/583) aged 2–3 years old, 8.6% (22/255) aged 3–4 years old, 4.2% (5/119) aged over 4 years, and 2.8% (24/855) of indeterminate age were positive for CSFV antibodies (Table 1). The CSF sero-positive rates in Gyeonggi (GG) increased continuously over the years: from 1.6% (5/302) in 2016 to 4.6% (6/129) in 2017, 9.2% (9/97) in 2018, and 14.3% (65/453) in 2019, as did the rates in Gangwon (GW) (from 0.6% (1/148) in 2016 to 4.7% (12/251) in 2017, 16.5% (33/200) in 2018, and 21.2% (129/608) in 2019) (Table 2). The number of CSF sero-positive wild boars of GW region in 2018 and 2019 was significantly different ($p < 0.01$ for 2018 and $p < 0.001$ for 2019), compared to that of other regions (Gyeongnam, Gyeongbuk, Jennam, Jenbuk, Chungnam, Chungbuk, Jeju, and Unknown), using two-way analysis of variance (ANOVA) with Bonferroni posttest (Table 2).

Table 1. CSF sero-positive, gender, and age of wild boars captured from 2016 to 2019.

Year	No. of AP[a] /No. of CWB[b]	Gender			Age (Months)					
		Male	Female	UK[c]	0–12	13–24	25–36	37–48	48–70	UK[c]
2016	7/1683	2/584	1/417	4/682	0/369	3/499	0/88	0/26	0/19	4/682
2017	20/1670	9/912	11/757	0/1	3/630	16/762	0/171	0/70	1/36	0/1
2018	47/1320	28/740	19/580	0/0	14/479	23/608	4/138	6/64	0/31	0/0
2019	200/2297	84/1126	101/1045	15/126	34/909	94/902	32/186	16/95	4/33	20/172
Total	3.9 [d] (274/ 6970)	3.6 (123/ 3362)	4.7 (132/ 2799)	2.3 (19/ 809)	2.1 (51/ 2387)	4.9 (136/ 2771)	6.1 (36/ 583)	8.6 (22/ 255)	4.2 (5/ 119)	2.8 (24/ 855)

Numbers in parenthesis denote CSF antibody-positive animals. AP[a]: antibody positive. CWB[b]: captured wild boar. UK[c]: unknown. [d]Positive percentage (%) (No. of antibody positive/No. of wild boars tested).

Table 2. CSF sero-positive and region in which wild boars were captured from 2016 to 2019.

Year	No. of AP[a] /No. of CWB[b]	Percentage (%) for Region (No. of Antibody Positive/No. of Wild Boars Tested)									
		GW	GG	GN	GB	JN	JB	CN	CB	JJ	UK[c]
2016	7/1683	0.6 (1/148)	1.6 (5/302)	0 (0/334)	0 (0/410)	0 (0/71)	0 (0/59)	0.3 (1/261)	0 (0/96)	0 (0/2)	0 (0/0)
2017	20/1670	4.7 (12/251)	4.6 (6/129)	0.5 (1/195)	0.3 (1/301)	0 (0/189)	0 (0/112)	0 (0/221)	0 (0/270)	0 (0/0)	0 (0/2)
2018	47/1320	16.5[d] (33/200)	9.2 (9/97)	0.5 (1/196)	0.8 (2/237)	0 (0/150)	0 (0/97)	0 (0/172)	1.3 (2/149)	0 (0/22)	0 (0/0)
2019	200/2297	21.2[e] (129/608)	14.3[f] (65/453)	0.3 (1/292)	0.3 (1/275)	1.4 (1/69)	0 (0/71)	0.3 (1/289)	0.9 (2/203)	0 (0/37)	0 (0/0)

GW: Gangwon; GG: Gyeonggi; GN: Gyeongnam; GB, Gyeongbuk; JN: Jennam; JB: Jenbuk; CN: Chungnam; CB: Chungbuk; JJ: Jeju. Numbers in parentheses denote CSF antibody-positive animals. AP[a]: antibody positive. CWB[b]: captured wild boar. UK[c]: unknown. [d]$p < 0.01$ and [e]$p < 0.001$: CSF sero-positive of GW region in 2018 and 2019 was compared with other regions (GN, GB, JN, JB, CN, CB, JJ, and UK) in 2018 and 2019. [f]$p < 0.05$: CSF sero-positive of GG region in 2019 was compared with other regions (GN, GB, JN, JB, CN, CB, JJ, and UK) in 2019.

2.2. Genetic Analysis of CSFVs Isolated from Wild Boars

Between 2017 and 2019, we isolated 16 CSFV strains from Korean wild boars: three (NYJ17WB01, NYJ17WB02, and CW17WB) in 2017, two (YW18WB and IJ18WB) in 2018, and 11 (HC19WB, CC19WB01, IJ19WB01, IJ19WB02, IJ19WB03, DH19WB01, PC19WB01, HC19WB02, HC19WB03, YP19WB02, and YP19WB03) in 2019. Phylogenetic analysis revealed that all strains belonged to sub-genotype 2.1d (Figure 1). The mean time of the most recent common ancestor (tMRCA) for the Korean wild-boar CSFV strains was estimated to be 26.231 years ago (95% highest posterior density (HPD) interval, 22.1806–17.6393), with an effective sample size (ESS) of 276.3935 on the maximum clade credibility (MCC) tree.

The clock rate ($\times 10^{-4}$ substitutions/site/year) was 6.19, with a 95% HPD interval of 5.2898–7.2025 (Figure 1). Genetic Analysis of the complete genomes of the 16 Korean strains isolated in 2017–2019 revealed 99.2%–99.5% identity. Analysis of complete E2 sequences among the 16 strains revealed 98.4%–99.3% identity at the nucleotide (nt) level and 98.1%–99.5% identity at the amino acid (aa) level. The 16 strains isolated in 2017–2019 were 95.3%–96.3% (nt) and 97.3%–98.7% (aa), similar to the complete E2 gene of the YC11WB strain isolated from Korean wild boars in 2011; however, they were 98.6%–99.8% (nt) and 98.9%–100% (aa), similar to the YC16CS strain isolated in 2016 from Korean domestic pigs (Yeoncheon region).

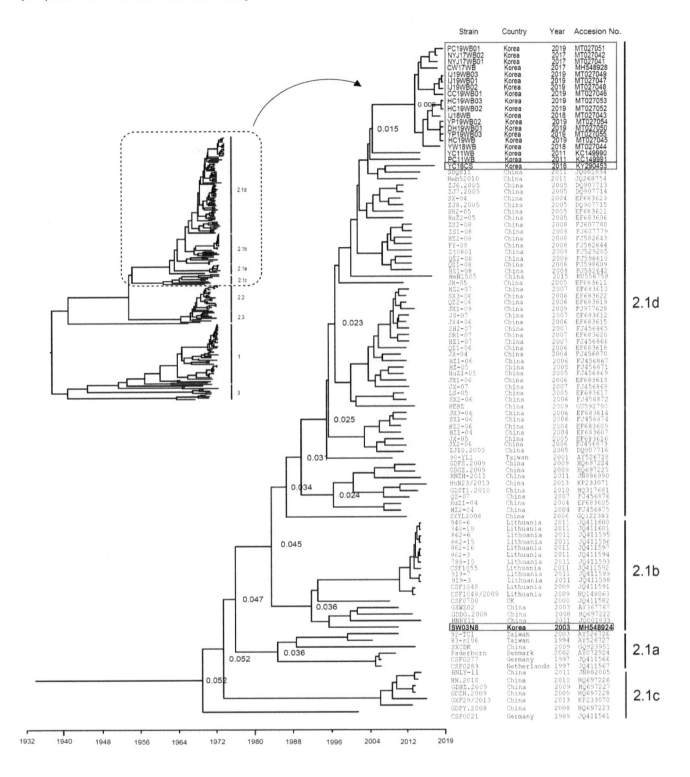

Figure 1. Phylogenetic analysis of the complete E2 gene sequence of 16 CSFV strains isolated from Korean wild boars (2017–2019). Complete E2 gene sequences (n = 197) were obtained from the NCBI GenBank database. Each dataset was simulated by using the following options: generation = 100,000,000; burn-in, 10%; and ESSs > 200. The confidence of the phylogenetic analysis-based timescale by factor (1.0) is represented by the numbers above the nodes representing branch length (time). Eighteen CSFV strains isolated from Korean wild boars (2011–2019) and two CSFV strains isolated from domestic pigs (2003 and 2016) are marked by red and blue boxes, respectively.

2.3. Space–Time Clusters

Space–time permutation analysis identified three significant space–time clusters ($p < 0.05$) across South Korea (Table 3 and Figure 2A,C–E). Cluster I was in an area located in the northern part of country (Pocheon), with a radius of 3.87 km in which five CSF sero-positive wild boars were captured from 30th September 2017 to 29th March 2018 (Table 3 and Figure 2C). Two pig farms raise 1420 pigs in Cluster I. Cluster II, about 4.45 km southeast from Cluster I, the 22 CSF antibody-positive cases were detected within a 23.05 km (Gapyeong and Chuncheon) radius from 1st March 2019 to 29th April 2019 (Table 3 and Figure 2D). The 103 pig farms raise 119,346 pigs in Cluster II. Cluster III, which lies east of Cluster II, had a radius of 24.49 km (Hongcheon); 34 CSF sero-positive cases were captured here from 30th December 2018 to 28th February 2019 (Table 3 and Figure 2E). The 49 pig farms raise 54,690 pigs in Cluster III.

Multi-distance spatial cluster analysis of the three Cluster regions estimated that the transmission time for CSFV among wild boars was about 46.7 days/km for cluster I, 2.6 days/km for Cluster II, and 2.49 days/km for Cluster III. Areas harboring boars with high CSFV antibody titers were also examined by using space–time permutation analysis (aggregate unit: one month). The data revealed one significant space–time cluster ($p < 0.05$); from 11th January 2017 to 31th October 2019, 107 cases were identified with high CSFV antibody titers within a 55.15 km (Cluster IV) radius (Figure 2A,F). The mean titer inside and outside $\log_2$ transformation of the Cluster IV were 6.94 and 7.99 $\log_2$, respectively, and standard deviation is 1.62 $\log_2$. The 395 pig farms raise 641,541 pigs in Cluster IV. Total of pig farms in Gangwon (n = 264) and Gyeonggi (n = 1249) is 1513 (Figure 2B). The number of pigs is approximately 485,875 in Gangwon and 1,913,234 in Gyeonggi, respectively. CSF antigen- and antibody-positive wild boars by year (2016–2019) were gradually expanded from west to east (Figure 3A). CSFV-infected wild boars are predicted to move along the mountain range (Figure 3B,C).

Table 3. Spatiotemporal cluster analysis of CSF antibody distribution in captured Korean wild boars. Aggregate unit: one month.

Cluster	Spatiotemporal Cluster Analysis of CSF Antibody Distribution		
	I	II	III
Observed notifications	5	22	34
Expected notifications	0.35	6.84	11.59
Duration (days)	181	60	61
Start date	30/11/2017	01/03/2019	30/12/2018
End date	29/05/2018	29/04/2019	28/02/2019
Radius (km)	3.87	23.05	24.49
p-value	0.038	0.0018	<0.001

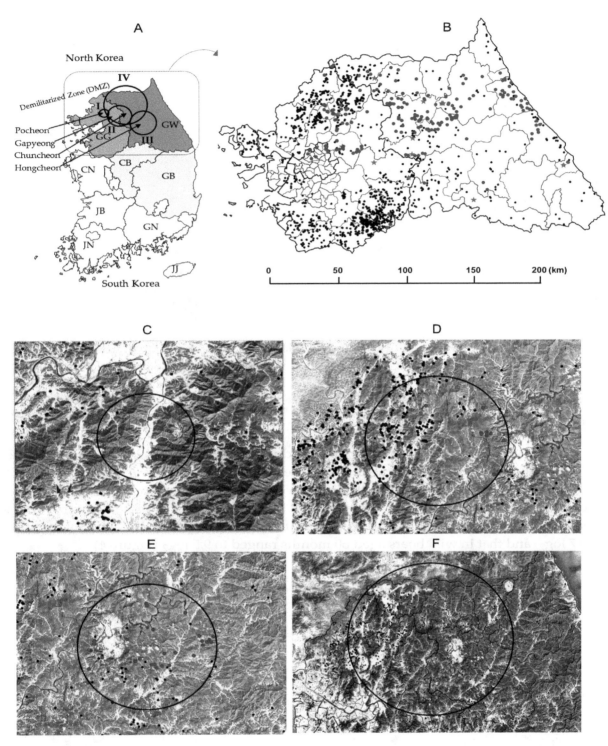

Figure 2. Space–time cluster analysis of CSF antibody-positive cases and antibody titers in wild boars. Positions of four clusters on the Korea map (**A**). Positions of pig farms (dark dot) and of CSF antibody (blue dot) and CSF antigen (red star) from captured wild boars between 2016 and 2019 (**B**). Space–time cluster analysis of CSF sero-positive wild boars was conducted, using SaTScan software (version 9.6), with the minimum time aggregation set as one month. Three clusters are marked with black circles (**C**: cluster I, **D**: cluster II, and **E**: cluster III). Space–time cluster analysis of CSF antibody titers was conducted by using data from the cluster IV marked with a black circle (**F**). Images (C,D, E,F) are marked dark dot (pig farm) and blue dot (CSF sero-positive wild boar). The nine regions (A) were as follows: GW: Gangwon; GG: Gyeonggi; GN: Gyeongnam; GB, Gyeongbu; JN: Jennam; JB: Jenbuk; CN: Chungnam; CB: Chungbuk; and JJ: Jeju.

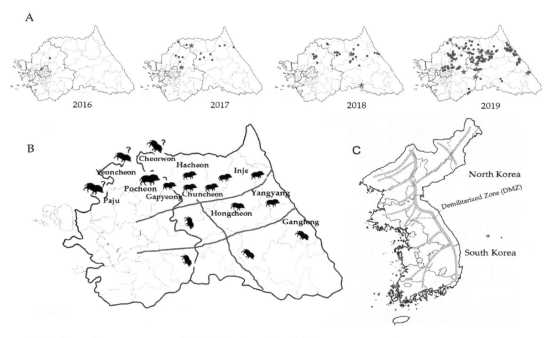

Figure 3. Predicted movements of CSFV-infected wild boars. Sites of capture of CSF antigen- and antibody-positive wild boars by year (2016–2019) are marked by a red star and blue circle, respectively (**A**). Expected routes and highways are marked by wild-boar pictures and blue lines (**B**). On the map of Korea, consecutive high mountains are marked by green lines (**C**).

2.4. Relationship among CSF Sero-Positive and Age

From January 2016 to December 2019, 274 wild boars were confirmed as CSF sero-positive (Figure 4). Age and antibody titer (calculated from the serum neutralization antibody test and CSFV AB B-ELISA results) of CSFV-positive wild boars showed a close relationship (Figure 4). PI values for all antibody-positive wild boars ranged from 65.5 to 111.5 in the antibody ELISA and from 4 to 10 $\log_2$ in the serum neutralization antibody test (Figure 4). In boars aged < 5 months, the SN titer ranged from 6 to 7 $\log_2$, and that in wild boars aged 60 months ranged to 9.5 $\log_2$ (Figure 4).

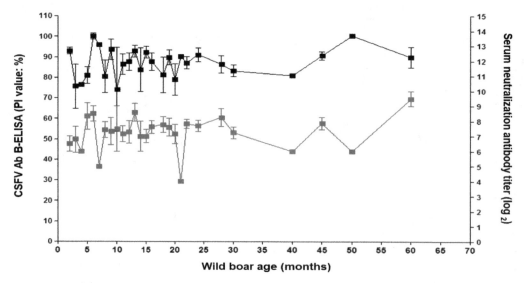

Figure 4. Relationship between CSF sero-positive and wild-boar age. CSFV antibodies were measured by PI value (≥ 40% positive and < 40% negative), using the CSFV Ab B-ELISA (black line) and titers ($\log_2$), using the serum neutralization antibody test (red line). Data are expressed as the mean ± SD (standard deviation).

3. Discussion

To investigate the increase of CSF among wild boars in Korea, we mainly used CSF antibody detection and consider that CSF sero-positive wild boars as CSFV affected animal. Two CSF sero-positive wild boars were identified in wild boars from the Pocheon region, in the second half of 2016; since then, the number of positive cases has increased rapidly, spreading from east to west, between 2017 and 2019. The temporal clustering of CSF infection in wild boars is consistent with animal movements during the mating and breeding seasons, mainly late autumn and early spring (i.e., November and March); this period involved increased contact between susceptible animals and infected hosts. In addition, the radius of spatial–temporal clusters is heavily influenced by habitat fragmentation caused by roads, railways, and pipelines [12]. The average CSF transmission time per km in Cluster I (Pocheon) was 46.7 days, compared with 2.6 days for Cluster II (Gapyeong and Chuncheon) and 2.49 days for Cluster III (Hongcheon). The differences are thought to be due to differences in wild-boar population density. The population density of wild boars in Pocheon increased sharply from 0.8 in 2016 to 3.9 in 2017, after which the density in neighboring Gapyeong to the east increased from 1.1 in 2017 to 5.3 in 2018, and that in Chuncheon increased from 3.3 in 2017 to 6.7 in 2018 [13]. As the number of wild boars within a certain habitat increased, CSF spread could be predicted indirectly based on animal movements. Paju, Yeoncheon, and Cheorwon are adjacent to the demilitarized zone (DMZ), meaning that North Korean wildlife can cross into these areas over the mountain range. Pocheon, which lies just below these three regions, is a good wild-boar habitat and can act as a reservoir of CSFV. The first CSF antigens were detected in wild boars from Yeoncheon and Pocheon in 2011; since then, antibody-positive cases have been detected continuously within the area [10]. Interestingly, the CSFV strain (YC16CS) isolated from a breeding pig farm in Yeoncheon in 2016 is genetically identical to the 16 CSFV strains isolated from wild boars in 2017–2019 [11]. This suggested that CSFV could be infected mutually between wild boars and breeding pigs [11]. The risk of spreading CSF from wild boars to breeding pigs is much higher west region because more pig farms were present inside Cluster II (west), rather than Cluster III, in the east region in this study. Generally, pig farms are more concentrated in Northern Gyeonggi Province (Paju, Yeoncheon, Pocheon, etc.) than in Gangwon province. Nevertheless, pig farms are also distributed in Hongcheon (Cluster III) and Chuncheon (east of Cluster II), and the risk of spread from wild boars to breeding pigs was present. In Japan, directional distribution of CSF notifications from September 2018 to June 2019 showed movement toward the northeast direction [9]. The 16 CSFVs from Korean wild boars spread from west to east between 2017 and 2019, and CSF sero-positive wild boars also showed similar pattern (west to east). Interestingly, of the 18 CSFV strains belonging to sub-genotype 2.1d detected since 2011, the two strains (YC11WB and PC11WB) identified in 2011 were slightly different from the 16 strains isolated between 2017 and 2019 [11]. This may be due to genetic mutations caused by self-circulating infection among Korean wild boars over six years; however, it could be due to the crossing of other strains from North Korea into the DMZ. A previous study suggested that the persistence of CSFV infection among wild boars is due to a combination of virus characteristics (e.g., pathogenicity) and the size of the wild-boar population [2]. It was known that, a small population (less than 2000) of wild boars would promote self-limit on the spread of CSFV within one year, whereas CSFV tends to persist and become endemic for years, in larger populations [7].

In September 2019, in South Korea, African swine fever virus (ASFV) was endemic in breeding pigs; the cause of the disease was believed to be wild boars [14]. For CSFV, South Korean experts also confirmed that the virus had spread from North Korean wild boars that had crossed the DMZ. To control transmission of ASF from wild boars, the wire fences running west to east were installed close to the DMZ, to prevent wild boars from crossing over. Between these two sets of wire fences, large-scale hunting was carried out, using firearms. As a result, 306 cases of ASFV were identified, with cases moving along the DMZ from west to east [14]. Because the Korean government began a large-scale hunting policy at the end of 2019, to control wild boars and reduce the risk of ASF, we expect that the number of CSFV antigen- and antibody-positive cases in 2020 will be less than that in

2019; this will tell us whether mass wild-boar hunting is an effective control measure for CSFV. The biggest obstacle to large-scale hunting in Korea is the inability to hunt in national parks. National parks have the possibility to act as uncontrolled disease reservoirs; therefore, controlling disease with different strategies, such as the installation of a protective fence in national parks, should be considered.

The effectiveness of using the hunting policy to control the disease spread was still controversial. Several reports suggested that hunting wild boars has reduced CSF occurrence [6,15]. In 1997, CSF was detected in wild boars in Northern Italy; therefore, the governments of Italy and Switzerland began a joint program to capture wild boars, leading to a marked reduction in the incidence CSF [6]. CSF sero-positive rates in these regions fell sharply, from 42.2% to 8.8%, suggesting no CSFV transmission between wild boars [6]. However, a recent study suggested that intensifying hunting or erecting fences has not been adequate for preventing disease spread or persistence [16] and also suggested that oral mass vaccine (OMV) has proved to be effective in maintaining herd immunity and achieving CSF control and it is the only available method for CSF eradication in large forested areas [16]. The European Food Safety Authority (EFSA) suggests that the reduction of the wild-boar population (targeted hunting of female wild boar) and carcass removal to stop the spread of ASFV in the wild-boar population are more effective when applied preventively in the infected area [17]. In order to decrease the spread of CSF among wild boars in Korea, we already try to reduce the wild-boar population by large-scale hunting policy and can install a fence to delay the transmission of CSF. In addition, CSF bait vaccine to maintain herd immunity will be sprayed in Gangwon and Gyenggi province from 2020. The CSF bait vaccine with DIVA function was developed to base the Flc-LOM-BE^{rns} vaccine strain [18]. Baiting of wild boars with the Flc-LOM-BE^{rns} vaccine will induce production of anti-CSF E2 antibodies and anti-BVDV E^{rns} antibodies simultaneously, but no anti-CSF E^{rns} antibodies [18], which make differential diagnosis of vaccinated animal from wild-type CSFV-infected animal.

After CSFV spread from west to east, we expected it to descend south along the mountains. We did not observe southward spread in 2018, although it did spread gradually in 2019. We suspect that the main reason for this spread pattern is physical obstacles, e.g., major roads crossing from west to east. The information obtained from wild-boar CSFV-surveillance studies will help to predict the path of spread in wild boars and protect domestic pig farms from CSFV. Moreover, studying the pattern of CSF occurrence in wild boars will be a valuable guide to predicting the route and direction of ASFV spread to the south from the nearby DMZ.

In conclusion, a rapid increase of CSF sero-positive in Korean wild boars may result from the circulating infections and increased population density within the hub area. In addition, the distribution of the CSFV in wild boars gradually spread from the west to the southeast and was affected by obstacles, such as small-scale hunting, geographical features, highways, and wire fences.

4. Materials and Methods

4.1. Sample Collection, RT-PCR, and Phylogenetic Analysis

From 2010, wild boars were hunted in co-operation with the Korean Pork Producers Association and the Korean government, to satisfy the OIE requirements for surveillance of wild boars and feral pigs in CSF-free countries. Blood samples were collected from 6970 wild boars hunted in nine provinces (Gangwon, Gyeonggi, Gyeongnam, Gyeongbuk, Jennam, Jenbuk, Chungnam, Chungbuk, and Jeju), in South Korea, between February 2016 and November 2019 (Table 1). Blood was collected in heparinized tubes. Total RNA was extracted by using a micro-column-based RNeasy Mini kit (Qiagen, CA, USA). The RT-PCR conditions and specific primers used to amplify the complete E2 gene have been reported previously [11,19]. Complete E2 gene sequences for CSFVs were obtained from the NCBI GenBank database and aligned by using the CLUSTAL X alignment program. A BEAST input file was then generated, using BEAUti within the BEAST package v1.8.1 [20]. Rates of nucleotide substitution per site and per year, and the tMRCA, were estimated by using a Bayesian MCMC approach. The exponential clock and expansion growth population model in the BEAST program was used to obtain the best-fit evolutionary model, and the MCC tree was visualized by using Figtree 1.4 [21].

4.2. Spatiotemporal Cluster Analysis

Space–time permutation scan statistics [22] were calculated retrospectively, to identify the presence of space–time clusters for geographical localities in which CSFV antibodies were detected in wild boars (*Sus scrofa*); there were 274 sites from 1st January 2016 to 31th December 2019. Space–time cluster analysis was conducted by using SaTScan software version 9.6 (Kulldor, Boston, MA, USA), with the minimum time aggregation set at 1 month (accounting for the minimum duration of CSFV antibody persistence), a maximum spatial cluster size set as 50% of the population at risk, and a maximum spatial cluster size set as 50% of the total study period [9]. Test statistics were calculated for 999 Monte Carlo replications, to identify candidate clusters with statistical significance ($p = 0.05$).

4.3. CSFV Ab B-ELISA and SN Tests

Serum samples from wild boars were tested in a CSFV E2 Antibody ELISA. The CSFV Ab B-ELISA (BioNote Co. Cat. No. EB4413PO, Korea) is a competition ELISA designed to detect the E2 protein; however, it also provides a PI value ($\geq$40% positive and <40% negative). Serum neutralization (SN) tests based on a neutralizing peroxidase-linked assay (NPLA) were performed to detect CSFV-specific neutralizing antibodies. Briefly, PK-15 cells inoculated with CSFV were incubated for 72 h, at 37 °C/5% CO_2, with serum samples (serially diluted 2-fold). PK-15 cells were fixed in prechilled 80% acetone and then reacted with a 3B6 monoclonal antibody specific for CSFV E2 3B6 (Median Diagnostics Co., South Korea). PK-15 cells were then stained, using a VECTOR kit (Vector Laboratories, Burlingame, CA, USA), biotinylated anti-mouse IgG (H+L) (Cat. No. BA-9200), ABC solution (Cat. No. PK-4000), and a DAB peroxidase substrate (Cat. No. SK-4100). Staining was observed under a microscope.

4.4. Statistical Analysis

All statistical analyses were performed by using GraphPad Prism software, version 6.0, for Windows. Data were analyzed by using two-way analysis of variance (ANOVA) with Bonferroni posttest.

Author Contributions: Conceptualization, S.C. and B.-K.P.; methodology, R.M.C., D.-S.Y., K.-S.K., S.S., B.-I.J., S.-H.C., and S.-I.L.; writing—review and editing, B.-H.H. and D.-J.A. All authors have read and agreed to the published version of the manuscript.

References

1. Edwards, S.; Fukusho, A.; Lefèvre, P.C.; Lipowski, A.; Pejsak, Z.; Roehe, P.; Westergaard, J. Classical swine fever: The global situation. *Vet. Microbiol.* **2000**, *73*, 103–119. [CrossRef]

2. Moennig, V. The control of classical swine fever in wild boar. *Front. Microbiol.* **2015**, *6*, 1211. [CrossRef] [PubMed]

3. Fritzemeier, J.; Teuffert, J.; Greiser-Wilke, I.; Staubach, C.; Schlüter, H.; Moennig, V. Epidemiology of classical swine fever in Germany in the 1990s. *Vet. Microbiol.* **2000**, *77*, 29–41. [CrossRef]

4. Postel, A.; Moennig, V.; Becher, P. Classical swine fever in Europe—The current situation. *Berl. Munch. Tierarztl. Wochenschr.* **2013**, *126*, 468–475. [PubMed]

5. Staubach, C.; Höreth-Böntgen, D.; Blome, S.; Fröhlich, A.; Blicke, J.; Jahn, B.; Teuffert, J.; Kramers, M. Descriptive summary of the classical swine fever control in wild boar in Germany since 2005. *Berl. Munch. Tierarztl. Wochenschr.* **2013**, *126*, 491–499. [PubMed]

6. Zanardi, G.; Macchi, C.; Sacchi, C.; Rutili, D. Classical swine fever in wild boar in the Lombardy region of Italy from 1997 to 2002. *Vet. Rec.* **2003**, *152*, 461–465. [CrossRef] [PubMed]

7.   Rossi, S.; Fromont, E.; Pontier, D.; Crucière, C.; Hars, J.; Barrat, J.; Pacholek, X.; Artois, M. Incidence and persistence of classical swine fever in free-ranging wild boar (*Sus scrofa*). *Epidemiol. Infect.* **2005**, *133*, 559–568. [CrossRef] [PubMed]

8.   Kameyama, K.I.; Nishi, T.; Yamada, M.; Masujin, K.; Morioka, K.; Kokuho, T.; Fukai, K. Experimental infection of pigs with a classical swine fever virus isolated in Japan for the first time in 26 years. *J. Vet. Med. Sci.* **2019**, *81*, 1277–1284. [CrossRef]

9.   Ito, S.; Jurado, C.; Bosch, J.; Ito, M.; Sanchez-Vizcaino, J.M.; Isoda, N.; Sakoda, A.Y. Role of Wild Boar in the Spread of Classical Swine Fever in Japan. *Pathogens* **2019**, *8*, 206. [CrossRef]

10. Kim, Y.K.; Lim, S.I.; Kim, J.J.; Cho, Y.Y.; Song, J.Y.; Cho, I.S.; Hyun, B.H.; Choi, S.H.; Kim, S.H.; Park, E.H.; et al. Surveillance of classical swine fever in wild boar in South Korea from 2010–2014. *J. Vet. Med. Sci.* **2016**, *77*, 1667–1671. [CrossRef] [PubMed]

11. An, D.J.; Lim, S.I.; Choe, S.; Kim, K.S.; Cha, R.M.; Cho, I.S.; Song, J.Y.; Hyun, B.H.; Park, B.K. Evolutionary dynamics of classical swine fever virus in South Korea: 1987–2017. *Vet. Microbiol.* **2018**, *225*, 79–88. [CrossRef] [PubMed]

12. Rho, P. Using habitat suitability model for the wild boar (*Sus scrofa* Linnaeus) to select wildlife passage sites in extensively disturbed temperate forests. *J. Ecol. Environ.* **2015**, *38*, 163–173. [CrossRef]

13. *2018 Korean Wildlife Survey*; Biological Resources Research Department, National Institute of Biological Resources: Incheon, Korea, 2018.

14. Food and Agriculture Organization of the United Nations (FAO). ASF Situation in Asia Update 5 March 2020. Available online: http://www.fao.org/ag/againfo/programmes/en/empres/ASF/Situation_update.html (accessed on 5 March 2020).

15. Schnyder, M.; Stärk, K.D.; Vanzetti, T.; Salman, M.D.; Thor, B.; Schleiss, W.; Griot, C. Epidemiology and control of an outbreak of classical swine fever in wild boar in Switzerland. *Vet. Rec.* **2002**, *150*, 102–109. [CrossRef] [PubMed]

16. Rossi, S.; Staubach, C.; Blome, S.; Guberti, V.; Thulke, H.H.; Vos, A.; Koenen, F.; LePotier, M.F. Controlling of CSFV in European wild boar using oral vaccination: A review. *Front. Microbiol.* **2015**, *6*, 1141. [CrossRef] [PubMed]

17. Depner, K.; Gortazar, C.; Guberti, V.; Masiulis, M.; More, S.; O_l_sevskis, E.; Thulke, H.H.; Viltrop, A.; Wo_zniakowski, G.; Abrahantes, J.C.; et al. Epidemiological analyses of African swine fever in the Baltic States and Poland. *EFSA J.* **2017**, *15*, 5068.

18. Lim, S.I.; Choe, S.; Kim, K.S.; Jeoung, H.Y.; Cha, R.M.; Park, G.S.; Shin, J.; Park, G.N.; Cho, I.S.; Song, J.Y.; et al. Assessment of the efficacy of an attenuated live marker classical swine fever vaccine (Flc-LOM-BE^{rns}) in pregnant sows. *Vaccine* **2019**, *37*, 3598–3604. [CrossRef] [PubMed]

19. Paton, D.J.; McGoldrick, A.; Greiser-Wilke, I.; Parchariyanon, S.; Song, J.Y.; Liou, P.P.; Stadejek, T.; Lowings, J.P.; Björklund, H.; Belák, S. Genetic typing of classical swine fever virus. *Vet. Microbiol.* **2000**, *73*, 137–157. [CrossRef]

20. Drummond, A.J.; Suchard, M.A.; Xie, D.; Rambaut, A. Bayesian phylogenetics with BEAUti and the BEAST 1.7. *Mol. Biol Evol.* **2012**, *29*, 1969–1973. [CrossRef] [PubMed]

21. Rambaut, A. FigFree v.1.4.0. 2012. Available online: http://tree.bio.ed.ac.uk/software/figtree (accessed on 20 November 2019).

22. Kulldorff, M.; Heffernan, R.; Hartman, J.; Assunção, R.; Mostashari, F. A space–time permutation scan statistic for disease outbreak detection. *PLoS Med.* **2005**, *2*, e59. [CrossRef] [PubMed]

6

Comparison of the Pathogenicity of Classical Swine Fever Virus Subgenotype 2.1c and 2.1d Strains from China

Genxi Hao [1,2], **Huawei Zhang** [1,2], **Huanchun Chen** [1,2,3,4], **Ping Qian** [1,2,3,4,*] and **Xiangmin Li** [1,2,3,4,*]

[1] State Key Laboratory of Agricultural Microbiology, Huazhong Agricultural University, Wuhan 430070, China; chzhx5210@webmail.hzau.edu.cn (G.H.); ZHW@mail.hzau.edu.cn (H.Z.); chenhch@mail.hzau.edu.cn (H.C.)

[2] Laboratory of Animal Virology, College of Veterinary Medicine, Huazhong Agricultural University, Wuhan 430070, China

[3] Key Laboratory of Development of Veterinary Diagnostic Products, Ministry of Agriculture, Wuhan 430070, China

[4] Key Laboratory of Preventive Veterinary Medicine in Hubei Province, The Cooperative Innovation Center for Sustainable Pig Production, Wuhan 430070, China

[*] Correspondence: qianp@mail.hzau.edu.cn (P.Q.); lixiangmin@mail.hzau.edu.cn (X.L.)

Abstract: Classical swine fever (CSF) caused by classical swine fever virus (CSFV) is a highly contagious and devastating disease. The traditional live attenuated C-strain vaccine is widely used to control disease outbreaks in China. Since 2000, subgenotype 2.1 has become dominant in China. Here, we isolated subgenotype 2.1c and 2.1d strains from CSF-suspected pigs. The genetic variations and pathogenesis of subgenotype 2.1c and 2.1d strains were investigated experimentally. We aimed to evaluate and compare the replication characteristics and clinical signs of subgenotype 2.1c and 2.1d strains with those of the typical highly virulent CSFV SM strain. In PK-15 cells, the three CSFV isolates exhibited similar replication levels but significantly lower replication levels compared with the CSFV SM strain. The experimental animal infection model showed that the pathogenicity of subgenotype 2.1c and 2.1d strains was less than that of the CSFV SM strain. According to the clinical scoring system, subgenotype 2.1c (GDGZ-2019) and 2.1d (HBXY-2019 and GXGG-2019) strains were moderately virulent. This study showed that the pathogenicity of CSFV field strains will aid in the understanding of CSFV biological characteristics and the related epidemiology.

Keywords: classical swine fever virus (CSFV); subgenotype 2.1c; subgenotype 2.1d; pathogenicity; China

1. Introduction

Classical swine fever (CSF) is a highly contagious disease of pigs caused by classical swine fever virus (CSFV) [1]. CSF also causes great harm to the pig industry. Pigs are the natural hosts of CSFV and pigs of various breeds or ages can be infected. CSFV is a positive sense single-stranded RNA virus and a member of the genus Pestivirus within the family Flaviviridae [2]. The CSFV genome contains a large open reading frame that encodes four structural proteins (C, Erns, E1 and E2) and eight nonstructural proteins (Npro, p7, NS2, NS3, NS4A, NS4B, NS5A and NS5B) [3].

The E2 protein is the main structural protein of CSFV and is highly variable among isolates; it induces the neutralizing antibodies and shows a relationship with virulence [4,5]. On the basis of the E2 gene, CSFV isolates can be divided into three genotypes (1, 2 and 3) and are further subdivided into 11 subgenotypes (1.1–1.4, 2.1–2.3 and 3.1–3.4) [6]. CSFV outbreaks caused by genotype 2 have been increasing in Europe and Asia [2,3,7,8]. Given this situation, the genetic evolution of CSFV has been analyzed in detail and subgenotype 2.1 isolates have been further classified into 10 clades (2.1a–2.1j). Phylogenetic analysis indicates that CSFV in pigs in China includes subgenotypes 1.1, 2.1, 2.2 and 2.3b [6,9]. Since 2000, subgenotype 2.1 has become dominant in China. Among all subgenotypes of 2.1, subgenotypes 2.1c and 2.1d are currently the most widely prevalent in China [1,6,10]. The field virulence of CSFV is inconsistent with its genotype [11,12]. No consensus has been reached with regard to the virulence of pandemic CSFV strains.

In this study, the characterization of the CSFV isolates from three farms in Hubei, Guangxi and Guangdong provinces were evaluated. To investigate the virulence of subgenotype 2.1c and 2.1d isolates, we compared the pathogenicity of subgenotype 2.1 strains and the subgenotype 1.1 SM strain that is the high-virulence strain in China.

2. Results

2.1. Virus Isolation

RT-PCR assays were performed with the amplified E2 gene fragments of CSFV to detect clinical samples. Positive clinical CSFV samples were inoculated into PK-15 cells. The inoculated cells were passaged successively for the fifth generation. RT-PCR assay and indirect IFA showed positive results (Figure 1). CSFV strains were isolated from positive samples. The three CSFV isolates, which were obtained from Hubei, Guangdong and Guangxi, were named as HBXY-2019, GDGZ-2019 and GXGG-2019, respectively.

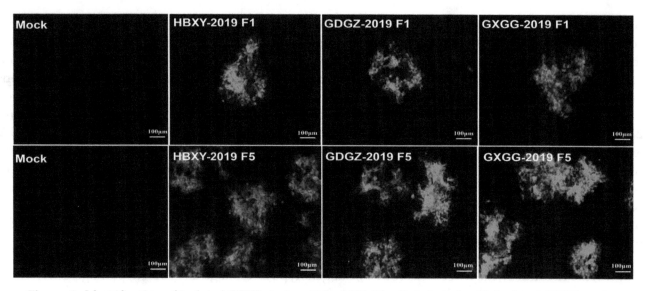

Figure 1. Identification of isolated CSFV strains. IFA of PK-15 cells infected with isolated CSFV strains at 36 h post-infection.

2.2. Phylogenetic Analysis of the E2 Gene

The nucleotide sequences of the three isolated CSFV strains were compared with those of the other CSFV strains in GenBank. Sequence analysis revealed that the E2 gene of the three isolated strains showed 81.1–98.4% nucleotide similarity with other Chinese strains. The E2 AA sequence homologies among three isolated strains ranged from 95.6% to 99.5% and all isolates shared high similarities of 96.4–99.7% with CSFV from subgenotype 2.1 and lower identities with genotype 1 (89.3–90.4%).

The phylogenetic trees of the full-length E2 gene were constructed by using MEGA7.0 (https://www.megasoftware.net/). Phylogenetic analysis indicated that the three isolated CSFV strains belonged to subgenotype 2.1. CSFV HBXY-2019 and GXGG-2019 isolates were grouped into subgenotype 2.1d and GDGZ-2019 was grouped into subgenotype 2.1c (Figure 2).

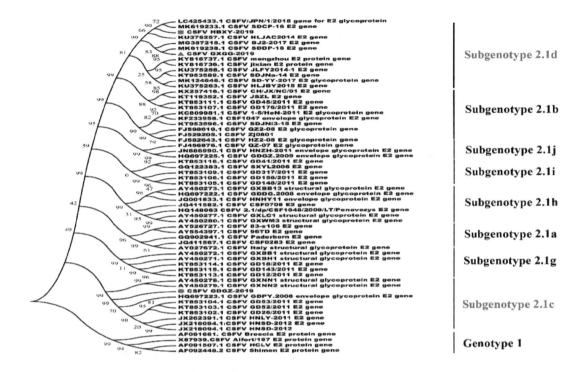

Figure 2. Phylogenetic analysis based on the full-length E2 gene of the isolated virus. Phylogenetic trees were constructed using MEGA 7.0.18 software with the neighbor-joining method (1000 bootstrap replicates). The isolated virus is marked in red.

2.3. Comparison of the AA Mutations of the E2 Gene in Three CSFV Isolated Strains

As shown in Figure 3, 44 mutated AAs were observed between the three CSFV isolated strains and subgenotype 1.1, and 15 mutated AAs were detected among GDGZ-2019, HBXY-2019 and GXGG-2019. Two AAs were mutated in HBXY-2019 and GXGG-2019 (K197M and R303K). The E2 proteins of different genotypes contained high levels of mutated AAs, indicating that E2 proteins were mutant viral proteins (Figure 3 and Table 1).

2.4. Virus Proliferation of CSFV Isolated Strains

We performed one-step growth experiments to analyze the replication characteristics of the three isolated CSFV strains. As shown in Figure 4A, no significant difference was observed among the three isolated CSFV strains. However, the CSFV SM strain exhibited a significantly higher replication level than the three isolated CSFV strains. At 72 hpi, the average CSFV SM viral titer was $10^{7.5}$ TCID$_{50}$/mL, whereas GDGZ-2019, HBXY-2019 and GXGG-2019 viral titers were $10^{6.3}$, $10^{6.7}$ and $10^{6.1}$ TCID$_{50}$/mL, respectively (Figure 4).

2.5. Pathogenicity Analysis of CSFV Isolated Strains

All pigs in the CSFV SM group showed typical high fever post-challenge. The average rectal temperature of pigs infected with CSFV SM exceeded 41.0 °C at 3 dpi and a high body temperature was continually observed until death. All the pigs in the CSFV SM group died at 7–13 dpi and displayed typical CSF symptoms. The average rectal temperature of pigs in the GDGZ-2019, HBXY-2019 and GXGG-2019 groups rose and exceeded 40.0 °C at 3 or 4 dpi (Figure 5A). The temperature of two pigs in the HBXY-2019 and GXGG-2019 groups exceeded 41 °C at 7 or 11 dpi. Three pigs in the GDGZ-2019 group had a fever temperature of more than 41 °C at 5, 8 and 11 dpi. The temperatures of all pigs normalized at 18 dpi. Two pigs in the HBXY-2019 and GXGG-2019 group died at the end of the experiment, whereas three dead pigs were noted in the GDGZ-2019 group (Figure 5B).

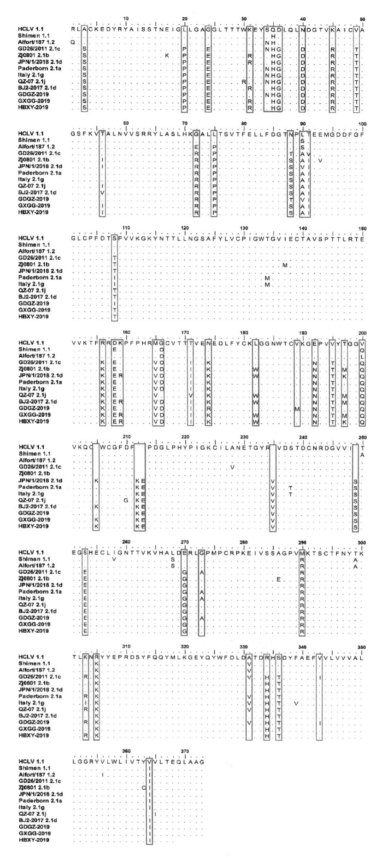

Figure 3. Amino acid sequence analysis of E2 genes of the three CSFV isolates. The special sites of AA mutation of these isolates are marked as red boxes.

Table 1. The difference in the amino acid of E2 gene of the isolated virus.

Positions (AA)	HCLV	GDGZ-2019	GXGG-2019	HBXY-2019
3	A	S	S	S
20	L	P	P	P
24	G	E	E	E
31	K	K	R	R
34	S	N	S	S
35	Q	H	H	H
36	D	G	G	G
40	N	D	D	D
45	K	R	R	R
49	V	T	T	T
56	T	T	I	I
72	G	R	R	R
75	L	P	P	P
88	N	T	S	S
90	L	V	A	A
91	T	I	I	I
108	S	I	T	T
156	R	K	K	K
158	D	E	E	E
159	K	K	R	R
165	M	V	V	V
166	G	D	D	D
171	T	I	I	I
174	N	R	K	K
182	L	L	W	W
192	E	N	N	N
195	V	T	T	T
197	T	T	M	K
200	V	Q	Q	Q
205	R	R	K	K
212	D	N	N	N
213	G	E	E	E
235	I	V	V	V
249	R	S	S	S
253	S	E	E	E
270	E	G	G	G
273	G	A	G	G
290	M	R	R	R
303	K	R	K	R
305	R	K	K	K
331	A	V	A	A
334	R	H	H	H
336	S	T	T	T
343	V	I	V	V

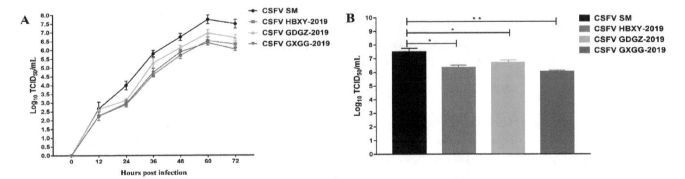

Figure 4. Comparison of the characteristics of the three CSFV isolates in PK15 cells. **(A)** One-step growth curves of the three CSFV isolates. **(B)** At 72 h post infection, the virus titers were determined in PK15 cells. Data represent the mean ± SEM from three independent experiments. * $p < 0.05$; ** $p < 0.01$.

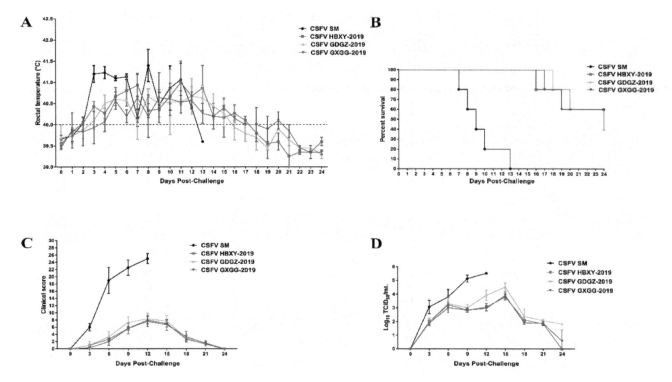

Figure 5. Rectal temperatures (**A**), survival rates (**B**), clinical scores (**C**) and viremia levels (**D**) of the pigs infected with the three CSFV isolates. Virus titers in blood are expressed as the mean $\log_{10}TCID_{50}/mL$. All data are expressed as mean ± SEM.

All pigs in the CSFV SM, GDGZ-2019, HBXY-2019 and GXGG-2019 groups displayed clinical signs of CSFV infection (Figure 5C). Clinical signs were the most severe in the CSFV SM group but developed slowly and were less severe in the GDGZ-2019, HBXY-2019 and GXGG-2019 groups. However, infected pigs with rectal temperatures over 41 °C displayed more clinical symptoms than those in the GDGZ-2019, HBXY-2019 and GXGG-2019 groups.

According to the CS system, the clinical score of the CSFV SM group was higher than that of the other group. The peak CS value of the pigs infected with CSFV SM was 26 and the CS value of each pig exceeded 15. The CS values of all pigs in the GDGZ-2019, HBXY-2019 and GXGG-2019 groups were all less than 15 (Figure 5C). Three out of five pigs in the GDGZ-2019 group had scores higher than 10 at 12 dpi and two out of five pigs in the HBXY-2019 and GXGG-2019 groups also had scores higher than 10. On the basis of mean clinical scores, the GDGZ-2019, HBXY-2019 and GXGG-2019 strains were defined as moderately virulent compared with the highly virulent CSFV SM strain.

Viremia was detected through virus isolation techniques. Viremia in blood was detected in all pigs of the CSFV SM, GDGZ-2019, HBXY-2019 and GXGG-2019 groups (Figure 5D). The viral titer of pigs infected with CSFV SM gradually increased throughout the experiment. The viral titer of pigs infected with the GDGZ-2019, HBXY-2019 and GXGG-2019 strains peaked at 15 dpi. Then, viremia rapidly declined in the GDGZ-2019, HBXY-2019 and GXGG-2019 groups.

2.6. Hematological Data

CSFV infection may induce leukopenia and immunosuppression. Blood samples were collected at different times post-challenge for the hematology test. The leukocyte and platelet counts were low in all CSFV-infected pigs (Figure 6). Leukopenia and thrombocytopenia were significantly severe at 6 and 12 dpi ($p < 0.05$) in CSFV SM-infected pigs. CSFV SM-infected pigs showed reduced leukocyte and PLT counts until death. However, the leukopenia and thrombocytopenia of GDGZ-2019, HBXY-2019 and GXGG-2019-infected pigs were significantly less than those in CSFV SM-infected pigs. Differences among the GDGZ-2019, HBXY-2019 and GXGG-2019 groups were not significant. Leukocyte counts and platelet counts in GDGZ-2019, HBXY-2019 and GXGG-2019-infected pigs were reduced to a minimum at 12 dpi. Then, the leukocyte counts and platelet counts of the pigs infected with the three strains gradually recovered and returned to normal at the end of the experiment.

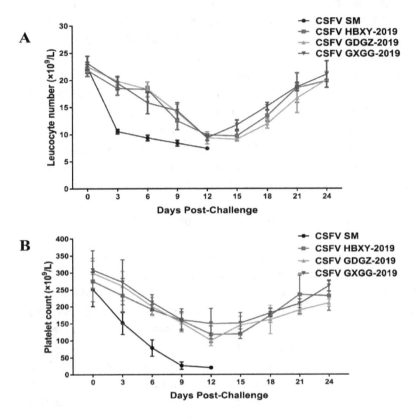

Figure 6. Hematological data of clinical samples from animals infected with the three new CSFV isolates. The leukocyte numbers (**A**) and platelet counts (**B**) are expressed as numbers/L of blood. Data are presented as the mean ± SEM.

3. Discussion

The traditional live attenuated C-strain vaccine is widely used in the world and plays a critical role in controlling CSF in multiple countries [13]. The immune effect of the C-strain is safe and effective. CSF has been controlled and eradicated in many countries. Vaccination and differential diagnosis are effective ways to eradicating CSF. However, the C-strain vaccine cannot serologically discriminate between vaccinated animals and infected animals [5,14]. Therefore, the classical attenuated vaccine encounters challenges in eradicating the CSF epidemic. At present, the C-strain is widely used to control disease outbreaks in China and frequent vaccinations are performed in pig farms. For the moment, the numbers of immunization failure and atypical clinical signs of CSF have been observed in clinical practice [1,6,9]. No mass outbreak of CSF has been recorded in recent years, whereas sporadic cases have been reported in C-strain-vaccinated farms in many regions of China.

In this study, three CSFV isolates were isolated from CSF-suspected pigs. The E2 sequences of isolated strains were compared with other CSFV strains in GenBank. One isolate was clustered into subgenotype 2.1c and the other two isolates were clustered into subgenotype 2.1d (Figure 2). These isolates shared high similarities of 96.4–99.7% with CSFV from subgenotype 2.1 and low identities with genotype 1 (89.3–90.4%). The E2 protein of these isolates had 44 mutated AAs compared with that of subgenotype 1.1. The WH303 epitope (TAVSPTTLR) of the E2 protein is an immunodominant epitope among CSFV strains. This epitope also exists in the three CSFV isolates, showing no genetic variability.

We compared the replication capability of subgenotypes 2.1c and 2.1d via one-step growth experiments and evaluated their pathogenicity in weaned piglets. Three CSFV isolates exhibited similar replication levels in PK-15 cells. However, these isolates exhibited significantly lower replication levels than the CSFV SM strain ($p < 0.05$). The results of animal experiments indicated that subgenotypes 2.1c (GDGZ-2019) and 2.1d (HBXY-2019 and GXGG-2019) were less pathogenic than the CSFV SM strain. No significant difference was noted among the three CSFV isolates. The virulence of subgenotypes 2.1c (GDGZ-2019) and 2.1d (HBXY-2019 and GXGG-2019) was assessed on the basis of the CS system. Subgenotypes 2.1c (GDGZ-2019) and 2.1d (HBXY-2019 and GXGG-2019) were moderately virulent ($5 < CS \leq 15$) compared with the highly virulent SM strain, a known reference strain that belongs to subgenotype 1.1. Several studies have reported that genotype 2 of CSFV is less virulent than genotype 1. We also observed that subgenotypes 2.1c (GDGZ-2019) and 2.1d (HBXY-2019 and GXGG-2019) had moderate pathogenicity; this observation is consistent with the findings of other studies [1,10,15,16]. The moderate clinical symptoms caused by the CSFV isolates observed in the present study were consistent with the atypical clinical signs of CSF observed in clinical practice. Previous studies have demonstrated that the E2 protein is a determinant of virulence [4,17,18]. The substitution or mutation of E2 leads to viral attenuation [18]. A recent study showed that AA T56I and M290K substitutions, especially the M290K mutation, in E2 protein increase virus pathogenicity [19]. A similar mutation was detected among three CSFV isolates (Figure 3). However, CSFV virulence is also affected by other gene mutations [20,21].

At present, subgenotype 2.1 strains are the dominant pandemic strains in China [6,10,22]. Three CSFV isolates were isolated from different provinces of China in the present study. These CSFV isolates belong to two different subgenotypes (2.1c and 2.1d). We compared the pathogenicity of subgenotype 2.1c and 2.1d strains via the intranasal route in weaned piglets. After pigs were infected with CSFV 2.1 isolates, there were some marked characteristic changes, such as hemocytopenia, especially leukopenia and thrombocytopenia. CSFV SM-infected pigs showed reduced leukocyte and PLT counts until death. However, leukopenia and thrombocytopenia of GDGZ-2019, HBXY-2019 and GXGG-2019-infected pigs were significantly less than those in CSFV SM-infected pigs and gradually recovered and went back to normal at the end of the experiment. CSFV 2.1c (GDGZ-2019) and 2.1d (HBXY-2019 and GXGG-2019) strains are moderate virulent strains, similar to the published results on subgenotype 2.1 strains. This study shows the necessity of monitoring the molecular epidemiology and the etiological characteristics of the epidemic CSFV 2.1 isolates, which may help us to understand the CSFV 2.1 isolates' biological characteristics and control the CSF outbreaks.

4. Materials and Methods

4.1. Sample Collection

Ten clinical samples (tonsils, lymph nodes and spleen) were collected from three pig farms in China (Hubei, Guangdong and Guangxi) in 2019. The RNA of clinical samples was isolated by using TRIzol reagent (Invitrogen, Carlsbad, California, USA) in accordance with the manufacturer's instructions. RNA was then quantified and reverse-transcribed by using a First Strand cDNA Synthesis Kit (TOYOBO, Osaka City, Osaka Prefecture, Japan) in accordance with the manufacturer's instructions. All samples were amplified by reverse transcription-polymerase chain reaction (RT-PCR) by using previously described specific primers, which were used for the CSFV E2 full-sequence gene [5]. The amplified gene segments were then ligated into a pEASY®-blunt cloning vector (Transgen Biotech, Beijing, China). Positive clones were sequenced by using Sanger Sequencing Technology and submitted to NCBI (GenBank accession number: MT422346, MT422347, MT422348).

4.2. Cells and Antibodies

Porcine kidney cells (PK-15; ATCC, CCL-33) were grown in Dulbecco's modified essential medium (DMEM; Invitrogen, Waltham, MA, USA) containing 10% fetal bovine serum (FBS) (Gibco, Waltham, MA, USA) at 37 °C in a humidified 5% CO_2 incubator. E2-specific monoclonal antibodies were prepared in our laboratory. Alexa Fluor 488 goat anti-mouse secondary antibody was obtained from Life Technologies, USA.

4.3. CSFV Isolation

Virus isolation was conducted in PK-15 cells maintained in DMEM (Invitrogen, Waltham, MA, USA) supplemented with 10% FBS (Invitrogen) at 37 °C. Clinical samples were ground into suspensions and clarified through centrifugation. The supernatant was passed through a sterile 0.22 μm filter and inoculated into PK-15 cells. After 60 h of incubation, the supernatant was harvested. RT-PCR with CSFV E2-specific primers verified that the viral isolate was CSFV.

4.4. Indirect Immunofluorescence Assay

PK-15 cells were seeded into 24-well plates and separately infected with the CSFV strains. At 36 h post-infection, the cells were fixed in 4% paraformaldehyde for 20 min, permeabilized with 0.1% Triton X-100 at room temperature for 10 min and blocked with 2% bovine serum albumin. The cells were subsequently incubated with AH09 E2-specific monoclonal antibodies (1:200 dilution in our laboratory) and the fixed cells were incubated with Alexa Fluor 488 goat anti-Mouse secondary antibodies (1:1000 dilution, Invitrogen). Fluorescence was observed under an Olympus IX73 fluorescent microscope.

4.5. Phylogenetic Analysis

The amino acid (AA) sequences of the three isolates were analyzed by using the Clustal W method of Lasergene (Version 7.1) (DNASTAR Inc., Madison, WI, USA). The phylogenetic trees of full-length E2 genes were constructed through the neighbor-joining method and the maximum composite likelihood model was established by using 1000 replicates with bootstrap values.

4.6. One-Step Growth Curve

The confluent monolayers of PK-15 cells in T25 flasks were inoculated with the CSFV SM, HBXY-2019, GDGZ-2019, or GXGG-2019 strains at a multiplicity of infection equal to 0.1. After incubation for 1 h at 37 °C, the inoculated cells were washed twice with phosphate-buffered saline. Then, a fresh medium containing 2% FBS was added. The infected cells were further cultured in an incubator at 37 °C. The culture supernatant was harvested by centrifugation at 0, 12, 24, 36, 48, 60 and 72 h. The viral titers were calculated as median tissue culture infective dose ($TCID_{50}$) and determined by IFA, which was performed as described above [1].

4.7. Animal Experiment

The animal experiment was approved by the Research Ethics Committee of College of Veterinary Medicine, Huazhong Agricultural University, Hubei, China (No.20190526). Twenty 8-week-old three-breed cross pigs were purchased from the experimental farm of Huazhong Agricultural University and randomly divided into four groups. All pigs were confirmed to be seronegative for CSFV by neutralization test and RT-PCR. The four groups of pigs were housed in the negative-pressure facility of Wuhan Keqian Biology Co., Ltd (Wuhan, China) and were placed in separate rooms to avoid cross infection.

Pigs in group A (control group) were inoculated intranasally with 2×10^6 $TCID_{50}$ of virulent CSFV SM strain. Pigs in group B were inoculated intranasally with 2×10^6 $TCID_{50}$ of HBXY-2019 strain. Pigs in group C were inoculated intranasally with 2×10^6 $TCID_{50}$ of GDGZ-2019 strain. Pigs in group D were inoculated intranasally with 2×10^6 $TCID_{50}$ of GXGG-2019 strain. Following challenge, the rectal temperature and clinical signs (liveliness, body tension, body shape, breathing, neurological signs, conjunctivitis, appetite, defecation and so on) were monitored daily. A rectal temperature above 40.0 °C is considered an indication of fever. The clinical scoring (CS) system was used to evaluate the virulence of CSFV in accordance with previously established standards [23]. Clinical scores were evaluated based on 10 clinical parameters [23]. Each parameter was calculated as follows: normal, 0 points; slightly altered, 1 point; distinct clinical signs, 2 points; severe CSF symptom, 3 points. The maximum total score per pig was 30.

4.8. Routine Blood Tests

Anticoagulated blood was collected every 3 days post-challenge until the trial ended. Leukocyte counts and platelet counts were determined using a Mindray BC-2800 Vet analyzer (Shenzhen Mindray Bio-Medical Electronics Co., Shenzhen, China).

4.9. Statistical Analysis

Statistical analyses were performed using one-way ANOVA in GraphPad Prism software (GraphPad Software Inc., La Jolla, CA, USA). $p < 0.05$ was considered statistically significant.

Author Contributions: Designed the experiments: P.Q., H.C. and X.L.; Performed the experiments: G.H. and H.Z.; Analyzed the data: G.H. and P.Q.; Wrote the paper: G.H. and H.Z.; Proofed the manuscript: P.Q., H.C. and X.L. All authors have read and agreed to the published version of the manuscript.

References

1. Luo, Y.; Ji, S.; Liu, Y.; Lei, J.-L.; Xia, S.-L.; Wang, Y.; Du, M.-L.; Shao, L.; Meng, X.; Zhou, M.; et al. Isolation and Characterization of a Moderately Virulent Classical Swine Fever Virus Emerging in China. *Transbound. Emerg. Dis.* **2016**, *64*, 1848–1857. [CrossRef] [PubMed]
2. Biagetti, M.; Greiser-Wilke, I.; Rutili, D. Molecular epidemiology of classical swine fever in Italy. *Vet. Microbiol.* **2001**, *83*, 205–215. [CrossRef]
3. Paton, D.J.; McGoldrick, A.; Greiser-Wilke, I.; Parchariyanon, S.; Song, J.-Y.; Liou, P.P.; Stadejek, T.; Lowings, J.P.; Björklund, H.; Belák, S. Genetic typing of classical swine fever virus. *Vet. Microbiol.* **2000**, *73*, 137–157. [CrossRef]
4. Risatti, G.R.; Holinka, L.; Carrillo, C.; Kutish, G.F.; Lu, Z.; Tulman, E.R.; Sainz, I.F.; Borca, M. Identification of a novel virulence determinant within the E2 structural glycoprotein of classical swine fever virus. *Virology* **2006**, *355*, 94–101. [CrossRef] [PubMed]
5. Chen, N.; Tong, C.; Li, D.; Wan, J.; Yuan, X.; Li, X.; Peng, J.; Fang, W. Antigenic analysis of classical swine fever virus E2 glycoprotein using pig antibodies identifies residues contributing to antigenic variation of the vaccine C-strain and group 2 strains circulating in China. *Virol. J.* **2010**, *7*, 378. [CrossRef] [PubMed]
6. Xing, C.; Lu, Z.; Jiang, J.; Huang, L.; Xu, J.; He, D.; Wei, Z.; Huang, H.; Zhang, H.; Murong, C.; et al. Sub-subgenotype 2.1c isolates of classical swine fever virus are dominant in Guangdong province of China, 2018. *Infect. Genet. Evol.* **2019**, *68*, 212–217. [CrossRef]
7. Sun, S.-Q.; Yin, S.-H.; Guo, H.-C.; Jin, Y.; Shang, Y.-J.; Liu, X.-T. Genetic Typing of Classical Swine Fever Virus Isolates from China. *Transbound. Emerg. Dis.* **2013**, *60*, 370–375. [CrossRef]
8. Khatoon, E.; Barman, N.N.; Deka, M.; Rajbongshi, G.; Baruah, K.; Deka, N.; Bora, D.P.; Kumar, S. Molecular characterization of classical swine fever virus isolates from India during 2012–14. *Acta Trop.* **2017**, *170*, 184–189. [CrossRef]
9. Zhang, H.; Leng, C.; Tian, Z.-J.; Liu, C.; Chen, J.; Bai, Y.; Li, Z.; Xiang, L.; Zhai, H.; Wang, Q.; et al. Complete genomic characteristics and pathogenic analysis of the newly emerged classical swine fever virus in China. *BMC Vet. Res.* **2018**, *14*, 204. [CrossRef]
10. Gong, W.; Li, J.; Wang, Z.; Sun, J.; Mi, S.; Lu, Z.; Cao, J.; Dou, Z.; Sun, Y.; Wang, P.; et al. Virulence evaluation of classical swine fever virus subgenotype 2.1 and 2.2 isolates circulating in China. *Vet. Microbiol.* **2019**, *232*, 114–120. [CrossRef]
11. Leifer, I.; Ruggli, N.; Blome, S. Approaches to define the viral genetic basis of classical swine fever virus virulence. *Virology* **2013**, *438*, 51–55. [CrossRef] [PubMed]
12. Huang, Y.-L.; Deng, M.-C.; Tsai, K.-J.; Liu, H.-M.; Huang, C.-C.; Wang, F.-I.; Chang, C.-Y. Competitive replication kinetics and pathogenicity in pigs co-infected with historical and newly invading classical swine fever viruses. *Virus Res.* **2017**, *228*, 39–45. [CrossRef] [PubMed]

13. Luo, Y.; Li, S.; Sun, Y.; Qiu, H.-J. Classical swine fever in China: A minireview. *Vet. Microbiol.* **2014**, *172*, 1–6. [CrossRef] [PubMed]

14. Blome, S.; Gabriel, C.; Schmeiser, S.; Meyer, D.; Meindl-Bohmer, A.; Koenen, F.; Beer, M. Efficacy of marker vaccine candidate CP7 _ E2alf against challenge with classical swine fever virus isolates of different genotypes. *Vet. Microbiol.* **2014**, *169*, 8–17. [CrossRef] [PubMed]

15. Everett, H.; Salguero, F.J.; Graham, S.P.; Haines, F.; Johns, H.; Clifford, D.; Nunez, A.; La Rocca, S.; Parchariyanon, S.; Steinbach, F.; et al. Characterisation of experimental infections of domestic pigs with genotype 2.1 and 3.3 isolates of classical swine fever virus. *Vet. Microbiol.* **2010**, *142*, 26–33. [CrossRef] [PubMed]

16. Choe, S.; Le, V.P.; Shin, J.; Kim, J.-H.; Kim, K.-S.; Song, S.; Cha, R.M.; Park, G.-N.; Nguyen, T.L.; Hyun, B.-H.; et al. Pathogenicity and Genetic Characterization of Vietnamese Classical Swine Fever Virus: 2014–2018. *Pathogens* **2020**, *9*, 169–172. [CrossRef] [PubMed]

17. Risatti, G.R.; Borca, M.; Kutish, G.F.; Lu, Z.; Holinka, L.G.; French, R.A.; Tulman, E.R.; Rock, D.L. The E2 Glycoprotein of Classical Swine Fever Virus Is a Virulence Determinant in Swine. *J. Virol.* **2005**, *79*, 3787–3796. [CrossRef]

18. Risatti, G.; Holinka, L.; Sainz, I.F.; Carrillo, C.; Kutish, G.; Lu, Z.; Zhu, J.; Rock, D.; Borca, M. Mutations in the carboxyl terminal region of E2 glycoprotein of classical swine fever virus are responsible for viral attenuation in swine. *Virology* **2007**, *364*, 371–382. [CrossRef]

19. Wu, R.; Li, L.; Zhao, Y.; Tu, J.; Pan, Z. Identification of two amino acids within E2 important for the pathogenicity of chimeric classical swine fever virus. *Virus Res.* **2016**, *211*, 79–85. [CrossRef]

20. Tamura, T.; Sakoda, Y.; Yoshino, F.; Nomura, T.; Yamamoto, N.; Sato, Y.; Okamatsu, M.; Ruggli, N.; Kida, H. Selection of Classical Swine Fever Virus with Enhanced Pathogenicity Reveals Synergistic Virulence Determinants in E2 and NS4B. *J. Virol.* **2012**, *86*, 8602–8613. [CrossRef]

21. Wu, R.; Li, L.; Lei, L.; Zhao, C.; Shen, X.; Zhao, H.; Pan, Z. Synergistic roles of the E2 glycoprotein and 3? untranslated region in the increased genomic stability of chimeric classical swine fever virus with attenuated phenotypes. *Arch. Virol.* **2017**, *162*, 2667–2678. [CrossRef] [PubMed]

22. Huang, Y.-L.; Tsai, K.-J.; Deng, M.-C.; Liu, H.-M.; Huang, C.-C.; Wang, F.-I.; Chang, C.-Y. In Vivo Demonstration of the Superior Replication and Infectivity of Genotype 2.1 with Respect to Genotype 3.4 of Classical Swine Fever Virus by Dual Infections. *Pathogens* **2020**, *9*, 261. [CrossRef] [PubMed]

23. Mittelholzer, C.; Moser, C.; Tratschin, J.-D.; Hofmann, M.A. Analysis of classical swine fever virus replication kinetics allows differentiation of highly virulent from avirulent strains. *Vet. Microbiol.* **2000**, *74*, 293–308. [CrossRef]

7

In Vivo Demonstration of the Superior Replication and Infectivity of Genotype 2.1 with Respect to Genotype 3.4 of Classical Swine Fever Virus by Dual Infections

Yu-Liang Huang [1], Kuo-Jung Tsai [1], Ming-Chung Deng [1], Hsin-Meng Liu [1], Chin-Cheng Huang [2], Fun-In Wang [3],* and Chia-Yi Chang [1],*

[1] Animal Health Research Institute, Council of Agriculture, Executive Yuan, 376 Chung-Cheng Road, Tansui, New Taipei City 25158, Taiwan; ylhuang@mail.nvri.gov.tw (Y.-L.H.); krtsai@mail.nvri.gov.tw (K.-J.T.); mcdeng@mail.nvri.gov.tw (M.-C.D.); hmliu@mail.nvri.gov.tw (H.-M.L.)
[2] Council of Agriculture, Executive Yuan, No. 37 Nanhai Road, Taipei 10014, Taiwan; cch@mail.coa.gov.tw
[3] School of Veterinary Medicine, National Taiwan University, No. 1, Section 4, Roosevelt Road, Taipei 10617, Taiwan
* Correspondence: fiwangvm@ntu.edu.tw (F.-I.W.); cychang@mail.nvri.gov.tw (C.-Y.C.)

Abstract: In Taiwan, the prevalent CSFV population has shifted from the historical genotype 3.4 (94.4 strain) to the newly invading genotype 2.1 (TD/96 strain) since 1996. This study analyzed the competition between these two virus genotypes in dual infection pigs with equal and different virus populations and with maternally derived neutralizing antibodies induced by a third genotype of modified live vaccine (MLV), to simulate that occurring in natural situations in the field. Experimentally, under various dual infection conditions, with or without the presence of maternal antibodies, with various specimens from blood, oral and fecal swabs, and internal organs at various time points, the TD/96 had consistently 1.51–3.08 log higher loads than those of 94.4. A second passage of competition in the same animals further widened the lead of TD/96 as indicated by viral loads. The maternally derived antibodies provided partial protection to both wild type CSFVs and was correlated with lower clinical scores, febrile reaction, and animal mortality. In the presence of maternal antibodies, pigs could be infected by both wild type CSFVs, with TD/96 dominating. These findings partially explain the CSFV shift observed, furthering our understanding of CSFV pathogenesis in the field, and are helpful for the control of CSF.

Keywords: classical swine fever virus; genotype; virus shift; viral replication; dual infections

1. Introduction

Classical swine fever virus (CSFV) is the etiological agent of classical swine fever (CSF), which is a highly contagious disease of swine. The CSFV is an enveloped positive-stranded RNA virus belonging to the genus *Pestivirus* of the family *Flaviviridae* [1]. The genome of CSFV is approximately 12.3 kb in length and contains a single open reading frame encoding for a polyprotein of 3,898 amino acids, which is flanked by 5′ and 3′ non-translated regions (NTR). The translated polyprotein is processed by cellular and viral proteases to the mature viral proteins of four structural (C, E^{rns}, E1, and E2) and eight nonstructural proteins (N^{pro}, p7, NS2, NS3, NS4A, NS4B, NS5A, and NS5B) [2].

The CSFV strains are divided into three genotypes, each with three to four subtypes—1.1, 1.2, 1.3, and 1.4; 2.1, 2.2, and 2.3; and 3.1, 3.2, 3.3, and 3.4—by analyzing three genomic regions: 5′-UTR, E2, and NS5B [3,4]. Genotype 1 comprises most of the historical strains including vaccine strains. Genotype 2 contains the most currently globally prevalent strains over the last two decades. Genotype 3 contains most of the strains with restricted distribution [3,5–7]. In recent years, there has been a shift in CSFV genotypes in the field, from genotypes 1 and 3 to genotype 2, which was observed in Europe and Asia [8–11]. The mechanisms for this shift remain unclear. In Taiwan, two CSFV populations coexist, namely the historical strain of genotype 3.4 (94.4 strain) prior to the 1920s and the newly invading strain of genotype 2.1 (TD/96 strain) since 1994, the latter of which became dominant in 1996 [12,13]. This means that in the field, pigs could be infected by two different genotypes of CSFV. In pig infections, the dominance of one strain, such as TD/96, over another strain, such as 94.4, could cause potential problems in the diagnosis, pathogenesis and epidemiological studies and control of CSF in the field, if not given special attention. From a clinical point of view, this replication advantage of genotype 2.1 could likely mask the detection, isolation and more aspects of genotype 3.4. The situation is further complicated by the routine use of modified live vaccines (MLV) to prevent and control CSF, in which all MLV strains used nowadays in different countries belong to genotype 1, a third genotype [3,14]. The MLVs offer protection from field viruses of different genotypes [14–16]. However, several factors, including viral loads of vaccines, routes and ages of vaccination, and co-presence of other pathogens, can interfere with the vaccine's efficacy [14,16,17].

To deepen our understanding of the characteristics of diverse CSFV genotypes, it is important to elucidate the mechanism of the virus shift in the field. Previous study revealed that the newly invading genotype 2.1 replicated more efficiently than genotype 3.4 did both in vitro and in vivo [18]. To further the understanding of pathogenesis that occurs in dual infections of CSFV, this study analyzed the competitions of the viruses of the two genotypes in co-infected pigs with equal and different virus populations without neutralizing antibodies and also in co-infected pigs with maternally derived neutralizing antibodies induced by MLV of a third genotype, with the goal of experimentally simulating the natural situations in the field.

2. Results

2.1. Clinical Manifestation

Pigs in Group 1 (co-infected_P1) were inoculated with equal amounts of the TD/96/TWN strain (designated TD/96 and belonging to genotype 2.1) and the 94.4/IL/94/TWN strain (designated 94.4 and belonging to genotype 3.4) simultaneously. Pigs in Group 2 (co-infected_P2) were inoculated with whole blood taken from a pig of Group 1 at 12 dpi. Pigs in Group 3 (co-infected with Ab) were inoculated with equal amounts of the TD/96 strain and the 94.4 strain simultaneously, born from a sow vaccinated with LPC vaccine, in which the maternal antibody response was in decline.

Clinical scores and temperature records of the experimental pigs are shown in Figure 1 and Table 1. The clinical signs were most numerous and significantly severe in co-infected_P2 (second passage of competition) pigs (Group 2; average maximum clinical score: 19.33 ± 0.58) and the first febrile reaction was detected as early as 2 or 3 days post-infection (dpi). The highest clinical score of Group 2 was the result of the pigs being inoculated with higher viral loads of the TD/96 strain than the pigs of the other two groups were (Table 1).

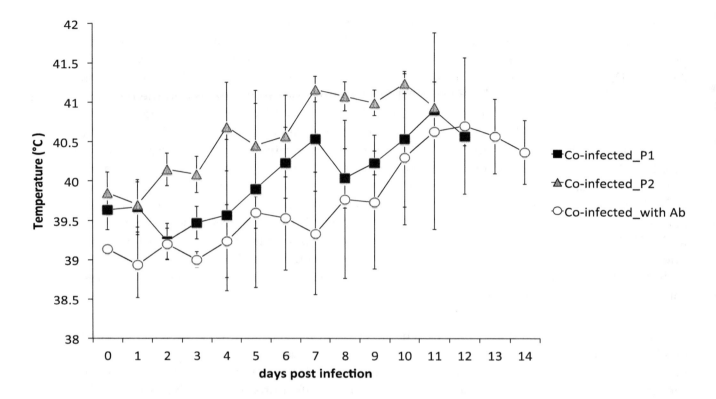

Figure 1. Body temperatures of pigs co-inoculated with classical swine fever viruses of two genotypes. Pigs in the group co-infected_P1 (square) were inoculated with TD/96 strain (genotype 2.1) and 94.4 strain (genotype 3.4). Pigs in the group co-infected_P2 (triangle) were inoculated with whole blood taken from a pig of group co-infected_P1 at 12 days post-infection. Pigs in the group co-infected with Ab (circle) were born from a sow vaccinated with LPC vaccine and were inoculated with the two virus strains. Each point represents the mean and standard deviation of the three pigs in the same group.

Those pigs in co-infected_P1 (first passage of competition) were less severe (Group 1; average maximum clinical score: 15.67 ± 1.53), and first febrile reaction was detected at 4 to 6 dpi. Clinical signs of those pigs co-infected with the presence of maternal antibodies developed more slowly and were significantly less severe (Group 3; average maximum clinical score: 4.67 ± 0.58) and all pigs survived until the end of experiment. First febrile reaction in pigs in Group 3 was detected at 6 to 12 dpi.

The febrile profile shown in Figure 1 was largely compatible with those of the averaged clinical scores shown in Table 1. In other words, Group 2, having higher clinical scores, also had higher febrile reactions, while Group 3, having lower clinical scores, also had lower febrile reaction.

2.2. Virus Titration of Viremia for Co-Infected_P2 Pigs Inoculation

Co-infected_P2 pigs were inoculated with whole blood taken from a pig of the co-infected_P1 group at 12 dpi (Group 2, Table 1). The virus titers of the TD/96 strain and the 94.4 strain from viremia at 12 dpi of a co-infected_P1 pig were $10^{8.3}$ TCID$_{50}$/mL (tissue culture infectious dose 50%) and $10^{5.87}$ TCID$_{50}$/mL, respectively, determined by CSFV genotype-specific monoclonal antibodies (mAbs) (Table 2).

Table 1. Clinical scores and virus detection of individual pigs co-inoculated with classical swine fever viruses.

Inoculated Group	Time (dpi) of the First Observation of Fever	Maximum Clinical Score	Time (dpi) of Death	Time (dpi) of the First Detection of Virus in Blood		Time (dpi) of the First Detection of Virus in Oral Swabs		Time (dpi) of the First Detection of Virus in Fecal Swabs	
				TD/96[†]	94.4	TD/96	94.4	TD/96	94.4
Group 1: Co-infected_P1	4	17	13	2	4	6	8	6	8
(TD/96 10^6 TCID$_{50}$ + 94.4 10^6 TCID$_{50}$)	6	16	13	2	4	6	8	8	10
	6	14 Average $15.67 \pm 1.53^{b*}$	13	2	4	6	8	6	8
Group 2: Co-infected_P2	2	19	9	2	6	4	ND§	4	ND
(blood of group 1 pig containing TD/96 $10^{8.3}$ TCID$_{50}$ and 94.4 $10^{5.87}$ TCID$_{50}$)	3	20	12	2	6	4	8	6	8
	2	19 Average 19.33 ± 0.58^{a}	11	2	6	6	8	6	8
Group 3: Co-infected with Ab	12	5	14¶	4	6	6	8	8	8
(TD/96 10^6 TCID$_{50}$ + 94.4 10^6 TCID$_{50}$)	10	5	14¶	4	6	6	8	6	8
	6	4 Average 4.67 ± 0.58^{c}	14¶	4	6	8	8	8	8

† TD/96 and 94.4 indicate the TD/96/TWN and 94.4/IL/94/TWN strains, respectively. * Values with different superscript letters, a–c, among the three groups of samples at the same dpi indicate a statistically significant difference ($p < 0.05$) from each other. The superscript letter "a" indicates the highest viral load and "c" indicates the lowest viral load among the compared groups. ¶ The pig was euthanized at the end of the experiment. § ND: not detected.

Table 2. Viral loads in blood from a pig of the co-infected_P1 group at 12 dpi.

Viral Loads	Log		Methods	
	TD/96[†]	94.4	TD/96	94.4
Viral titer (TCID$_{50}$/mL)	8.3	5.87	By IFA* using mAb T6 specific for TD/96	By IFA using mAb L71 specific for 94.4
Viral genome (copies/μL)	7.64	5.23	By RT-MRT-PCR[¶] using specific TaqMan probe for TD/96	By RT-MRT-PCR using specific TaqMan probe for 94.4

[†] TD/96 and 94.4 indicate the TD/96/TWN and 94.4/IL/94/TWN strains, respectively. * IFA indicates indirect fluorescent assay. [¶] RT-MRT-PCR indicates reverse transcription multiplex real-time polymerase chain reaction.

2.3. Cross-Neutralizing Antibodies against Three Genotypes of CSFVs

The role of maternal antibodies during dual infections was further investigated (Table 3). The pigs' sera of co-infected_P1 (Group 1) and co-infected_P2 (Group 2) at 0 dpi to the end of the experimental period showed no neutralizing antibodies against genotypes 1.1 (LPC/AHRI strain), 2.1 (TD/96 strain) or 3.4 (94.4 strain), consistent with the more severe clinical scores and animal mortalities at 9–13 dpi observed in both groups (Table 1).

Table 3. Cross-neutralizing antibodies of three pigs co-inoculated with classical swine fever viruses with maternally derived neutralizing antibodies (Group 3).

Time (dpi) of the Collected Pig Sera	Cross-Neutralizing Antibodies Against (log$_2$)			Time (dpi) of the Collected Pig Sera	Cross-neutralizing Antibodies Against (log$_2$)		
	LPC[†]	TD/96	94.4		LPC	TD/96	94.4
0	4.5	2.5	2.5	8	2.5	<2	<2
	4.5	3.5	3.5		3.5	<2	<2
	5	3.5	2.5		<2	<2	<2
	Average 4.7 ± 0.3^{a*}	Average 3.2 ± 0.6^b	Average 2.8 ± 0.6^b				
2	4	2	2	10	<2	<2	<2
	4.5	3	3		<2	<2	<2
	5	3.5	2.5		<2	<2	<2
	Average 4.5 ± 0.5^a	Average 2.8 ± 0.8^b	Average 2.5 ± 0.5^b				
4	3	2.5	2	12	<2	<2	<2
	5	3.5	3		<2	<2	<2
	5	3	2.5		<2	<2	<2
	Average 4.3 ± 1.2^a	Average 3 ± 0.5^{ab}	Average 2.5 ± 0.5^b				
6	3	2.5	2	14	<2	<2	<2
	4.5	3.5	3		<2	<2	<2
	5	2.5	2		<2	<2	<2
	Average 4.2 ± 1^a	Average 2.8 ± 0.6^{ab}	Average 2.3 ± 0.6^b				

[†] LPC, TD/96 and 94.4 indicate the LPC/AHRI, TD/96/TWN and 94.4/IL/94/TWN strains, respectively. * Values with different superscript letters, a–b, among the three groups of samples at the same dpi indicate a statistically significant difference ($p < 0.05$) from each other. The superscript letter "a" indicates the highest viral load, and "b" indicates the lowest viral load among the compared groups, while "ab" indicates a viral load in between categories "a" and "b". No significant difference exists between values containing the same letter. The absence of a superscript letter indicates no statistical analysis.

The neutralizing antibodies against the LPC strain in the sera of co-infected pigs with maternal antibodies (Group 3) before inoculation indicated that these pigs were in a declining phase of maternal antibody response (data not shown). Sera of co-infected pigs at 0–6 dpi did show cross-neutralizing antibodies against three genotypes (Table 3), consistent with the much milder clinical scores seen in this group. A critical time window was noted at 6–8 dpi, when the cross-neutralizing antibody titers against TD/96 and 94.4 CSFVs dropped from log$_2$ 2.3–2.8 to < 2.0 (Table 3), and yet the animals survived until 14 dpi (Table 1). The neutralizing antibody titers against the LPC strain were significantly higher than those against the TD/96 strain and the 94.4 strain at 0 and 2 dpi and significantly higher than those against the 94.4 strain at 4 and 6 dpi. There was no significant difference between the neutralizing antibody titer against the TD/96 strain and the 94.4 strain. From 8 or 10 dpi to 14 dpi, sera of co-infected with Ab pigs did not show detectable neutralizing antibodies against any of the three genotypes (Table 3).

2.4. Viral Loads in Bloods

Primary viremia of TD/96 strain was first detected in both co-infected_P1 pigs and co-infected_P2 pigs at 2 dpi, and in co-infected with Ab pigs at 4 dpi, earlier than that of 94.4 strain, which was first detected in co-infected_P1 pigs at 4 dpi and in both co-infected_P2 pigs and co-infected with Ab pigs at 6 dpi (Figures 2A and 3A, Table 1). The viral loads of the TD/96 strain were always significantly higher than those of the 94.4 strain ($p < 0.05$) (Figures 2A and 3A) in all the co-infected pigs. The viral loads of the TD/96 strain were on average 1.89, 2.93, and 1.51 log higher than that of the 94.4 strain at all dpi in co-infected_P1 pigs, co-infected_P2 pigs and co-infected with Ab pigs, respectively. Comparing the three groups, the co-infected_P2 pigs had the highest lead of TD/96 at all dpi; the viral loads were above 3 log higher than that of the 94.4 strain at 4 and 6 dpi. The highest lead of TD/96 was observed at 4 dpi, when it was on average 3.96 log higher than that of the 94.4 strain. No lead of TD/96 was above 3 log in co-infected_P1 pigs or co-infected with Ab pigs.

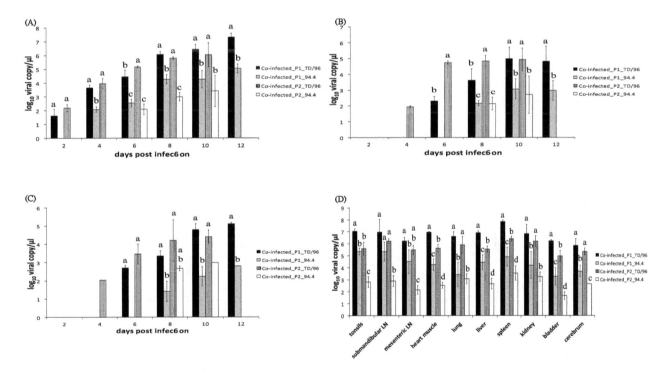

Figure 2. Comparison of viral loads of co-infected_P1 (Group 1) and co-infected_P2 pigs (Group 2). Viral loads in (**A**) blood, (**B**) oral swabs, (**C**) fecal swabs, and (**D**) organs of co-infected_P1 and co-infected_P2 pigs were quantified by reverse transcription multiplex real-time polymerase chain reaction. The data represent the mean and standard deviation from three pigs. Values with different superscript letters, a–d, among the four groups of samples at the same dpi (**A–C**) or the same organ (**D**) indicate a statistically significant difference ($p < 0.05$) from each other. The superscript letter "a" indicates the highest viral load and "d" indicates the lowest viral load among the compared groups, while "ab" indicates a viral load in between categories "a" and "b". No significant differences exist between values containing the same letter. The absence of a superscript letter indicates no statistical analysis due to only one sample of a group or only one group within the same dpi.

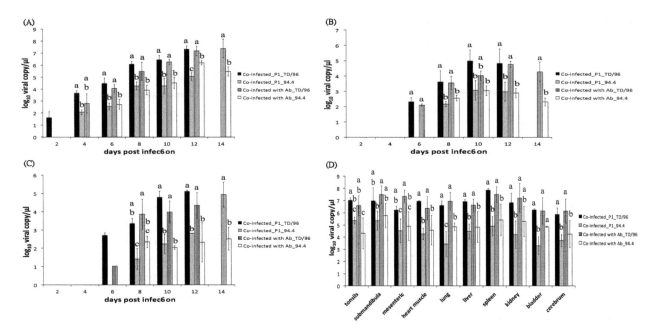

Figure 3. Comparison of viral loads of co-infected_P1 (Group 1) and co-infected with Ab pigs (Group 3). Viral loads in (**A**) blood, (**B**) oral swabs, (**C**) fecal swabs, and (**D**) organs of co-infected_P1 and co-infected with Ab pigs were quantified by reverse transcription multiplex real-time polymerase chain reaction. The data represent the mean and standard deviation from three pigs. Values with different superscript letters, a–d, among the four groups of samples at the same dpi (**A–C**) or the same organ (**D**) indicate a statistically significant difference ($p < 0.05$) from each other. The superscript letter "a" indicates the highest viral load and "d" indicates the lowest viral load among the compared groups, while "ab" indicates a viral load in between categories "a" and "b". No significant differences exist between values containing the same letter. The absence of a superscript letter labeled indicates no statistical analysis due to only one sample of a group or only one group within the same dpi.

2.5. Viral Loads in Secretions and Excretions

In co-infected_P2 pigs, the TD/96 strain was first detected in oral swabs and fecal swabs at 4 to 6 dpi, whereas in co-infected_P1 pigs and co-infected with Ab pigs, the TD/96 strain first presented at 6 to 8 dpi (Table 1). The 94.4 strain was first detected in oral swabs and fecal swabs at 8 to 10 dpi in all co-infected pigs, except one co-infected_P2 pig that died at 9 dpi, in which the virus was not detected (Table 1).

In oral swabs, the viral loads of the TD/96 strain were always significantly higher than those of the 94.4 strain in all the co-infected pigs ($p < 0.05$) (Figures 2B and 3B), with only one exception at 10 dpi of co-infected with Ab pigs. The viral loads of the TD/96 strain were on average 1.88, 3.08 and 1.59 log higher than that of the 94.4 strain at all dpi in co-infected_P1 pigs, co-infected_P2 pigs and co-infected with Ab pigs, respectively. Comparing the three groups, the co-infected_P2 pigs had the highest lead of TD/96 at all dpi, in which the viral loads were above 3 log higher than that of the 94.4 strain at 6 and 8 dpi. The highest lead of TD/96 was observed at 6 dpi, when it was on average 4.74 log higher than that of the 94.4 strain. No lead of TD/96 was above 3 log in co-infected_P1 pigs or co-infected with Ab pigs.

In fecal swabs, the viral loads of the TD/96 strain were always significantly higher than those of the 94.4 strain in all co-infected pigs ($p < 0.05$) (Figures 2C and 3C), with only one exception at 8 dpi of co-infected_P2. The viral loads of the TD/96 strain were on average 2.49, 2.7 and 1.84 log higher than that of the 94.4 strain at all dpi in co-infected_P1 pigs, co-infected_P2 pigs and co-infected with Ab pigs, respectively. Comparing the three groups, the co-infected_P2 pigs had the highest lead of TD/96 at all dpi; the highest lead of TD/96, with on average 3.45 log higher than that of the 94.4 strain, was observed at 6 dpi. No lead of TD/96 was above 3 log in co-infected_P1 pigs or co-infected with Ab pigs.

2.6. Viral Loads in Visceral Organs

The viral loads of the TD/96 strain were consistently significantly higher than those of the 94.4 strain in most tested organs ($p < 0.05$) (Figures 2D and 3D) in all pigs. The viral loads of the TD/96 strain were on average 2.39, 3.00, and 2.09 log higher than those of the 94.4 strain in co-infected_P1 pigs, co-infected_P2 pigs, and co-infected with Ab pigs, respectively. Comparing the three groups, the co-infected_P2 pigs had the highest lead of TD/96 in most tested organs; the viral loads were above 2.5 log higher than that of the 94.4 strain. The highest lead of TD/96 was observed in lymph nodes, where it was on average 3.33 log higher than that of the 94.4 strain.

3. Discussion

The shift in CSFV populations in the field, from genotypes 1 and 3 to genotype 2, was observed worldwide [8–12]. However, the mechanisms responsible for the shift remain unclear. A previous study hypothesized that genotype 2 had higher genetic diversity than genotypes 1 and 3 did, which might explain why it is the most prevalent endemic situation [19]. Three hypotheses were proposed: First, virus strains of genotype 2.1 may have higher replication efficiency than the genotype 3.4 strains in pigs; second, the strains of genotype 2.1 may have higher affinity and competitiveness to cellular receptors than those of genotype 3.4; and third, the strains of genotype 2.1 may have better ability than those of genotype 3.4 to escape from antibody neutralization induced by the attenuated lapinized vaccine strain LPC of genotype 1.1, which has been used to protect pigs against the 3.4 strains since the 1950s in Taiwan [12]. To test the first two hypotheses, Huang et al. [18] allowed two viruses belonging to genotypes 2.1 and 3.4, respectively, to compete in vivo and in vitro, and the results revealed that the virus of genotype 2.1 replicated more efficiently than that of genotype 3.4. To further explore and to simulate the field situation, this study analyzed the competitions of the viruses of the two genotypes in co-infected pigs for two passages without neutralizing antibodies (Groups 1 and 2). Moreover, we also examined the dynamics of virus replication and disease development of the infected pigs in the presence of maternally derived neutralizing antibodies induced by LPC vaccine (Group 3). To the best of our knowledge, this study is the first attempt to test the competitions of CSFV in this way.

The new CSFV strain of genotype 2.1 has higher replication efficiency than the historical genotype 3.4 strain in pigs. Indeed, when given equal opportunity to compete in the same animal for the first passage of competition, the genotype 2.1 CSFV (represented by TD/96) had 2.43 log (8.3–5.87) higher $TCID_{50}$ titer over that of genotype 3.4 (represented by 94.4) in the blood (Group 2 inoculum, Table 1). This advantage of TD/96 in blood was also amply supported by quantifications of viral loads using quantitative reverse transcription multiplex real-time polymerase chain reaction (RT-MRT-PCR) (Table 2). Under various dual infection conditions with or without the presence of maternal antibodies, the TD/96 strain had consistently 1.51–3.08 log higher loads than those of 94.4. The 2.43 log $TCID_{50}$ replication advantage of TD/96 in the first passage of competition in an animal body falls within the range of 1.51–3.08 log, as estimated by RT-MRT-PCR. Given a second passage of competition, the lead of TD/96 was widened further. The TD/96 strain was first detected in oral swabs and fecal swabs of co-infected_P2 pigs 2–4 days earlier than in those of co-infected_P1 pigs. On the other hand, the 94.4 strain was first detected in viremia of co-infected_P2 pigs 2 days later than in those of co-infected_P1 pigs, despite the two groups having been inoculated with similar amounts of the 94.4 strain (10^6 $TCID_{50}$/mL in co-infected_P1 pigs and $10^{5.87}$ $TCID_{50}$/mL in co-infected_P2 pigs). The results revealed that when the viruses of genotype 2.1 are dominant in the field, the viruses replicate more efficiently and shed earlier than the viruses of genotype 3.4 do. Therefore, the genotype of CSFV in the pig population shifted from genotype 3.4 to 2.1. Given further passages of dual infection in pigs, the competition edge of genotype 2.1 would likely lead to the disappearance of genotype 3.4 in pigs.

Colostrum maternal antibodies offer partial protection for dually infected pigs, despite the genotype difference of the LPC vaccine virus (of genotype 1.1) from those of genotype 2.1 and 3.4 of dually infected viruses (Group 3). The TD/96 and 94.4 strains were first detected in the blood of co-infected with Ab pigs 2 days later than in co-infected_P1 pigs, although pigs in these two groups were inoculated with the same amounts of the TD/96 and 94.4 strains. The maternal antibodies protection was ineffective when the genotypic heterologous neutralizing titer dropped to below 1:4 during dpi 8–14 (Table 3), for febrile reactions were observed after 10 dpi (Figure 1). This finding suggests that the protection offered by the maternal antibodies is not limited to the initial engagement to neutralize incoming virus but also allows for the host to launch immune responses before the system is overwhelmed.

Antigenic variations among various genotypes of CSFVs certainly render the currently available vaccines more effective in neutralizing historical viruses, while allowing the newly invading virus to escape. This hypothesis has been amply addressed in several previous studies [20–23]. The neutralizing antibodies of co-infected with Ab pigs against the LPC/AHRI strain were higher than those against the TD/96 strain and the 94.4 strain. However, there was no significant difference between the neutralizing antibodies against the TD/96 strain and those against the 94.4 strain. This evidence supported previous studies that antibodies induced by live virus neutralize genotypically homologous strains better than heterologous strains [17,24,25]. In co-infected with Ab pigs, similarly to Group 1, the TD/96 strain was shed by infected pigs earlier than the 94.4 strain was. In addition, the viral loads of the TD/96 strain were significantly higher than those of the 94.4 strain. The results indicated that the presence of maternally derived antibodies induced by modified live virus of genotype 1.1 might not influence the competition between viruses of genotypes 2.1 and 3.4. Previous study demonstrated that the LPC vaccine could offer pigs protection from challenges of field viruses of genotypes 2.1 and 3.4 [26]. This study revealed that when pigs or piglets infected by CSFV field viruses of genotypes 2.1 and 3.4 were vaccinated, the vaccine's efficacy was interfered with, and also that when the maternally derived antibodies declined in piglets before vaccination, the pigs produced lower neutralizing antibodies and had delayed clinical signs. However, the CSFVs were detected in those infected pigs, in which the genotype 2.1 viruses were released earlier and replicated more efficiently than did genotype 3.4 viruses. These results may suggest that the newly invading strains dominated in the field under vaccination.

Contact infection may present another aspect of virus competition. To investigate how the competition occurs between viruses of genotypes 2.1 and 3.4, in this study we employed the intramuscular route for the co-infection. This route can ensure that both viruses enter the hosts with the same amount of virus simultaneously to allow comparison of their replication efficiency and pathogenicity. However, when the virus is introduced through natural routes, the influencing factors could be more numerous and much complicated. To further explore the natural situations and to evaluate the possible effect of the superinfection exclusion phenomenon of CSFV [27] in the field in terms of the competence of these two genotypes, cohabitation infection with 2.1 virus infected pigs and 3.4 virus infected pigs is warranted.

In conclusion, examining the competition of the historical and newly invading genotypes of CSFV in co-infected pigs with different virus populations and with maternally derived neutralizing antibodies revealed that the new CSFV genotype 2.1 replicates more efficiently, at 1.51–3.08 log higher than that of the historical genotype 3.4. The maternally derived antibodies provide partial protection to both wild type CSFVs and correlate with lower clinical scores, febrile reaction, and animal mortality. In the presence of maternal antibodies, pigs could be infected by both wild type CSFVs, with the genotype 2.1 dominating. These results could further our understanding of the prevalence of genotype 2 in the field, which is widely observed in Asia and Europe. This is the first time that the higher replication capacity of genotype 2.1 than that of genotype 3.4 has been demonstrated in vivo with this design.

4. Materials and Methods

4.1. Cells and Viruses

Porcine kidney-15 (PK-15) cells were maintained in minimum essential medium supplemented with 10% fetal bovine serum and incubated at 37 °C in 5% CO_2. The three CSFV strains used in this study, comprised the two representative CSFV strains TD/96 and 94.4 and an attenuated lapinized vaccine strain LPC/AHRI, were propagated in the PK-15 cells [3,12,13].

4.2. mAbs Specific for CSFV

Three mAbs against CSFVs were used in this study. The mAbs T6 and L71 were produced by the Animal Health Research Institute, Taiwan, and the mAb WH303 by the Animal and Plant Health Agency, the United Kingdom. The mAb T6 recognizes the TD/96 strain of genotype 2.1 but not the 94.4 strain of genotype 3.4. In contrast, the mAb L71 recognizes the 94.4 strain but not the TD/96 strain [18]. The mAb WH303 reacts with most CSFV strains tested [28], including the three strains used in this study.

4.3. Experimental Infections

Six 4-week-old specific pathogen-free (SPF) pigs were randomly separated into two groups of three pigs: Groups 1 and 2 (Table 1). Pigs in Group 1 (co-infected_P1) were inoculated intramuscularly with 1 mL of the TD/96 strain and 1 mL of the 94.4 strain simultaneously, each at a virus amount of 10^6 $TCID_{50}$/mL, to ensure that both strains could enter the hosts simultaneously. The concept of the Group 1 co-infection experiment design was similar to that described in Group 3 of Huang et al. [18] and was repeated here, in separate pigs, for comparison with Groups 2 and 3 (see below). Pigs in Group 2 (co-infected_P2) were inoculated intramuscularly with 1 mL of whole blood taken from a pig of Group 1 at 12 dpi. This inoculum contained TD/96 $10^{8.3}$ $TCID_{50}$ and 94.4 $10^{5.87}$ $TCID_{50}$ as titrated later (Table 1). Group 3 (co-infected with Ab) included three 4-week-old pigs born from a sow vaccinated with LPC vaccine, in which the maternal antibody response was in decline. These animals were chosen in order to examine the effect of antibody drop on co-infection. These pigs were inoculated intramuscularly with 1 mL of the TD/96 strain and 1 mL of the 94.4 strain simultaneously, as in Group 1, at 10^6 $TCID_{50}$/mL. The three groups were housed separately in three negative air-pressure isolation units. For animal welfare reasons, pigs were euthanized when they were moribund and unable to stand up. All surviving pigs were euthanized at 14 dpi, the end of the experimental period. This animal experiment was approved by the Institutional Animal Care and Use Committee of the Animal Health Research Institute (Approval number A02040).

4.4. Clinical Signs, Body Temperature, and Sampling Procedures

Rectal temperature was recorded daily during the experimental period. Fever was defined as a temperature higher than 40 °C. For evaluation of clinical signs, the ten parameters described by Mittelholzer et al. [29] were scored from 0 to 3 to represent normal to severe CSF symptoms. The scores of each pig were summed into a total score for each day. Blood, oral swabs, and fecal swabs were collected prior to inoculation at 0 dpi and then at 2-day intervals post infection. Swabs were weighed before and after sampling to normalize the viral loads. Each swab was immersed in 2 mL of phosphate buffered saline (PBS) and centrifuged at 3,000 × g for 10 min, and the harvested supernatant was stored at −70 °C. Necropsies were performed after euthanasia or death, and tissue samples of tonsil, submandibular and mesenteric lymph nodes, heart muscle, lung, liver, spleen, kidney, bladder, and cerebrum were collected from all pigs.

4.5. Virus Titration

Ten-fold serial diluted blood (inoculum of Group 2) at 12 dpi from a pig of co-infected_P1 was added into eight wells each of 96-well plates duplicated and seeded with PK-15 cells. Whether the cells were infected was observed using indirect fluorescent assay (IFA) at 72 hours post infection (hpi). The mAbs T6 and L71 were used for virus titration. One 96-well plate was stained with mAb T6, which recognizes the TD/96 strain but not the 94.4 strain; the other 96-well plate was stained with mAb L71, which recognizes the 94.4 strain but not the TD/96 strain [18]. Virus titers were calculated as $TCID_{50}$ using the Reed-Muench method [30].

4.6. Quantitative Reverse Transcription Multiplex Real-Time Polymerase Chain Reaction (RT-MRT-PCR)

Viral RNAs were extracted using the QIAamp® Viral RNA Mini Kit (QIAGEN, Hilden, Germany). The specific RT-MRT-PCR was performed to detect and genotype CSFV as described by Huang et al. [31], who demonstrated no inter-genotypic cross-reactivity among different CSFV strains using the universal primers and specific TaqMan probes for each of the three genotypes, genotypes 1, 2, and 3. The viral loads, determined by the RT-MRT-PCR, are expressed as log viral genome copies/μL.

4.7. Cross-Neutralizing Antibodies against Three Genotypes of CSFV

The genotype-specific neutralizing antibodies were cross-neutralized with sera from pigs at 0 dpi (before inoculation) to 14 dpi (or the end of the experimental period) against CSFV strains of genotypes 1.1 (LPC/AHRI strain), 2.1 (TD/96 strain) and 3.4 (94.4 strain). Two-fold serial diluted 56 °C heat-inactivated sera were mixed with equal volumes of 100 TCID$_{50}$ of the viruses, incubated at 37 °C for 1 h, and subsequently transferred to PK-15 cells in 96-well plates. The starting dilution of each serum was 1:4. At 72 hpi, the cells were fixed and stained for the presence CSFV antigen by the IFA. Neutralizing titer is the log$_2$ of the antibody dilution factor (reciprocal of dilution) when 50% of the wells are protected from infection.

4.8. Indirect Fluorescent Assay (IFA)

The inoculated cells in 96-well plates were fixed with 10% formaldehyde at room temperature for 10 min and washed three times with PBS. Each mAb against CSFV was diluted 1:100 in PBS, and 50 μL of the diluted mAb was added per well (mAb T6 for virus titration of the TD/96 strain and mAb L71 for virus titration of the 94.4 strain; mAb WH303 for detection of cross-neutralizing antibodies). The cells were then incubated at 37 °C for 1 h and washed three times with PBS. Fluorescein isothiocyanate-conjugated goat anti-mouse IgG (Jackson ImmunoResearch Laboratories, West Grove, PA, USA) diluted 1:100 in PBS was added, 50 μL per well. The cells were incubated at 37 °C for 1 h and then washed three times with PBS. Fluorescence of the stained cells was observed under a fluorescence microscope (Olympus Imaging America, Center Valley, PA, USA).

4.9. Statistical Analysis

Differences in the values between two groups and among various groups were statistically analyzed using the Student's t-test and one-way analysis of variance (ANOVA), respectively. ANOVA was combined with the Duncan multiple range test. The statistical analysis was carried out in Statistical Analysis System (SAS) Enterprise Guide 7.1 (SAS Institute Inc., Cary, NC, USA). Mean differences were considered statistically significant when the p-value was <0.05.

Author Contributions: Conceptualization, Y.-L.H., C.-C.H., and C.-Y.C.; Methodology, Y.-L.H., H.-M.L., and C.-Y.C.; Validation, Y.-L.H. and C.-Y.C.; Formal Analysis, Y.-L.H. and H.-M.L.; Investigation, Y.-L.H., K.-J.T., M.-C.D., H.-M.L., and C.-Y.C.; Resources, Y.-L.H., K.-J.T., M.-C.D., and C.-Y.C.; Data Curation, K.-J.T., M.-C.D., and F.-I.W.; Writing—Original Draft Preparation, C.-Y.C.; Writing—Review & Editing, F.-I.W.; Supervision, F.-I.W.; Project Administration, C.-Y.C.; Funding Acquisition, C.-Y.C. All authors have read and agreed to the published version of the manuscript.

Acknowledgments: We particularly thank Yi-Hsieng Samuel Wu, Department of Animal Science and Technology, National Taiwan University, for his assistance in the statistical analysis. We thank Fan Lee, Animal Health Research Institute, for his critical comments on the manuscript.

References

1.   Simmonds, P.; Becher, P.; Collett, M.; Gould, E.; Heinz, F.; Meyers, G.; Monath, T.; Pletnev, A.; Rice, C.; Stiasny, K.; et al. Family Flaviviridae. In *Virus Taxonomy: Ninth Report of the International Committee on Taxonomy of Viruses*; King, A.M.Q., Adams, M.J., Carstens, E.B., Eds.; Elsevier Academic Press: San Diego, CA, USA, 2011; pp. 1003–1020.

2. Lindenbach, B.D.; Murray, C.L.; Thiel, H.J.; Rice, C.M. Flaviviridae: The viruses and their replication. In *Fields Virology*, 6th ed.; Knipe, D.M., Howley, P.M., Eds.; Lippincott Williams&Wilkins: Philadelphia, PA, USA, 2013; pp. 712–747.

3. Paton, D.J.; McGoldrick, A.; Greiser-Wilke, I.; Parchariyanon, S.; Song, J.Y.; Liou, P.P.; Stadejek, T.; Lowings, J.P.; Björklund, H.; Belák, S. Genetic typing of classical swine fever virus. *Vet. Microbiol.* **2000**, *73*, 137–157. [CrossRef]

4. Postel, A.; Schmeiser, S.; Perera, C.L.; Rodríguez, L.J.P.; Frias-Lepoureau, M.T.; Becher, P. Classical swine fever virus isolates from Cuba form a new subgenotype 1.4. *Vet. Microbiol.* **2013**, *161*, 334–338. [CrossRef]

5. Beer, M.; Goller, K.V.; Staubach, C.; Blome, S. Genetic variability and distribution of classical swine fever virus. *Anim. Health Res. Rev.* **2015**, *16*, 33–39. [CrossRef] [PubMed]

6. Everett, H.; Salguero, F.J.; Graham, S.P.; Haines, F.; Johns, H.; Clifford, D.; Nunez, A.; La Rocca, S.A.; Parchariyanon, S.; Steinbach, F.; et al. Characterisation of experimental infections of domestic pigs with genotype 2.1 and 3.3 isolates of classical swine fever virus. *Vet. Microbiol.* **2010**, *142*, 26–33. [CrossRef] [PubMed]

7. Sakoda, Y.; Ozawa, S.; Damrongwatanopokin, S.; Sato, M.; Ishikawa, K.; Fukusho, A. Genetic heterogeneity of porcine and ruminant pestiviruses mainly isolated in Japan. *Vet. Microbiol.* **1999**, *65*, 75–86. [CrossRef]

8. Cha, S.H.; Choi, E.J.; Park, J.H.; Yoon, S.R.; Kwon, J.H.; Yoon, K.J.; Song, J.Y. Phylogenetic characterization of classical swine fever viruses isolated in Korea between 1988 and 2003. *Virus Res.* **2007**, *126*, 256–261. [CrossRef] [PubMed]

9. Greiser-Wilke, I.; Fritzemeier, J.; Koenen, F.; Vanderhallen, H.; Rutili, D.; De Mia, G.M.; Romero, L.; Rosell, R.; Sanchez-Vizcaino, J.M.; San Gabriel, A. Molecular epidemiology of a large classical swine fever epidemic in the European Union in 1997–1998. *Vet. Microbiol.* **2000**, *77*, 17–27. [CrossRef]

10. Shivaraj, D.B.; Patil, S.S.; Rathnamma, D.; Hemadri, D.; Isloor, S.; Geetha, S.; Manjunathareddy, G.B.; Gajendragad, M.R.; Rahman, H. Genetic clustering of recent classical swine fever virus isolates from Karnataka, India revealed the emergence of subtype 2.2 replacing subtype 1.1. *Virus Dis.* **2015**, *26*, 170–179. [CrossRef]

11. Tu, C.; Lu, Z.; Li, H.; Yu, X.; Liu, X.; Li, Y.; Zhang, H.; Yin, Z. Phylogenetic comparison of classical swine fever virus in China. *Virus Res.* **2001**, *81*, 29–37. [CrossRef]

12. Deng, M.C.; Huang, C.C.; Huang, T.S.; Chang, C.Y.; Lin, Y.J.; Chien, M.S.; Jong, M.H. Phylogenetic analysis of classical swine fever virus isolated from Taiwan. *Vet. Microbiol.* **2005**, *106*, 187–193. [CrossRef]

13. Lin, Y.J.; Chien, M.S.; Deng, M.C.; Huang, C.C. Complete sequence of a subgroup 3.4 strain of classical swine fever virus from Taiwan. *Virus Genes* **2007**, *35*, 737–744. [CrossRef]

14. Suradhat, S.; Damrongwatanapokin, S.; Thanawongnuwech, R. Factors critical for successful vaccination against classical swine fever in endemic areas. *Vet. Microbiol.* **2007**, *119*, 1–9. [CrossRef] [PubMed]

15. Graham, S.P.; Everett, H.E.; Haines, F.J.; Johns, H.L.; Sosan, O.A.; Salguero, F.J.; Clifford, D.J.; Steinbach, F.; Drew, T.W.; Crooke, H.R. Challenge of pigs with classical swine fever viruses after C-strain vaccination reveals remarkably rapid protection and insights into early immunity. *PLoS ONE* **2012**, *7*, e29310. [CrossRef] [PubMed]

16. van Oirschot, J.T. Vaccinology of classical swine fever: From lab to field. *Vet. Microbiol.* **2003**, *96*, 367–384. [CrossRef] [PubMed]

17. Huang, Y.L.; Deng, M.C.; Wang, F.I.; Huang, C.C.; Chang, C.Y. The challenges of classical swine fever control: Modified live and E2 subunit vaccines. *Virus Res.* **2014**, *179*, 1–11. [CrossRef]

18. Huang, Y.L.; Deng, M.C.; Tsai, K.J.; Liu, H.M.; Huang, C.C.; Wang, F.I.; Chang, C.Y. Competitive replication kinetics and pathogenicity in pigs co-infected with historical and newly invading classical swine fever viruses. *Virus Res.* **2017**, *228*, 39–45. [CrossRef]

19. Rios, L.; Coronado, L.; Naranjo-Feliciano, D.; Martínez-Pérez, O.; Perera, C.L.; Hernandez-Alvarez, L.; Díaz de Arce, H.; Núñez, J.I.; Ganges, L.; Pérez, L.J. Deciphering the emergence, genetic diversity and evolution of classical swine fever virus. *Sci. Rep.* **2017**, *7*, 17887. [CrossRef]

20. Chen, N.; Hu, H.; Zhang, Z.; Shuai, J.; Jiang, L.; Fang, W. Genetic diversity of the envelope glycoprotein E2 of classical swine fever virus: Recent isolates branched away from historical and vaccine strains. *Vet. Microbiol.* **2008**, *127*, 286–299. [CrossRef]

21. Coronado, L.; Rios, L.; Frías, M.T.; Amarán, L.; Naranjo, P.; Percedo, M.I.; Perera, C.L.; Prieto, F.; Fonseca-Rodriguez, O.; Perez, L.J. Positive selection pressure on E2 protein of classical swine fever virus drives variations in virulence, pathogenesis and antigenicity: Implication for epidemiological surveillance in endemic areas. *Transbound. Emerg. Dis.* **2019**, *66*, 2362–2382. [CrossRef]

22. Ji, W.; Niu, D.D.; Si, H.L.; Ding, N.Z.; He, C.Q. Vaccination influences the evolution of classical swine fever virus. *Infect. Genet. Evol.* **2014**, *25*, 69–77. [CrossRef]

23. Yoo, S.J.; Kwon, T.; Kang, K.; Kim, H.; Kang, S.C.; Richt, J.A.; Lyoo, Y.S. Genetic evolution of classical swine fever virus under immune environments conditioned by genotype 1-based modified live virus vaccine. *Transbound. Emerg. Dis.* **2018**, *65*, 735–745. [CrossRef] [PubMed]

24. Chen, N.; Tong, C.; Li, D.; Wan, J.; Yuan, X.; Li, X.; Peng, J.; Fang, W. Antigenic analysis of classical swine fever virus E2 glycoprotein using pig antibodies identifies residues contributing to antigenic variation of the vaccine C-strain and group 2 strains circulating in China. *Virol. J.* **2010**, *7*, 378. [CrossRef] [PubMed]

25. Oleksiewicz, M.B.; Rasmussen, T.B.; Normann, P.; Uttenthal, Å. Determination of the sequence of the complete open reading frame and the 5'NTR of the Paderborn isolate of classical swine fever virus. *Vet. Microbiol.* **2003**, *92*, 311–325. [CrossRef]

26. Deng, M.C. Molecular Analysis of Classical Swine Fever Viruses in Taiwan and the Development of Rapid Diagnostic Method. Ph.D. Thesis, Department of Veterinary Medicine, National Chung Shing University, Taichung, Taiwan, 2008.

27. Muñoz-González, S.; Pérez-Simó, M.; Colom-Cadena, A.; Cabezón, O.; Bohórquez, J.A.; Rosell, R.; Pérez, L.J.; Marco, I.; Lavín, S.; Domingo, M.; et al. Classical swine fever virus vs. classical swine fever virus: The superinfection exclusion phenomenon in experimentally infected wild boar. *PLoS ONE* **2016**, *11*, e0149469. [CrossRef] [PubMed]

28. Edwards, S.; Moennig, V.; Wensvoort, G. The development of an international reference panel of monoclonal antibodies for the differentiation of hog cholera virus from other pestiviruses. *Vet. Microbiol.* **1991**, *29*, 101–108. [CrossRef]

29. Mittelholzer, C.; Moser, C.; Tratschin, J.D.; Hofmann, M.A. Analysis of classical swine fever virus replication kinetics allows differentiation of highly virulent from avirulent strains. *Vet. Microbiol.* **2000**, *74*, 293–308. [CrossRef]

30. Reed, L.J.; Muench, H.A. A simple method of estimating fifty percent endpoints. *Am. J. Epidemiol.* **1938**, *27*, 493–497. [CrossRef]

31. Huang, Y.L.; Pang, V.F.; Pan, C.H.; Chen, T.H.; Jong, M.H.; Huang, T.S.; Jeng, C.R. Development of a reverse transcription multiplex real-time PCR for the detection and genotyping of classical swine fever virus. *J. Virol. Methods* **2009**, *160*, 111–118. [CrossRef]

8

Dynamics of Classical Swine Fever Spread in Wild Boar in 2018–2019, Japan

Norikazu Isoda [1,2,†], Kairi Baba [3,†], Satoshi Ito [1], Mitsugi Ito [4], Yoshihiro Sakoda [2,5] and Kohei Makita [3,*]

[1] Unit of Risk Analysis and Management, Research Center for Zoonosis Control, Hokkaido University, Kita 20, Nishi 10, Kita-Ku, Sapporo 001-0020, Japan; isoda@czc.hokudai.ac.jp (N.I.); satoshi125@czc.hokudai.ac.jp (S.I.)

[2] Global Station for Zoonosis Control, Global Institute for Collaborative Research and Education (GI-CoRE), Hokkaido University, Sapporo 001-0020, Japan; sakoda@vetmed.hokudai.ac.jp

[3] Veterinary Epidemiology Unit, School of Veterinary Medicine, Rakuno Gakuen University, 582, Bunkyodai Midorimachi, Ebetsu 069-8501, Japan; s21561088@stu.rakuno.ac.jp

[4] Akabane Animal Clinic, Co. Ltd., 55 Ishizoe, Akabane-Cho, Tahara 441-3502, Japan; m-ito@oasis.ocn.ne.jp

[5] Laboratory of Microbiology, Department of Disease Control, Faculty of Veterinary Medicine, Hokkaido University, Kita 18, Nishi 9, Kita-Ku, Sapporo 060-0818, Japan

* Correspondence: kmakita@rakuno.ac.jp

† Co-first author.

Abstract: The prolongation of the classic swine fever (CSF) outbreak in Japan in 2018 was highly associated with the persistence and widespread of the CSF virus (CSFV) in the wild boar population. To investigate the dynamics of the CSF outbreak in wild boar, spatiotemporal analyses were performed. The positive rate of CSFV in wild boar fluctuated dramatically from March to June 2019, but finally stabilized at approximately 10%. The Euclidean distance from the initial CSF notified farm to the farthest infected wild boar of the day constantly increased over time since the initial outbreak except in the cases reported from Gunma and Saitama prefectures. The two-month-period prevalence, estimated using integrated nested Laplace approximation, reached >80% in half of the infected areas in March–April 2019. The area affected continued to expand despite the period prevalence decreasing up to October 2019. A large difference in the shapes of standard deviational ellipses and in the location of their centroids when including or excluding cases in Gunma and Saitama prefectures indicates that infections there were unlikely to have been caused simply by wild boar activities, and anthropogenic factors were likely involved. The emergence of concurrent space–time clusters in these areas after July 2019 indicated that CSF outbreaks were scattered by this point in time. The results of this epidemiological analysis help explain the dynamics of the spread of CSF and will aid in the implementation of control measures, including bait vaccination.

Keywords: classical swine fever; Japan; space–time analysis; wild boar

---

1. Introduction

Classical swine fever (CSF) is a highly contagious disease causing a multisystemic infection in domestic and wild pigs. CSF is distributed worldwide and causes enormous economic losses in husbandry due to its high virulence in domestic pigs [1]. The causative agent of CSF is the CSF virus (CSFV), which belongs to the genus *Pestivirus* and the family *Flaviviridae*. CSFV exhibits a variety of disease modes in host animals with infections that may be acute, subacute, chronic, late-onset, or asymptomatic. It is known that disease severity depends on the virulence of the CSFV, age and species of a host animal, and status of individual or herd immunity. CSFVs with moderate virulence have recently been isolated in Mongolia and China [2,3].

Japan once achieved the elimination of CSF through the application of the attenuated CSFV vaccine [4]. Since 1992, no notifications of CSF had been reported, and Japan was designated as a CSF-free country by the World Organisation for Animal Health (OIE) in 2007 [4]. However, in September 2018, CSF reemerged in Gifu Prefecture, and despite strenuous control efforts, the outbreak was not successfully contained. Detection and culling and movement restriction, which are all basic control measures for CSF outbreaks in domestic pigs, were implemented. However, due to the wider spread of the disease, the government decided to apply preventive vaccination in domestic pigs in the affected prefectures in October 2019 to inhibit further CSF spread.

The current CSF outbreaks were indicated to be driven by the circulation of a CSFV with a moderate pathogenicity that most closely matched in identity in two regions of CSFVs recently isolated in China and Mongolia, thereby further complicating the outbreak situation [4,5]. A high proportion of dead wild boars found in the affected areas were positive for CSFV infection, even in the early phase of the current CSF outbreak [6]. For this reason, prefectural offices in and around the affected area decided to implement an intensive program to capture wild boar for CSFV testing and to erect fencing to control wild boar movements. Moreover, due to the further spread of CSF from the prefectures affected, the Japanese government decided to apply oral bait vaccination in selected areas of the affected prefectures in three seasons of 2019. The initial batch of bait was disseminated twice between March and May 2019 in two prefectures (Aichi and Gifu). The second batch of bait was disseminated twice (in most prefectures) between July and September 2019 in nine prefectures (Gifu, Aichi, Mie, Fukui, Nagano, Toyama, Ishikawa, Shizuoka, and Shiga). Despite the control measures targeting wild boar, the trend of CSF infection was not terminated. As of the end of November 2019, there were 50 CSF outbreaks in pig farms, leading to the death of approximately 120,000 animals in seven prefectures, along with 1470 cases in wild boar in 12 prefectures [6,7].

One year after the initial CSF notification, the lack of success in controlling the outbreak is concerning. To provide another perspective that could be of assistance, we investigated the dynamics of CSF spread in wild boar by analyzing the transmission pattern of CSFV in wild boar temporally and spatially. The identification of CSF cases which were unlikely to have been transmitted via wild boar would suggest important opportunities for biosecurity measures in farms and a disease containment strategy.

2. Results

2.1. Temporal Trend of CSF Cases in Wild Boar

From September 2018 to the middle of November 2019, a total of 6,594 wild boars, including 826 dead and 5768 captured animals were tested for CSF infection (Figure 1). After the utilization of bait vaccination, no wild boars positive for a CSFV strain used for the oral vaccine were reported. During the early phase of the CSF outbreak, from the initial notification to the end of 2018, in which cases were limited in two prefectures, the positive rates ranged mostly between 10% and 20%. The fluctuation was larger in the first half of 2019 and, especially between March and June 2019, the ratio increased to between 40% and 60%. However, as the number of tested animals increased, the CSFV-positive rates decreased gradually to approximately 10% in the second half of 2019.

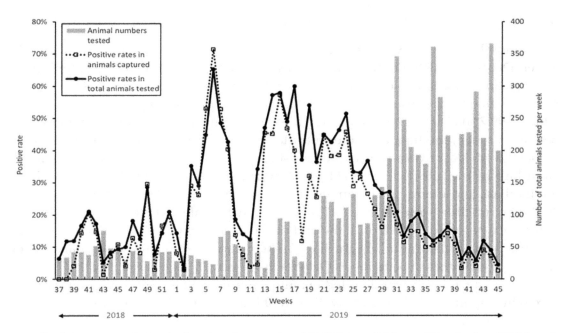

Figure 1. Positive rates of classical swine fever virus (CSFV) in wild boar. Results for CSFV antigen detection in wild boar in 12 prefectures were combined. Solid line: CSFV-positive rates in total animals tested in each week. Dashed line: CSFV-positive rates in animals captured in each week. Bar chart: The number of dead and captured wild boars tested in each week.

2.2. Distance of CSF Cases in Wild Boar from the Initial Outbreak Point

In general, the direct distance between the locations of the initial CSF notification and cases in wild boar increased proportionally with time (Figure 2). However, many of the notifications reported in the second half of 2019 did not correspond with the general trend, with those from Saitama and Gunma prefectures in particular appearing unexpectedly distant from the initial location in a rather short time.

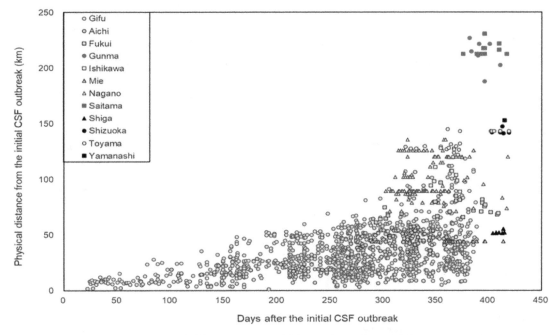

Figure 2. Distances of CSF cases in wild boar from the initial case over time.

For each case of CSF notified in wild boar, the distance from the initial CSF case and time since the initial case was plotted.

2.3. Spatial Change of CSF Period Prevalence Over Time

The two-month-period prevalence showed the first peak around the area of the initial farm case in November–December 2018 (Figure 3A). The mean period prevalence in 10 infected municipalities was 32.5% (median = 21.2%, 95% credible interval: CI of median posterior = 9.0%–42.0%), and distinct high period-prevalence was observed in two municipalities: 90.0% (95% CI: 68.0%–99.7%) and 81.6% (95% CI: 40.7%–99.7%). The expanded infected areas (19 municipalities) had moderate homogeneous prevalence, with mean, median, and interquartile ranges of period-prevalence estimates at 44.0%, 45.0%, and 44.9%–45.1%, respectively, in January–February 2019 (Figure 3B). The prevalence reached over 80% in half of the infected areas (11 of 22 municipalities) in March–April 2019 (Figure 3C). The mean, median, and interquartile ranges of the estimates were 73.7%, 79.3%, and 59.0%–88.4%, and the 95% CI of median posterior was 52.7%–95.5%. As the infected areas continued to expand, the period prevalence began to reduce until the end of the period of observation in September–October 2019 (72 municipalities maximum, Figure 3D–F). The mean, median, and interquartile ranges of the period prevalence estimates in September–October 2019 were 27.4%, 24.8%, and 15.7%–35.4%. In this period, the disease in wild boar was detected in remote municipalities (not contiguous with the existing infected area) in Saitama and Gunma, as well as in Shizuoka prefecture (Figure 3F).

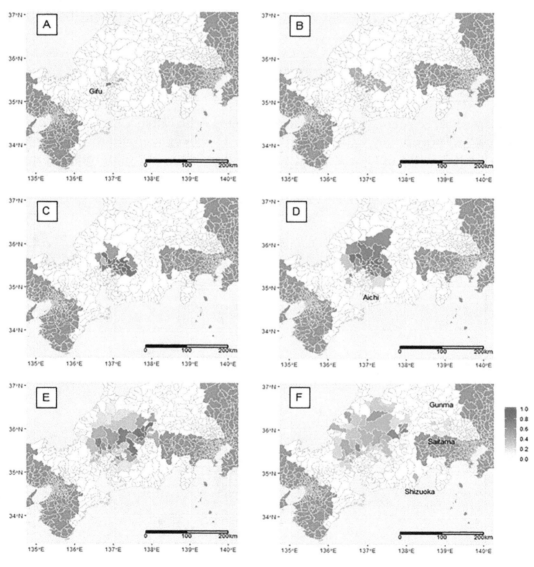

Figure 3. Spatial change of two-month-period prevalence of CSF in wild boar.

The intensity of the red color indicates the estimated two-month-prevalence of CSF in wild boar at the municipality level, with an intensity of 1.0 indicating a prevalence of 100%. A: November–December 2018, B: January–February 2019, C: March–April 2019, D: May–June 2019, E: July–August 2019, F: September–October 2019.

2.4. Standard Deviational Ellipse Analysis

Standard deviational ellipses (SDEs) for the three phases were overlaid on a map with CSF-positive notifications to illustrate the directional trends and dispersion of CSF notifications (Figure 4). The position of the centroids of the ellipses in the two early phases did not differ on the map, whereas the centroid of the third ellipse was positioned approximately 100 km away from the other two and toward the northeast. The forms of the ellipses for the second and third periods, excluding disease notifications in Gunma and Saitama prefectures, differed from those that included these notifications. The centroids of the ellipses for the second and third periods, excluding the notifications in the two eastern provinces, were located relatively close to the centroid for the first period.

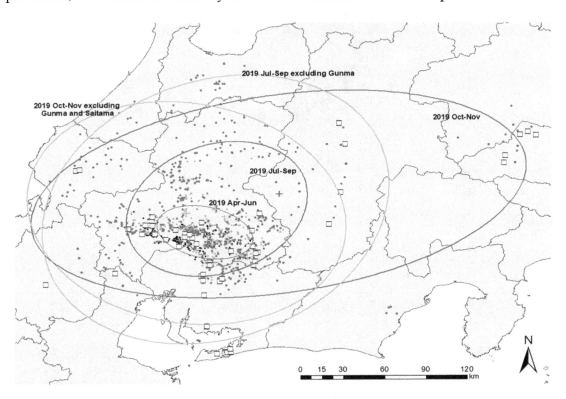

Figure 4. Spatiotemporal distribution of classical swine fever notifications from April to November 2019.

Standard deviational ellipses for three time periods (April–June 2019, July–September 2019, October–November 2019). Ellipses and their centroids (green and pink plus signs) were overlaid with CSF notifications distinguishing domestic pig (white square) and wild boar (dot) cases. Black dot: CSF notification of wild boar in September 2018–March 2019, green dot: April–June 2019, blue dot: July–September 2019, red dot: October–November 2019. For the last two periods, standard deviational ellipses that exclude the notification data in Gunma and Saitama prefectures are shown.

2.5. Space–Time Cluster Analysis

A total of 13 significant space–time clusters were identified from the CSF notification dataset by space–time permutation analysis based on the 26-km upper limit on cluster size set in the software (Figure 5). Clusters 1 and 2 equate to the periods September 2018 to February 2019 and February to June 2019, respectively, and their timings did not overlap (Table 1). However, after June 2019, several clusters appeared concurrently in different areas with the disease scattered widely, including in the two eastern provinces. Compared to Cluster 1, the radii of the clusters identified after June 2019 were greater but the durations were shorter, indicating that the disease was being disseminated rapidly and widely even within the cluster areas. The habitats of each of the 13 clusters were visually assessed with the guide of Global Map Specifications [8]. Most of the areas in the clusters comprised several types of forests and croplands.

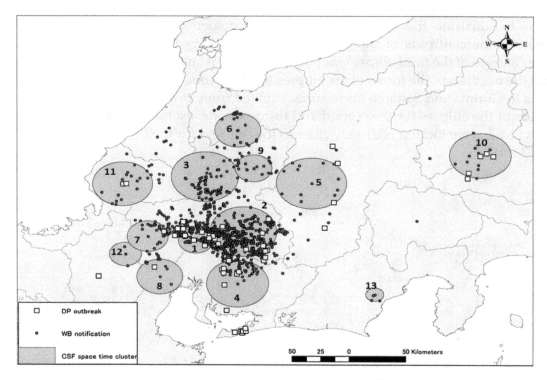

Figure 5. Locations of the significant space–time clusters of CSF.

Table 1. Details of each space-time cluster detected ($p < 0.05$) in CSF notification.

Cluster	Duration (Days)	Start Date	End Date	Radius (km)	Main Land Covers *
1	148	2018/9/9	2019/2/4	12.53	Closed shrublands, Cropland/Natural vegetation mosaic
2	132	2019/2/12	2019/6/24	24.41	Mixed forest
3	69	2019/6/25	2019/9/2	24.33	Mixed forest, Deciduous broadleaf forest, Cropland/Natural vegetation mosaic
4	48	2019/7/2	2019/8/19	22.88	Mixed forest, Deciduous broadleaf forest
5	48	2019/7/16	2019/9/2	24.89	Cropland/Natural vegetation mosaic, Mixed forest
6	13	2019/9/3	2019/9/16	16.59	Deciduous broadleaf forest
7	27	2019/9/3	2019/9/30	15.11	Mixed forest, Deciduous broadleaf forest
8	55	2019/9/3	2019/10/28	16.99	Closed shrublands, Mixed forest, Croplands
9	20	2019/9/3	2019/9/23	13.30	Cropland/Natural vegetation mosaic, Mixed forest
10	41	2019/10/1	2019/11/11	21.87	Closed shrublands, Croplands, Mixed forest
11	27	2019/10/1	2019/10/28	21.46	Croplands, Deciduous broadleaf forest
12	20	2019/10/15	2019/11/4	11.61	Water bodies, Croplands, Mixed forest
13	20	2019/10/15	2019/11/4	6.52	Mixed forest

*: Types of main land covers in the cluster were visually assessed with Global Map Version 1.2.1 Specifications [8] and sorted in descending order of types.

During the study period, from September 2018 to November 2019, 13 significant clusters were observed in or around the disease notification area. Detailed information for each cluster is given in

Table 1. Yellow squares indicate the locations of CSF-positive farms. Red circles indicate the locations of CSFV-positive wild boar either captured or found dead.

3. Discussion

At the time of writing, November 2019, more than one year has passed since the initial CSF notification in September 2018, and the outbreak has still not been terminated. In this period, 46 CSF outbreaks in pig farms were reported with approximately 120,000 killed animals, but the wild boar population was considered to play a critical role in the spread of the disease. Disease notifications were concentrated at locations near the initial cases in the early phase of the current outbreaks and then became more widespread over time. The results from the present study indicate that the disease could have spread via the movement of wild boar to nearby contiguous areas was confirmed from spring 2019 onward through spatial changes in period prevalence. The risk of CSFV infection at a farm located at a 5-km distance from a CSFV-positive wild boar within 28 days was estimated at more than 5% in Hayama et al. [9]. It is noteworthy that the disease became dispersed to remote municipalities in Gunma and Saitama prefectures (areas that were not contiguous with the main outbreak), which was unexpected given the occurrence and spread patterns of CSFV in wild boar. In the SDE analysis, this unexpected dispersion of CSFV to two distant prefectures was demonstrated by a shift in the centroids and shape distortion of the ellipses between October and November 2019. In the Gunma and Saitama area, the first CSFV infection was confirmed in a pig farm before the detection of CSF cases in wild boar. Given the epidemiological situation, as well as the results of the epidemiological analysis in the present study, it seems likely that CSF jumped to Gunma and Saitama prefectures by factors other than transmission by wild boar without being detected. The phylogenetic analysis also supports that the CSFVs isolated in the current outbreak indicated that the CSFV isolated in the first farm in Saitama prefecture was most close to the strain isolated in Aichi prefecture, which was adjacent to neither the Gunma nor Saitama prefecture [6]. At this time, no epidemiological relevance between the CSF positive farms in these two prefectures and ones in other prefectures, including the introduction of potentially infected pigs, have been revealed. The spontaneous introduction of infectious pathogens by the movement of fomites, including humans and vehicles from the high-risk areas, might be a possible pathway of the CSF jump. Though the details will be revealed in the further epidemiological investigation, these would be associated with poor biosecurity measures in farms to introduce the contagious pathogens, or with low compliance in wild boar trapping to acquire the pathogens. Poor biosecurity measures in farms, including imperfect change of clothes and shoes and incomplete disinfection, as well as imperfect installation of fencing with large mesh that allow small animals passing, could also contribute to the introduction of the pathogen agent inside the farm. Furthermore, when wild boars are trapped for sample collection for laboratory diagnosis, adequate hygienic sampling and animal transportation, as well as intensive disinfection of clothes, equipment, and environment around the captured animal, are critical to minimize the level of contamination of the environment in order to prevent secondary infections in wild boar during capturing activities. Biosecurity measures in farms and wildlife management activities against CSFV should be reviewed to prevent careless facilitation of transmissions in both and between domestic pig and wild boar populations.

Since the 1990s, wild boar has been recognized as an important reservoir of CSFV due to a change in pathogenicity from high to moderate virulence in wild boar as well as domestic pigs. Transmission routes of CSFV are comparable in wild boar and domestic pigs, and occur either through direct contact between diseased animals or indirectly via feces, food, and carcasses [10]. During the 1993–1998 CSF outbreak in Germany, an indirect transmission of CSFV to domestic pigs from wild boar was indicated [11]. The infection of wild boar with moderately virulent CSFV enables a more effective transmission to other animals, and once a CSFV with moderate virulence crosses into the wild boar population, the disease becomes prevalent and persistent among unmonitored populations. It was also reported that CSFV tended to persist and become endemic for years in larger wildlife populations [12]. As population size and density are considered crucial factors for CSFV survival in wild boar populations [13], much effort has been focused toward population management, including hunting and trapping. However, it has also been demonstrated that a depopulation strategy is not effective for CSF control in wildlife because of the low probability of achieving depopulation to the desired low level, high uncertainty in the estimation of the number of wild boar, and low acceptability for depopulation among hunters [14]. Furthermore, hunting has been reported to play a negative role in CSF control in wild boar because excessive hunting pressure might increase population turnover, enabling the maintenance of pathogens among younger naïve animals and causing population mixing, leading to more frequent contact among animals. Delivery of bait vaccines has been considered effective as a control measure to limit CSF spread in wildlife by decreasing the proportion of susceptible animals. Although prophylactic vaccination is banned in Europe, the application of preventive vaccination is allowed in domestic pigs and wild boar if the spread of disease appears to be uncontrollable [10]. Bait vaccines for wild boar were employed during CSF outbreaks in Germany and France [15,16]. The estimations of the ideal vaccination rate in wild boar for the control of CSF were reported as 41% using a deterministic model, or from 9% to 52% using a stochastic model based on an outbreak of CSF in Pakistan [17,18].

Bait vaccination with the commercial vaccine (Pestiporc, Oral, IDT Biologika GmbH, Dessau-Rosslau, Germany) for wild boar was utilized twice between March and May 2019 in selected areas in Aichi and Gifu prefectures where CSF positive cases were found [19]. Oral vaccination of wild boar is an effective tool to decrease the number of susceptible animals against CSFV in the affected area with relatively low costs. Oral mass vaccination of wild boar against CSF has been conducted since the late 1990s in some European countries [14]. Thirty or forty baits each were delivered at 660 (in March) and 1,011 (April to May) locations, respectively, in these two prefectures. The overall bait collection rate after five days was 41.4%, and wild boar bite-mark traces were observed in approximately 25% of the remaining collected baits. On this basis, it was estimated that the intake rate of bait vaccine in the wild boar population was, at maximum, approximately 70%. The positive rate for CSFV antibodies increased from 50% before baiting to 70% after baiting within the vaccinated area in Aichi prefecture and from 40% to 62% in Gifu prefecture. However, care needs to be taken for a comparative interpretation of the effectiveness of the vaccination in two prefectures due to differences in the diagnosis and sampling methods (personal communication). The results of the spatial change of CSF period prevalence in wild boar in May–June 2019 when there was an expansion in the area of CSFV-positive wild boar demonstrated that the oral vaccination program was not able to prevent the spread of CSF, but worked on reducing prevalence in heavily affected areas. According to the results of the present study, CSFV might have been circulating at the early phase of the outbreak (from the initial case to April 2019) among wild boar in a limited area (Figure 3). From January to April 2019, the disease did not spread to a wider area, but was transmitted to more sensitive animals inside the existing area, resulting in CSFV infection of over 80% of the wild boar. Because the movement of wild boar is restricted mainly by snowfall in winter, and most Japanese wild boar (*Sus scrofa leucomystax*) breed piglet in April-June, especially in May, it would have been necessary to complete bait vaccination in the affected areas no later than May 2019 when the CSFV spread further by the movement of the wild boar [20–22]. In addition, comprehensive guideline for the vaccination of wild boar against CSFV at a national level, describing the methods of sample size calculation, sampling, and diagnosis for the evaluation, should be established. Since decreasing the sensitive wild boar to prevalent CSFV is so critical to achieving the containment of a CSF outbreak in domestic pigs, the development of an effective vaccination strategy for wildlife with practical and effective guidelines and adequate implementation should be highly prioritized. The sampling and diagnostic strategies for CSFV detection in wild boar are currently varied among prefectures. The lack of unified comprehensive guideline might also influence the interpretation of the results of CSFV detection from wild boar, like the cases in the Shizuoka prefecture. Though in Figure 5, all the CSF cases in wild boar in Shizuoka prefectures were geographically isolated and clustered, it seems likely that the CSF was transmitted to the Shizuoka prefecture by wild boar.

This is because, in Figure 1, the CSF cases in wild boar in Shizuoka prefecture mostly corresponded with the associations between the direct distance from the location of the initial CSF notification and cases in wild boar. Sampling and diagnostic bias would conceal the dynamics of disease spread by expressing "non-positive" results.

4. Conclusions

CSFV infection in domestic pigs was continuously notified in Japan since September 2018 and spread more widely mainly through wild boar movement. The implementation of effective control measures in wildlife, such as bait vaccination under a well-planned strategy and the involvement of a surveillance program using hunting or a capture scheme, is essential for successful containment. Though biosecurity measures were strengthened at pig farms to prevent CSF introduction, unexpected outbreaks occurred in pig farms in areas where the wild boar were unlikely to have been infected with CSFV. The current control measures both for domestic pigs and wild boar should be intensively reviewed.

5. Materials and Methods

5.1. Data and Data Sources

Epidemiological data of CSF notification and reverse transcription polymerase chain reaction (RT-PCR) test results of CSFV detection in domestic pigs and wild boar between September 9, 2018, and November 15, 2019, were collected from the websites of 15 prefectures. In Japan, the RT-PCR based on the Vilcek et al., using a positive control of the attenuated CSFV strain GPE$^-$, is performed in Livestock Hygiene Service Centers under the direction of the National Institute of Animal Hygiene as one of the diagnostics of CSFV detection [23,24]. The coordinates (latitude and longitude) of the CSF notifications were obtained from the website of the OIE [7]. A total of 1418 CSF notifications, 48 outbreaks on domestic pig farms, and 1370 cases in wild boar were confirmed during this period [7], as well as 5324 wild boars that were negative for CSFV infection. As we focused on the local spread of CSFV, notifications of CSF by slaughtering or in facilities through which CSF-affected pigs had been transported were not included in the present study.

5.2. Temporal Trend and Linear Distance of CSF Cases in Wild Boar from the Initial Case

The dates and locations of CSFV detection from both dead-found and captured wild boars were used to investigate the relationship between the time elapsed and distance from the location of the initial CSF notification in the domestic pig farm to each of the CSF cases in wild boar. The dates and locations of wild boars tested for CSFV, including those produced negative results, were used for the calculation of weekly positive rates of CSFV among both dead-found and captured animals, and among only captured animals, respectively, to describe the temporal trend of CSF positive rates in wild boar in expanding infected areas.

5.3. Description of Spatial Change of CSF Prevalence Over Time

Two-month-period wild boar diagnostic positive and negative results based on PCR tests were aggregated at the municipality level for the period between September 2018 and October 2019, and the period prevalence in each administrative unit was estimated using an integrated nested Laplace approximation (INLA) with zero-inflated binomial errors using the package R-INLA in the statistics software R version 3.6.1 (R Core Team, 2019) [25]. Intrinsic conditional autoregression (CAR) was selected to deal with spatial autocorrelation, based on the lowest value of deviance information criteria among the latent models in R-INLA.

5.4. SDE Analysis

SDE analysis was performed to describe the trend and spatial characteristics of CSF notifications in the study area using ArcGIS v10.6.1 software (ESRI Inc., Redlands, CA, USA). This provided the orientation and shape of a distribution, and dispersion of the diseases in domestic pigs and wild boar, following an approach similar to those in previous studies [5,26,27]. The ratio of the long and short ellipse axes was used to identify the degree of clustering or dispersion. To analyze the temporal changes in CSF notifications since July 2019, the study period was divided into three phases: (i) April to June 2019, (ii) July to September 2019, and (iii) October to November 2019.

5.5. Multi-Distance Spatial Cluster Analysis and Space–Time Cluster Analysis

A multi-distance spatial cluster analysis tool in ArcGIS v10.6.1 was used to identify the maximum distance of the relationships between CSF notifications by applying the common transformation of Ripley's *K* function. Detailed information on the method for calculating the maximum distance of relationships, which yielded the highest Diff *K* value, was described in a previous study [5]. A space–time permutation technique was applied to examine the presence of space–time clusters in the area affected by CSF. The upper limit on the geographical size of the cluster was set to 26 km, the minimum time aggregation to seven days, and the maximum temporal cluster size to 50% of the total study period (default setting) [28]. A Monte Carlo process was implemented using 999 replications to test for the presence of candidate clusters ($p < 0.05$). Analyses were conducted in SaTScan software v9.6 (Kulldorff, Boston, MA, USA) [29]. The habitat of each cluster was visually assessed with the guide of Global Map Specifications to assess the pattern of land cover in the cluster identified [8].

Author Contributions: Conceptualization, N.I., M.I., Y.S., and K.M.; Methodology, N.I., S.I., and K.M.; Validation, Y.S., and K.M.; Formal Analysis, K.B. and S.I.; Data Curation, N.I., K.B., S.I., M.I., and K.M.; Writing—Original Draft Preparation, N.I. and K.B.; Writing—Review and Editing, M.I., Y.S., and K.M.; Supervision, K.M. All authors have read and agree to the published version of the manuscript.

References

1. Edwards, S.; Fukusho, A.; Lefevre, P.C.; Lipowski, A.; Pejsak, Z.; Roehe, P.; Westergaard, J. Classical swine fever: The global situation. *Vet. Microbiol.* **2000**, *73*, 103–119. [CrossRef]
2. Enkhbold, B.; Shatar, M.; Wakamori, S.; Tamura, T.; Hiono, T.; Matsuno, K.; Okamatsu, M.; Umemura, T.; Damdinjav, B.; Sakoda, Y. Genetic and virulence characterization of classical swine fever viruses isolated in Mongolia from 2007 to 2015. *Virus Genes* **2017**, *53*, 418–425. [CrossRef] [PubMed]
3. Luo, Y.; Ji, S.; Liu, Y.; Lei, J.L.; Xia, S.L.; Wang, Y.; Du, M.L.; Shao, L.; Meng, X.Y.; Zhou, M.; et al. Isolation and Characterization of a Moderately Virulent Classical Swine Fever Virus Emerging in China. *Transbound. Emerg. Dis.* **2017**, *64*, 1848–1857. [CrossRef] [PubMed]
4. Kameyama, K.I.; Nishi, T.; Yamada, M.; Masujin, K.; Morioka, K.; Kokuho, T.; Fukai, K. Experimental infection of pigs with a classical swine fever virus isolated in Japan for the first time in 26 years. *J. Vet. Med. Sci.* **2019**. [CrossRef] [PubMed]
5. Ito, S.; Jurado, C.; Bosch, J.; Ito, M.; Sanchez-Vizcaino, J.M.; Isoda, N.; Sakoda, A.Y. Role of Wild Boar in the Spread of Classical Swine Fever in Japan. *Pathogens* **2019**, *8*, 206. [CrossRef]
6. Ministry of Agriculture, Forestry and Fisheries, Japan (MAFF). Update of Classical Swine Fever in Japan. Available online: http://www.maff.go.jp/j/syouan/douei/csf/index.html (accessed on 10 February 2020).
7. OIE. World Animal Health Information System. Available online: http://www.oie.int/wahis_2/public/wahid.php/Diseaseinformation/Diseasetimelines (accessed on 10 February 2020).
8. International Steering Committee for Global Mapping. Global Map Version 1.2.1. Specifications. Available online: https://www.geospatial.jp/ckan/dataset/a5424d4b-dba5-4e68-83c3-0a6c29faf734/resource/a8f375d5-ed82-4fca-b77d-19205a972960/download/1.x.pdf (accessed on 10 February 2020).
9. Hayama, Y.; Shimizu, Y.; Murato, Y.; Sawai, K.; Yamamoto, T. Estimation of infection risk on pig farms in infected wild boar areas-Epidemiological analysis for the reemergence of classical swine fever in Japan in 2018. *Prev. Vet. Med.* **2019**, *175*, 104873. [CrossRef] [PubMed]
10. Moennig, V. The control of classical swine fever in wild boar. *Front. Microbiol.* **2015**, *6*, 1211. [CrossRef]

11. Fritzemeier, J.; Teuffert, J.; Greiser-Wilke, I.; Staubach, C.; Schluter, H.; Moennig, V. Epidemiology of classical swine fever in Germany in the 1990s. *Vet. Microbiol.* **2000**, *77*, 29–41. [CrossRef]

12. Rossi, S.; Fromont, E.; Pontier, D.; Cruciere, C.; Hars, J.; Barrat, J.; Pacholek, X.; Artois, M. Incidence and persistence of classical swine fever in free-ranging wild boar (Sus scrofa). *Epidemiol. Infect.* **2005**, *133*, 559–568. [CrossRef]

13. Artois, M.; Depner, K.R.; Guberti, V.; Hars, J.; Rossi, S.; Rutili, D. Classical swine fever (hog cholera) in wild boar in Europe. *Revue Scientifique et Technique* **2002**, *21*, 287–303. [CrossRef]

14. Rossi, S.; Staubach, C.; Blome, S.; Guberti, V.; Thulke, H.H.; Vos, A.; Koenen, F.; Le Potier, M.F. Controlling of CSFV in European wild boar using oral vaccination: A review. *Front. Microbiol.* **2015**, *6*, 1141. [CrossRef]

15. Kaden, V.; Lange, E.; Fischer, U.; Strebelow, G. Oral immunisation of wild boar against classical swine fever: Evaluation of the first field study in Germany. *Vet. Microbiol.* **2000**, *73*, 239–252. [CrossRef]

16. Rossi, S.; Pol, F.; Forot, B.; Masse-Provin, N.; Rigaux, S.; Bronner, A.; Le Potier, M.F. Preventive vaccination contributes to control classical swine fever in wild boar (Sus scrofa sp.). *Vet. Microbiol.* **2010**, *142*, 99–107. [CrossRef] [PubMed]

17. Hone, J.; Pech, R.; Yip, P. Estimation of the dynamics and rate of transmission of classical swine fever (hog cholera) in wild pigs. *Epidemiol. Infect.* **1992**, *108*, 377–386. [CrossRef] [PubMed]

18. Inayatullah, C. *Wild boar in West Pakistan*; Pakistan Forest Institute, Peshawar, Division of Forestry Research, Wildlife Management Branch: Peshawar, Pakistan, 1973; 17p.

19. Ministry of Agriculture, Forestry and Fisheries, Japan (MAFF). Summary of 1st Meeting of Oral Vaccination to Classical Swine Fever (In Japanese). Available online: http://www.maff.go.jp/j/syouan/douei/csf/attach/pdf/domestic-26.pdf. (accessed on 10 February 2020).

20. Takao, Y. Wild Boars and the Protection of Farm Crops at the Foot of Mt. Hakusan in Gifu Prefecture, Japan. *Res. Rep. Hakusan Nat. Conserv. Cent. Ishikawa* **1997**, *24*, 57–66. (In Japanese)

21. Mauget, R. *Seasonality of Reproduction in the Wild Boar*; Butterworth Scientific: London, UK, 1982; pp. 509–526.

22. Kodera, Y.; Takeda, T.; Tomaru, S.; Sugita, S. The estimation of birth periods in wild boar by detailed aging. *Mamm. Sci.* **2012**, *52*, 185–191. (In Japanese)

23. Shimizu, Y.; Furuuchi, S.; Kumagai, T.; Sasahara, J. A mutant of hog cholera virus inducing interference in swine testicle cell cultures. *Am. J. Vet. Res.* **1970**, *31*, 1787–1794.

24. Vilcek, S.; Herring, A.J.; Herring, J.A.; Nettleton, P.F.; Lowings, J.P.; Paton, D.J. Pestiviruses isolated from pigs, cattle and sheep can be allocated into at least three genogroups using polymerase chain reaction and restriction endonuclease analysis. *Arch. Virol.* **1994**, *136*, 309–323. [CrossRef]

25. Bivand, R.S.; Gomez-Rubio, V.; Rue, H. Spatial Data Analysis with R-INLA with Some Extensions. *J. Stat. Softw.* **2015**, *63*, 1–31. [CrossRef]

26. Fonseca, O.; Coronado, L.; Amaran, L.; Perera, C.L.; Centelles, Y.; Montano, D.N.; Alfonso, P.; Fernandex, O.; Santoro, K.R.; Frias-Lepoureau, M.T.; et al. Descriptive epidemiology of endemic Classical Swine Fever in Cuba. *Span. J. Agric. Res.* **2018**, *16*, e0508. [CrossRef]

27. Lu, Y.; Deng, X.J.; Chen, J.H.; Wang, J.Y.; Chen, Q.; Niu, B. Risk analysis of African swine fever in Poland based on spatio-temporal pattern and Latin hypercube sampling, 2014–2017. *BMC Vet. Res.* **2019**, *15*, 160. [CrossRef] [PubMed]

28. Iglesias, I.; Rodriguez, A.; Feliziani, F.; Rolesu, S.; de la Torre, A. Spatio-temporal Analysis of African Swine Fever in Sardinia (2012-2014): Trends in Domestic Pigs and Wild Boar. *Transbound. Emerg. Dis.* **2017**, *64*, 656–662. [CrossRef] [PubMed]

29. Kulldorff, M.; Heffernan, R.; Hartman, J.; Assuncao, R.; Mostashari, F. A space-time permutation scan statistic for disease outbreak detection. *PLoS Med.* **2005**, *2*, e59. [CrossRef] [PubMed]

9

Serodynamic Analysis of the Piglets Born from Sows Vaccinated with Modified Live Vaccine or E2 Subunit Vaccine for Classical Swine Fever

Yi-Chia Li [1,2], **Ming-Tang Chiou** [1,2,*] and **Chao-Nan Lin** [1,2,*]

[1]   Animal Disease Diagnostic Center, College of Veterinary Medicine, National Pingtung University of Science and Technology, Pingtung 91201, Taiwan; yichavet@gmail.com

[2]   Department of Veterinary Medicine, College of Veterinary Medicine, National Pingtung University of Science and Technology, Pingtung 91201, Taiwan

*   Correspondence: mtchiou@mail.npust.edu.tw (M.-T.C.); cnlin6@mail.npust.edu.tw (C.-N.L.)

Abstract: Classical swine fever (CSF) caused by the CSF virus (CSFV) is one of the most important swine diseases, resulting in huge economic losses to the pig industry worldwide. Systematic vaccination is one of the most effective strategies for the prevention and control of this disease. Two main CSFV vaccines, the modified live vaccine (MLV) and the subunit E2 vaccine, are recommended. In Taiwan, CSF cases have not been reported since 2006, although systemic vaccination has been practiced for 70 years. Here, we examined the sero-dynamics of the piglets born from sows that received either the CSFV MLV or the E2 vaccine and investigated in the field the correlation between the porcine reproductive and respiratory syndrome virus (PRRSV) loads and levels of CSFV antibody. A total of 1398 serum samples from 42 PRRSV-positive farms were evaluated to determine the PRRSV loads by real-time PCR and to detect CSFV antibody levels by commercial ELISA. Upon comparing the two sow vaccination protocols (CSFV MLV vaccination at 4 weeks post-farrowing versus E2 vaccination at 4–5 weeks pre-farrowing), the lowest levels of CSFV antibody were found in piglets at 5–8 and 9–12 weeks of age for the MLV and E2 groups, respectively. Meanwhile, the appropriate time window for CSFV vaccination of offspring was at 5–8 and 9–12 weeks of age in the MLV and E2 groups, respectively. There was a very highly significant negative correlation between the PRRSV load and the level of CSFV antibody in the CSFV MLV vaccination group ($P < 0.0001$). The PRRSV detection rate in the pigs from the MLV group (27.78%) was significantly higher than that in pigs from the E2 group (21.32%) ($P = 0.011$). In addition, there was a significant difference ($P = 0.019$) in the PRRSV detection rate at 5–8 weeks of age between the MLV (42.15%) and E2 groups (29.79%). Our findings indicate that the vaccination of CSFV MLV in piglets during the PRRSV susceptibility period at 5–8 weeks of age may be overloading the piglet's immune system and should be a critical concern for industrial pork production in the field.

Keywords: classical swine fever; porcine reproductive and respiratory syndrome virus; quantitative PCR; antibody; modified live vaccine; E2 subunit vaccine

1. Introduction

Classical swine fever (CSF) caused by the CSF virus (CSFV) is one of the most important swine diseases, resulting in huge economic losses to the pig industry worldwide, and it is a World Organization for Animal Health (OIE)-listed disease. CSFV (previously called hog cholera virus) belongs to the genus *Pestivirus* within the family *Flaviviridae* together with bovine viral diarrhea virus 1, bovine viral diarrhea virus 2 and border disease virus [1]. Recently, CSFV has been redesignated as *Pestivirus C* [1].

CSF is an immunosuppressive disease in which several immune escape mechanisms of CSFV have been reported, such as apoptosis, autophagy and pyroptosis in bone marrow hematopoietic cells, lymphocytes and lymphoid organs [2]. A low CD4/CD8 ratio has been observed in the peripheral blood mononuclear cells of infected fetuses and piglets challenged with either high- or low-virulence CSFV strains. A low CD4/CD8 ratio indicates dysregulation of the immune response [3]. During CSFV infection, the clinical signs mainly depend on the ages of pigs and the virulence of the viral strains. The clinical forms of CSFV can show acute, chronic and persistent courses. The persistent course usually requires infection of sows at approximately 50–70 days of pregnancy [4–6]. In general, the acute form of CSF leads to clinical and pathological features that are very similar to those of African swine fever [5,6]. In addition, CSF must also be considered in the differential diagnosis of erysipelas, porcine circovirus type 2 (PCV2)-associated diseases (PCVAD), salmonellosis and porcine reproductive and respiratory syndrome (PRRS) [6]. The overlapping of the clinical presentations may lead to a misdiagnosis of CSF as PRRS virus (PRRSV) infection. PRRSV infection also causes reproductive symptoms in gestational sows and respiratory problems in young pigs [7,8]. PRRSV infection can induce several immunosuppressive responses [9], such as: i) dysregulation of NK cell cytotoxic activity [10]; ii) poor production of IFN-alpha [11]; and iii) promotion of the secretion of immunosuppressive cytokines such as interleukin-10 (IL-10) and transforming growth factor-beta [10,12,13].

Systematic vaccination and non-vaccination stamping-out are the two main strategies to control CSF [6,14]. Due to the enormous costs of stamping-out, systematic vaccination is a more effective strategy for CSF control in CSF endemic areas [6]. Two major kinds of CSFV vaccines, the modified live vaccine (MLV) and the subunit vaccine, are widely used in many countries [6,14]. The MLV vaccine can induce not only humoral immune responses but also cell-mediated immune responses against virulent CSFV. Subunit vaccines, such as E2 vaccines, usually only induce antibody responses [14]. However, the disadvantages of CSFV MLV vaccines are that their efficacy is inhibited by maternal-derived antibody (MDA) [14–19] and they lack differentiation with infection from vaccinated animals (DIVA) according to serological assays [16,20]. The CSFV subunit vaccines based on the E2 protein allow DIVA by E^{rns} enzyme-linked immunosorbent assays and provide good protection [21–23]. The drawbacks of E2 subunit marker vaccines are that they induce protection later than MLV vaccines, and their efficacy also interferes with maternal antibodies [21,24].

Transplacental transmission of CSFV occurred before the onset of the antibody response when sows were challenged with either high- or low-virulence CSFV strains. Therefore, rapid and solid immunity after sow vaccination is required for the prevention of congenital viral persistence [3]. In Taiwan, CSFV MLV has been used since the 1950s and proven to be sufficiently protective. CSFV MLV vaccination is only recommended in sows at 4 weeks post-farrowing (nonpregnancy stage) to overcome persistent infection. To avoid MDA, which interferes with the efficacy of CSFV MLV in the clinic, piglets should be vaccinated at 6 and 9 weeks old when sows are vaccinated in the nonpregnancy stage. However, PRRSV is still a major problem and difficult to control in the nursery stage, which overlaps with the CSFV MLV vaccination period in Taiwan. Certain severe PRRS cases in the nursery were observed just after CSFV MLV vaccination (data from the Animal Diseases Diagnostic Center of National Pingtung University of Science and Technology, not shown). The most reasonable explanation for PRRS and porcine respiratory disease complex induction is stress, which would be caused not only by vaccination but also by the side effects of CSFV MLV, pathogens spread by needles, the synergistic effects of bacterial pathogens such as *Glaesserella parasuis* (*G. parasuis*, previously called *Hemophilus parasuis*) and other factors [25]. In contrast, the E2 vaccine is recommended for application in sows at 4–5 weeks pre-farrowing and elicits a high level of neutralizing antibody [26–28], whereas the vaccination of offspring can be delayed until they are 10–12 weeks old [28], which is when most piglets have recovered from PRRS. Therefore, the level of MDA is very important for CSFV vaccination programs in piglets. Previous research findings showed that PRRSV infection prior to CSFV vaccination significantly suppressed the antibody response [29,30]. In addition, CSFV immunization during the acute phase of PRRSV infection could result in vaccination failure [31]. However, the correlation between the CSFV MDA levels produced in response to different types of CSFV vaccines and the PRRSV load in the field remains to be investigated. Herein, this retrospective study aimed to elucidate the sero-dynamics of the CSFV and PRRSV loads in piglets born from sows immunized with different types of CSFV vaccines to further the understanding of the interactions between the CSFV vaccine and the PRRSV, which is still prevalent in most areas of intense pork production in the field.

2. Results

2.1. Levels of CSFV Antibody in Pigs of Different Ages from Sows Immunized with Different Types of CSFV Vaccines

A total of 1398 blood samples from 42 PRRSV-positive commercial herds were included in this study that were obtained from 943 cases (from 29 pig herds) from the MLV group together with 455 cases (from 13 pig herds) from the E2 group. The evaluation of CSFV antibody levels at different ages in pigs revealed that the level of CSFV antibody was very highly significant ($P < 0.001$), higher in the E2 group than in the MLV group when pigs were less than 4 weeks old and 5–8 weeks old (Figure 1). However, the level of CSFV antibody in the MLV group was significantly higher than that in the E2 group at 9–12 weeks of age ($P < 0.01$), but the difference between the two groups was not statistically significant after 13 weeks of age (Figure 1).

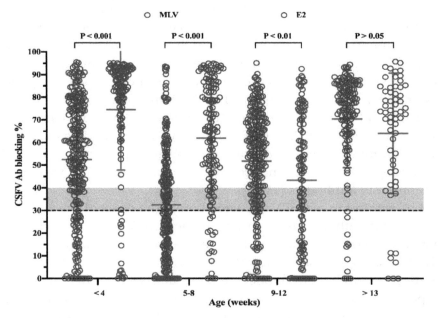

Figure 1. The humoral responses based on ELISA in piglets born in the classical swine fever virus modified live vaccine, (CSFV MLV) and E2 vaccine groups. The results are expressed as blocking %. The dashed line indicates a blocking %, the threshold below which the samples were considered negative. A blocking % between 30 and 40 was interpreted as suspected (gray area). A blocking % greater than or equal to 40 was interpreted as positive. The error bars show the standard deviation (SD). P values < 0.05, < 0.01 and < 0.001 were considered statistically significant, highly significant and very highly significant, respectively.

2.2. Correlation of the PRRSV Load and Level of CSFV MDA in the Piglets without CSFV Vaccination from Different Groups

To examine the correlation of the PRRSV load and level of CSFV MDA in different groups, the PRRSV load of all serum samples was quantitated by real-time polymerase chain reaction (PCR). The presence of PRRSV was calculated only in the piglets without CSFV vaccination. A total of 802 samples fit this criterion. The correlation between the PRRSV load and the level of CSFV antibody in piglets without CSFV vaccination was calculated using a linear regression analysis. The results of MLV group showed that there was a very highly significant negative correlation between the PRRSV load and the level of CSFV antibody ($P < 0.0001$) (Figure 2a). Surprisingly, there was no significant correlation between the PRRSV load and the level of CSFV antibody in piglets from E2 group ($P > 0.05$) (Figure 2b).

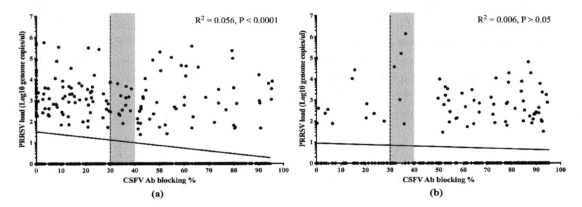

Figure 2. Linear regression analysis was used to calculate the porcine reproductive and respiratory virus (PRRSV) loads and levels of CSFV maternal-derived antibody (MDA) in piglets without CSFV vaccination in the MLV (**a**) and E2 (**b**) groups. The dashed line indicates a blocking %, the threshold below which the samples were considered negative. A blocking % between 30 and 40 was interpreted as suspected (gray area). A blocking % greater than or equal to 40 was interpreted as positive. P values < 0.05, < 0.01 and < 0.001 were considered statistically significant, highly significant and very highly significant, respectively.

2.3. Viral Load and Detection Rate of PRRSV in the Piglets without CSFV Vaccination from Different Groups

In the piglets without CSFV vaccination in different groups, 152 of 517 samples (29.40%) from the MLV group and 72 of the 285 samples (25.26%) from the E2 group were positive for PRRSV. The difference in the detection rate of PRRSV in the piglets without CSFV vaccination between both groups was not statistically significant ($P = 0.24$). However, the PRRSV load was significantly higher (ranging from 1.38 to 5.75 log10 PRRSV genome/μL, median 3.09 log10) in the MLV group than in the E2 group (ranging from 1.46 to 6.15 log10 PRRSV genome/μL, median 2.66 log10) ($P = 0.03$) (Figure 3).

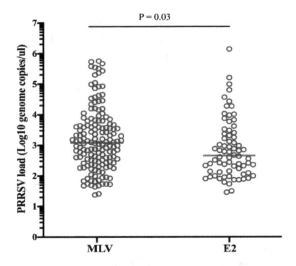

Figure 3. PRRSV loads in the serum samples from both the CSFV MLV and E2 vaccinated groups. The red horizontal lines represent the median concentrations for each group. Unpaired, 2-tailed Student's t-tests were used to compare the PRRSV loads between the MLV and E2 groups. P values < 0.05, < 0.01 and < 0.001 were considered statistically significant, highly significant and very highly significant, respectively.

2.4. Viral Load and Detection Rate of PRRSV in Different Age Groups

The evaluation of the PRRSV load at different ages revealed that the mean PRRSV load was not significantly different for both vaccine types in piglets that were less than 4 weeks old, 5–8 weeks old and 9–12 weeks old (Figure 4). Surprisingly, no PRRSV viremia was found in pigs aged more than 13 weeks in the E2 group (Figure 4 and Table 1). Furthermore, we compared the detection rate of PRRSV at different ages for different types of CSFV vaccines. The details of the detection rate of PRRSV for different types of CSFV vaccines are shown in Table 1. The highest detection rate of PRRSV in pigs was found at 5–8 weeks old (37.81%) compared to that found at other ages (Table 1). At 5–8 weeks old, the detection rate of PRRSV was significantly higher in the pigs from the MLV group (42.15%) compared with that in pigs from the E2 group (29.79%) ($P = 0.019$). The overall detection rate of PRRSV was significantly higher in the pigs from the MLV group than in that in pigs from the E2 group ($P = 0.011$) (Table 1).

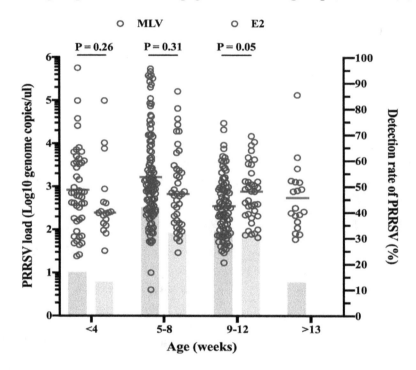

Figure 4. PRRSV loads (dot, left Y axis) and detection rates of PRRSV (bar chart, right Y axis) in serum samples from pigs of different ages from both the CSFV MLV and E2 groups. The dots represent the individual PRRSV load of each pig. The red horizontal lines represent the median concentrations for each group. The bar represents the detection rate of PRRS in pigs of different ages. An unpaired, 2-tailed Student's *t*-test was used to compare the PRRSV loads between the MLV and E2 groups. *P* values < 0.05, < 0.01 and < 0.001 were considered statistically significant, highly significant and very highly significant, respectively.

Table 1. Detection rates of PRRSV in the serum samples from pigs at different ages from both the CSFV MLV and E2 groups.

Age (Weeks)	CSFV Vaccine Type		Total	P Value [†]
	MLV	E2		
<4	47/276 (17.03)	18/135 (13.33)	65/411 (15.82)	0.412
5–8	110/261 (42.15)	42/141 (29.79)	152/402 (37.81)	0.019
9–12	86/261 (32.95)	37/119 (31.09)	123/380 (32.37)	0.081
>13	19/145 (13.10)	0/60 (0)	19/205 (9.27)	N/A *
Total	262/943 (27.78)	97/455 (21.32)	359/1398 (25.68)	0.011

[†] *P* values < 0.05, < 0.01 and < 0.001 were considered statistically significant, highly significant and very highly significant, respectively. * N/A, not applicable; the chi-square calculation does not support cell values that are zero.

3. Discussion

In industrial pork production, multiple viral infections, either in an individual pig or in a herd, with or without bacterial complications have occurred regularly. The systemic application of CSFV MLV further complicates the situation. In order to avoid this background noise, a total of 1398 cases were collected from commercial pig herds for statistical analysis. This study explored the intersectional plane of the interaction between PRRSV and CSFV to shed light on the day-to-day situation in the field.

In areas without CSFV eradication, such as Taiwan, routine vaccination is one of the most effective strategies for the prevention and control of this disease. Two major CSFV vaccines, the MLV and E2 vaccines, are recommended [6,14]. The CSFV MLV vaccine can induce not only humoral immune responses but also cell-mediated immune responses against virulent CSFV [14]. However, several disadvantages of CSFV MLV vaccines have been identified: i) a lack of DIVA according to serological assays [16,20]; ii) the adverse effects of the CSFV MLV vaccine in vaccinated pigs [32,33]; iii) pig-to-pig transmission of MLV [32]; and iv) farm-to-farm transmission of MLV by vehicles [32]. Additionally, the influence of MDA on the efficacy of CSFV MLV in the field has been well discussed [14–19]. Therefore, there is a negative correlation between the levels of MDA and CSFV MLV efficacy [16,17,19]. In Taiwan, CSFV MLV vaccination is only recommended in sows at 4 weeks post-farrowing to overcome persistent infection. Our results showed that the lowest level of CSFV antibody in piglets was found at 5–8 weeks of age in the MLV group (Figure 1), which suggests a time window that may be appropriate for CSFV vaccination. In addition to MDA, several other immunosuppressive viruses, such as PRRSV [29–31], PCV2 [34–36] and pseudorabies virus [37], can potentially interfere with the efficacy of the CSFV MLV vaccine.

The immunosuppression caused by PRRSV is related to IL-10 stimulation and inflammatory cytokine downregulation [10,12,13,30]. It has also been shown that vaccine failure can occur when CSFV MLV vaccine strain replication is inhibited by tumor necrosis factor-alpha induced by PRRSV [30]. Previous studies demonstrated that CSFV MLV immunization during the acute phase of PRRSV infection could suppress the efficacy of CSFV vaccination [29–31]. Thus, the CSFV vaccination time should not overlap with the PRRSV infection period. The efficacy of the CSFV MLV vaccine in the field is worthy of further investigation for the purpose of CSF eradication. According to the diagnostic reports of the Animal Diseases Diagnostic Center of National Pingtung University of Science and Technology, some severe PRRS cases in nursery pigs occurred just after CSFV MLV vaccination (data not shown). In industrial pork production, pigs often have multiple viral infections (e.g., PRRSV + PCV2) together with complicated bacterial infections such as G. parasuis [38]. A study revealed that infection with multiple viruses, such as PRRS and PCV2, may affect the replication or viral activity of the CSFV MLV virus [39]. PCVAD cause multifactorial syndromes that have been be a major problem in Taiwan [40,41]. Fortunately, the problems caused by PCV2 have resolved significantly since the PCV2 vaccine became available in Taiwan [42]. Currently, PRRSV remains a major problem and is difficult to control in the nursery stage, as indicated by the overall detection rate of PRRSV in pigs being the highest at 5–8 weeks of age (37.81%) compared to that at other ages (Table 1). Taken together, it should be further considered that the efficacy of CSFV MLV and stress caused by CSFV MLV vaccination during the PRRSV susceptibility period may induce clinical signs of PRRSV infection.

In the E2 group, the lowest level of CSFV antibody was observed at 9–12 weeks of age (Figure 1). To enhance CSFV vaccine efficacy, this time window may be more appropriate for CSFV vaccination in piglets. Based on the results of E2 vaccination in sows at 4–5 weeks pre-farrowing, the vaccination time of the offspring can be delayed until they are 10–12 weeks old [28], which is when they are less susceptible to PRRSV, as observed in most Taiwanese pig herds. In addition, the level of CSFV antibody was significantly higher at the suckling stage (less than 4 weeks old) in the E2 group than in the MLV group (Figure 1), reflecting the different levels of CSFV antibody in sows. This difference was due to sows being vaccinated with E2 at 4–5 weeks pre-farrowing, which elicited a sufficiently high level of CSFV antibody (Figure 1) [27,28]. However, decreases in CSFV antibody titers should be considered when sows are vaccinated with the MLV vaccine post-farrowing and/or when some sows have returned several times. Although the E2 vaccine can only induce antibody responses without inducing cellular immunity, the shedding of vaccine antigens in the field should not be a concern. In addition, the E2 vaccine induces E2-specific neutralizing antibodies to protect different genotypes from highly virulent CSFV challenge [23]. Although there may be other background issues (such as hygiene status and management of the herds) which co-influence the piglets' health state according to previous studies, CSFV E2 subunit vaccine on sows has shown several benefits, such as: (i) the detection rate of CSFV nucleic acid in saliva in their offspring was dramatically decreased [43]; (ii) the efficient induction of high levels of CSFV antibody until slaughter when their offspring only received a single shot of CSFV immunization [26]; and (iii) increase in the survival rate of the nursery pigs in our analyzed herds (herd practitioners' observation), which are consistent with our interpretation of the results in this study. Finally, and most importantly, the major difference between CSFV MLV vaccine and E2 subunit vaccine or inactivated vaccine is that only CSFV MLV provides replicating antigen [14].

In conclusion, our study revealed the sero-dynamics of piglets born from sows vaccinated with the CSFV MLV and E2 vaccines. There was a very highly significant negative correlation between the PRRSV load and the level of CSFV antibody in the CSFV MLV group. The lowest level of CSFV antibody was observed in the CSFV MLV group at 5–8 weeks of age, during which pigs are highly susceptible to PRRSV and CSFV MLV vaccination should be avoided. In contrast, after E2 vaccination of sows at 4–5 weeks pre-farrowing, the level of CSFV antibody remained positive at 9–12 weeks, which allowed CSFV vaccination with MLV to be postponed to avoid an overlap with the PRRS susceptibility period at 5–8 weeks of age. Additionally, our findings indicate that the vaccination of CSFV MLV in piglets during the PRRSV susceptibility period at 5–8 weeks of age may be overloading the piglet's immune system and should be a critical concern for industrial pork production in the field. Thus, using vaccines that provide non-replicating antigen such as E2 subunit vaccines is recommended.

4. Materials and Methods

4.1. Sample Source and Processing

Blood samples were collected in BD Vacutainer tubes with clot activator and gel (BD Diagnostics, Plymouth, UK) from piglets and submitted to the Animal Diseases Diagnostic Center of National Pingtung University of Science and Technology, Taiwan. All piglets were divided into two groups, the MLV and E2 groups. Piglets in the MLV group were born from sows vaccinated with the CSFV MLV vaccine at 4 weeks post-farrowing, whereas piglets in the E2 group were born from sows vaccinated with the CSFV E2 subunit vaccine (Bayovac® CSF-E2, Bayer Animal Health) at 4–5 weeks pre-farrowing. The blood samples were centrifuged at 2150× g for 15 min with a Himac CF 9RX (Hitachi Koki, Tokyo, Japan), and then the sera were carefully transferred into 1.5 mL centrifuge tubes. The stock serum was kept at −80 °C until needed.

4.2. Sample Preparation and PRRSV Real-Time PCR

Nucleic acid extraction was performed with a MagNA Pure LC 2.0 instrument by using the MagNA Pure LC total nucleic acid isolation kit (Roche Applied Science, IN, USA). cDNA synthesis was performed using PrimeScriptTM RT reagent kits (Takara, Kyoto, Japan). To quantify the PRRSV load in serum samples, a ZNA probe-based real-time PCR assay was tested and performed with a LightCycler® 96 System (Roche Applied Science, Basel, Switzerland) [44].

4.3. Serologic Assessment

The serum concentration of CSFV antibody was evaluated by a commercial ELISA (HerdChek CSFV antibody ELISA test kit, IDEXX, ME, USA). After measuring the optical density at a wavelength of 450 nm (OD450) with a Biochrom Anthos Zenyth 200st spectrophotometer (Anthos Labtec Instruments, Salzburg, Austria), if the mean OD450 of the duplicate negative controls (NC$\overline{x}$) was more than 0.5 and the mean blocking % of the duplicate positive controls was greater than 50, the assay was considered valid.

The blocking % was calculated with the equation, Blocking % $= 100 \times \frac{\text{NC}\bar{x} - \text{Sample OD450}}{\text{NC}\bar{x}}$. A blocking % less than or equal to 30 was interpreted as negative. A blocking % between 30 and 40 was interpreted as suspected. A blocking % greater than or equal to 40 was interpreted as positive.

4.4. Statistical Analysis

Student's *t*-test was applied to assess differences in the PRRSV load in the different conditions between the two groups. The relationship between the PRRSV load and the blocking percentage of the CSFV antibody was analyzed by linear regression. Positive rates of PRRSV in different age groups were determined with the chi-square test with Yate's correction. *P* values < 0.05, < 0.01 and < 0.001 were considered statistically significant, highly significant and very highly significant, respectively.

Author Contributions: Conceptualization, C.-N.L., and M.-T.C.; methodology, C.-N.L.; validation, C.-N.L.; formal analysis, C.-N.L.; resources, M.-T.C.; writing—original draft preparation, Y.-C.L.; writing—review and editing, C.-N.L., and M.-T.C. All authors have read and agreed to the published version of the manuscript.

Acknowledgments: We thank Wei-Hao Lin for many helpful discussions. We also thank Pao-Cheng Su for assisting sample collection.

References

1. Smith, D.B.; Meyers, G.; Bukh, J.; Gould, E.A.; Monath, T.; Muerhoff, A.S.; Pletnev, A.; Rico-Hesse, R.; Stapleton, J.T.; Simmonds, P.; et al. Proposed revision to the taxonomy of the genus Pestivirus, family Flaviviridae. *J. Gen. Virol.* **2017**, *98*, 2106–2112. [CrossRef]

2. Ma, S.M.; Mao, Q.; Yi, L.; Zhao, M.Q.; Chen, J.D. Apoptosis, Autophagy, and Pyroptosis: Immune Escape Strategies for Persistent Infection and Pathogenesis of Classical Swine Fever Virus. *Pathogens* **2019**, *8*, 239. [CrossRef] [PubMed]

3. Bohorquez, J.A.; Munoz-Gonzalez, S.; Perez-Simo, M.; Munoz, I.; Rosell, R.; Coronado, L.; Domingo, M.; Ganges, L. Foetal Immune Response Activation and High Replication Rate during Generation of Classical Swine Fever Congenital Infection. *Pathogens* **2020**, *9*, 285. [CrossRef] [PubMed]

4. Blome, S.; Staubach, C.; Henke, J.; Carlson, J.; Beer, M. Classical Swine Fever-An Updated Review. *Viruses* **2017**, *9*, 86. [CrossRef]

5. Moennig, V.; Floegel-Niesmann, G.; Greiser-Wilke, I. Clinical signs and epidemiology of classical swine fever: A review of new knowledge. *Vet. J.* **2003**, *165*, 11–20. [CrossRef]

6. Postel, A.; Austermann-Busch, S.; Petrov, A.; Moennig, V.; Becher, P. Epidemiology, diagnosis and control of classical swine fever: Recent developments and future challenges. *Transbound. Emerg. Dis.* **2018**, *65* (Suppl. S1), 248–261. [CrossRef]

7. Lin, W.H.; Kaewprom, K.; Wang, S.Y.; Lin, C.F.; Yang, C.Y.; Chiou, M.T.; Lin, C.N. Outbreak of Porcine Reproductive and Respiratory Syndrome Virus 1 in Taiwan. *Viruses* **2020**, *12*, 316. [CrossRef]

8. Lin, W.H.; Shih, H.C.; Wang, S.Y.; Lin, C.F.; Yang, C.Y.; Chiou, M.T.; Lin, C.N. Emergence of a virulent porcine reproductive and respiratory syndrome virus in Taiwan in 2018. *Transbound. Emerg. Dis.* **2019**, *66*, 1138–1141. [CrossRef]

9. Lunney, J.K.; Fang, Y.; Ladinig, A.; Chen, N.; Li, Y.; Rowland, B.; Renukaradhya, G.J. Porcine Reproductive and Respiratory Syndrome Virus (PRRSV): Pathogenesis and Interaction with the Immune System. *Annu. Rev. Anim. Biosci.* **2016**, *4*, 129–154. [CrossRef]

10. Renukaradhya, G.J.; Alekseev, K.; Jung, K.; Fang, Y.; Saif, L.J. Porcine reproductive and respiratory syndrome virus-induced immunosuppression exacerbates the inflammatory response to porcine respiratory coronavirus in pigs. *Viral. Immunol.* **2010**, *23*, 457–466. [CrossRef]

11. Albina, E.; Carrat, C.; Charley, B. Interferon-alpha response to swine arterivirus (PoAV), the porcine reproductive and respiratory syndrome virus. *J. Interferon Cytokine Res.* **1998**, *18*, 485–490. [CrossRef]

12. Dwivedi, V.; Manickam, C.; Patterson, R.; Dodson, K.; Murtaugh, M.; Torrelles, J.B.; Schlesinger, L.S.; Renukaradhya, G.J. Cross-protective immunity to porcine reproductive and respiratory syndrome virus by intranasal delivery of a live virus vaccine with a potent adjuvant. *Vaccine* **2011**, *29*, 4058–4066. [CrossRef]

13. Suradhat, S.; Thanawongnuwech, R.; Poovorawan, Y. Upregulation of IL-10 gene expression in porcine peripheral blood mononuclear cells by porcine reproductive and respiratory syndrome virus. *J. Gen. Virol.* **2003**, *84*, 453–459. [CrossRef]

14. Huang, Y.L.; Deng, M.C.; Wang, F.I.; Huang, C.C.; Chang, C.Y. The challenges of classical swine fever control: Modified live and E2 subunit vaccines. *Virus Res.* **2014**, *179*, 1–11. [CrossRef]

15. Huang, Y.L.; Tsai, K.J.; Deng, M.C.; Liu, H.M.; Huang, C.C.; Wang, F.I.; Chang, C.Y. In Vivo Demonstration of the Superior Replication and Infectivity of Genotype 2.1 with Respect to Genotype 3.4 of Classical Swine Fever Virus by Dual Infections. *Pathogens* **2020**, *9*, 261. [CrossRef]

16. Suradhat, S.; Damrongwatanapokin, S. The influence of maternal immunity on the efficacy of a classical swine fever vaccine against classical swine fever virus, genogroup 2.2, infection. *Vet. Microbiol.* **2003**, *92*, 187–194. [CrossRef]

17. Suradhat, S.; Damrongwatanapokin, S.; Thanawongnuwech, R. Factors critical for successful vaccination against classical swine fever in endemic areas. *Vet. Microbiol.* **2007**, *119*, 1–9. [CrossRef]

18. van Oirschot, J.T. Vaccinology of classical swine fever: From lab to field. *Vet. Microbiol.* **2003**, *96*, 367–384. [CrossRef]

19. Vandeputte, J.; Too, H.L.; Ng, F.K.; Chen, C.; Chai, K.K.; Liao, G.A. Adsorption of colostral antibodies against classical swine fever, persistence of maternal antibodies, and effect on response to vaccination in baby pigs. *Am. J. Vet. Res.* **2001**, *62*, 1805–1811. [CrossRef]

20. Blome, S.; Moss, C.; Reimann, I.; Konig, P.; Beer, M. Classical swine fever vaccines-State-of-the-art. *Vet. Microbiol.* **2017**, *206*, 10–20. [CrossRef]

21. Dewulf, J.; Laevens, H.; Koenen, F.; Vanderhallen, H.; Mintiens, K.; Deluyker, H.; de Kruif, A. An experimental infection with classical swine fever in E2 sub-unit marker-vaccine vaccinated and in non-vaccinated pigs. *Vaccine* **2000**, *19*, 475–482. [CrossRef]

22. Floegel-Niesmann, G. Classical swine fever (CSF) marker vaccine. Trial III. Evaluation of discriminatory ELISAs. *Vet. Microbiol.* **2001**, *83*, 121–136. [CrossRef]

23. Tran, H.T.T.; Truong, D.A.; Ly, V.D.; Vu, H.T.; Hoang, T.V.; Nguyen, C.T.; Chu, N.T.; Nguyen, V.T.; Nguyen, D.T.; Miyazawa, K.; et al. The potential efficacy of the E2-subunit vaccine to protect pigs against different genotypes of classical swine fever virus circulating in Vietnam. *Clin. Exp. Vaccine Res.* **2020**, *9*, 26–39. [CrossRef]

24. Klinkenberg, D.; Moormann, R.J.; de Smit, A.J.; Bouma, A.; de Jong, M.C. Influence of maternal antibodies on efficacy of a subunit vaccine: Transmission of classical swine fever virus between pigs vaccinated at 2 weeks of age. *Vaccine* **2002**, *20*, 3005–3013. [CrossRef]

25. Kavanova, L.; Matiaskova, K.; Leva, L.; Nedbalcova, K.; Matiasovic, J.; Faldyna, M.; Salat, J. Concurrent infection of monocyte-derived macrophages with porcine reproductive and respiratory syndrome virus and Haemophilus parasuis: A role of IFNalpha in pathogenesis of co-infections. *Vet. Microbiol.* **2018**, *225*, 64–71. [CrossRef]

26. Tsai, K.Y. Classical Swine Fever E2 Subunit Marker Vaccine: Field Trial and Assessment of Protective Efficacy. Master's Thesis, National Chung Hsing University, Taichung, Taiwan, 2002.

27. Lipowski, A.; Drexler, C.; Pejsak, Z. Safety and efficacy of a classical swine fever subunit vaccine in pregnant sows and their offspring. *Vet. Microbiol.* **2000**, *77*, 99–108. [CrossRef]

28. Lin, Y.C.; Lai, Y.C.; Wang, H.C.; Chien, M.S.; Lee, W.C. Monitoring maternal antibody from sows boosted with classical swine fever E2 subunit vaccine. In Proceedings of the 6th Asian Pig Veterinary Society Congress, Ho Chi Minh City, Vietnam, 23–25 September 2013.

29. Li, H.; Yang, H. Infection of porcine reproductive and respiratory syndrome virus suppresses the antibody response to classical swine fever virus vaccination. *Vet. Microbiol.* **2003**, *95*, 295–301. [CrossRef]

30. Wang, X.; Mu, G.; Dang, R.; Yang, Z. Up-regulation of IL-10 upon PRRSV vaccination impacts on the immune response against CSFV. *Vet. Microbiol.* **2016**, *197*, 68–71. [CrossRef]

31. Suradhat, S.; Kesdangsakonwut, S.; Sada, W.; Buranapraditkun, S.; Wongsawang, S.; Thanawongnuwech, R. Negative impact of porcine reproductive and respiratory syndrome virus infection on the efficacy of classical swine fever vaccine. *Vaccine* **2006**, *24*, 2634–2642. [CrossRef]

32. Choe, S.; Kim, J.H.; Kim, K.S.; Song, S.; Cha, R.M.; Kang, W.C.; Kim, H.J.; Park, G.N.; Shin, J.; Jo, H.N.; et al. Adverse Effects of Classical Swine Fever Virus LOM Vaccine and Jeju LOM Strains in Pregnant Sows and Specific Pathogen-Free Pigs. *Pathogens* **2019**, *9*, 18. [CrossRef]

33. Choe, S.; Le, V.P.; Shin, J.; Kim, J.H.; Kim, K.S.; Song, S.; Cha, R.M.; Park, G.N.; Nguyen, T.L.; Hyun, B.H.; et al. Pathogenicity and Genetic Characterization of Vietnamese Classical Swine Fever Virus: 2014-2018. *Pathogens* **2020**, *9*, 169. [CrossRef]

34. Chen, J.Y.; Wu, C.M.; Liao, C.M.; Chen, K.C.; You, C.C.; Wang, Y.W.; Huang, C.; Chien, M.S. The impact of porcine circovirus associated diseases on live attenuated classical swine fever vaccine in field farm applications. *Vaccine* **2019**, *37*, 6535–6542. [CrossRef] [PubMed]

35. Huang, Y.L.; Pang, V.F.; Deng, M.C.; Chang, C.Y.; Jeng, C.R. Porcine circovirus type 2 decreases the infection and replication of attenuated classical swine fever virus in porcine alveolar macrophages. *Res. Vet. Sci.* **2014**, *96*, 187–195. [CrossRef] [PubMed]

36. Huang, Y.L.; Pang, V.F.; Lin, C.M.; Tsai, Y.C.; Chia, M.Y.; Deng, M.C.; Chang, C.Y.; Jeng, C.R. Porcine circovirus type 2 (PCV2) infection decreases the efficacy of an attenuated classical swine fever virus (CSFV) vaccine. *Vet. Res.* **2011**, *42*, 115. [CrossRef]

37. Chinsakchai, S.; Molitor, T.W. Immunobiology of pseudorabies virus infection in swine. *Vet. Immunol. Immunopathol.* **1994**, *43*, 107–116. [CrossRef]

38. Lin, W.H.; Shih, H.C.; Lin, C.F.; Yang, C.Y.; Lin, C.N.; Chiou, M.T. Genotypic analyses and virulence characterization of Glaesserella parasuis isolates from Taiwan. *PeerJ* **2019**, *7*, e6960. [CrossRef]

39. Lim, S.I.; Jeoung, H.Y.; Kim, B.; Song, J.Y.; Kim, J.; Kim, H.Y.; Cho, I.S.; Woo, G.H.; Lee, J.B.; An, D.J. Impact of porcine reproductive and respiratory syndrome virus and porcine circovirus-2 infection on the potency of the classical swine fever vaccine (LOM strain). *Vet. Microbiol.* **2016**, *193*, 36–41. [CrossRef]

40. Chiou, M.T.; Su, P.C.; Chuang, M.S.; Lin, C.N. Porcine circovirus type 2 infection status in sick or moribund pigs in Taiwan. *Taiwan Vet. J.* **2004**, *30*, 163–168.

41. Yang, C.Y.; Chang, T.C.; Lin, C.N.; Tsai, C.P.; Chiou, M.T. Study of infectious agents involved in porcine respiratory disease complex in Taiwan. *Taiwan Vet. J.* **2007**, *33*, 40–46.

42. Tsai, G.T.; Lin, Y.C.; Lin, W.H.; Lin, J.H.; Chiou, M.T.; Liu, H.F.; Lin, C.N. Phylogeographic and genetic characterization of porcine circovirus type 2 in Taiwan from 2001–2017. *Sci. Rep.* **2019**, *9*, 10782. [CrossRef]

43. Lin, Y.C. Mornitoring Wild Classical Swine Fever Virus Persistent Infection and Antibody Responses of Different Vaccination Programs in Taiwan. Master's Thesis, National Chung Hsing University, Taichung, Taiwan, 2014.

44. Lin, C.N.; Lin, W.H.; Hung, L.N.; Wang, S.Y.; Chiou, M.T. Comparison of viremia of type II porcine reproductive and respiratory syndrome virus in naturally infected pigs by zip nucleic acid probe-based real-time PCR. *BMC Vet. Res.* **2013**, *9*, 181. [CrossRef] [PubMed]

Foetal Immune Response Activation and High Replication Rate during Generation of Classical Swine Fever Congenital Infection

José Alejandro Bohórquez [1,†], Sara Muñoz-González [1,†], Marta Pérez-Simó [1], Iván Muñoz [1], Rosa Rosell [1,2], Liani Coronado [1,3], Mariano Domingo [1,4] and Llilianne Ganges [1,*]

[1]   OIE Reference Laboratory for Classical Swine Fever, IRTA-CReSA, 08193 Barcelona, Spain; josealejandro.bohorquez@irta.cat (J.A.B.); sara.vets.11@gmail.com (S.M.-G.); marta.perez@irta.cat (M.P.-S.); ivan.munoz@irta.cat (I.M.); rosa.rosell@irta.cat (R.R.); lianicoronado@gmail.com (L.C.); mariano.domingo@uab.cat (M.D.)

[2]   Departament d'Agricultura, Ramadería, Pesca, Alimentació I Medi Natural i Rural (DAAM), 08007 Generalitat de Catalunya, Spain

[3]   Centro Nacional de Sanidad Agropecuaria (CENSA), Mayabeque 32700, Cuba

[4]   Servei de Diagnòstic de Patologia Veterinària (SDPV), Departament de Sanitat I d'Anatomia Animals, Universitat Autònoma de Barcelona, Bellaterra, 08193 Barcelona, Spain

*   Correspondence: llilianne.ganges@irta.cat

†   These two authors contributed equally.

Abstract: Classical swine fever virus (CSFV) induces trans-placental transmission and congenital viral persistence; however, the available information is not updated. Three groups of sows were infected at mid-gestation with either a high, moderate or low virulence CSFV strains. Foetuses from sows infected with high or low virulence strain were obtained before delivery and piglets from sows infected with the moderate virulence strain were studied for 32 days after birth. The low virulence strain generated lower CSFV RNA load and the lowest proportion of trans-placental transmission. Severe lesions and mummifications were observed in foetuses infected with the high virulence strain. Sows infected with the moderately virulence strain showed stillbirths and mummifications, one of them delivered live piglets, all CSFV persistently infected. Efficient trans-placental transmission was detected in sows infected with the high and moderate virulence strain. The trans-placental transmission occurred before the onset of antibody response, which started at 14 days after infection in these sows and was influenced by replication efficacy of the infecting strain. Fast and solid immunity after sow vaccination is required for prevention of congenital viral persistence. An increase in the CD8+ T-cell subset and IFN-alpha response was found in viremic foetuses, or in those that showed higher viral replication in tissue, showing the CSFV recognition capacity by the foetal immune system after trans-placental infection.

Keywords: classical swine fever; virulence; trans-placental transmission; persistent congenital infection; foetal immune response; classical swine fever virus; replication; sows

---

1. Introduction

Classical swine fever virus (CSFV) is one of the most relevant viruses in the Pestivirus genus, being the causative agent of classical swine fever (CSF), a highly impactful disease for the porcine industry worldwide [1]. The capacity of pestiviruses to generate persistent infection by trans-placental transmission has already been described [2–6]. Particularly, low virulence CSFV strains have been related to the development of congenital viral persistence in their offspring when infection of the sows occurs between 50 and 90 days of gestation [1–5]. Piglets that develop this form of infection are born infected, showing high viral replication and shedding in the absence of specific antibody response [3,4,7]. This type of viral persistence has been explained by the immunotolerance mechanism, due to a lack of CSFV recognition by the immature immune system of the foetus [5].

CSF still remains endemic in countries in Asia, the Caribbean, and Central and South America [1]. Previous studies have demonstrated the evolutionary capacity of CSFV towards less virulent strains in endemic situations under inefficient vaccination programs [8,9]. In this type of scenario, a recent study showed that CSF persistence was the predominant form, favoring virus prevalence and hampering the control tools [10].

CSFV also has the ability to generate viral persistence after postnatal infection, although unlike the congenital persistence forms, the generation of postnatal persistence has been associated with the CSFV moderate virulence strains [11,12]. Previous studies have also shown that moderate virulence strains are widely distributed [13–15]. In this regard, the strain of CSFV that recently caused an epidemic in Japan after 26 years has been characterised to be of moderate virulence [16,17].

Despite the known capacity of CSFV to be transmitted by the trans-placental route and to induce persistent congenital infection, few scientific works have dealt with the immunopathogenesis of this form of the disease, especially from a virus–host interaction standpoint. Considering this background, the aim of this work is to evaluate the capacity of CSFV strains with different virulence degrees to infect pregnant sows and its relation with the vertical transmission by trans-placental infection of fetuses. Likewise, the implication of the virulence degree in the generation of CSFV congenital persistent infection is also assessed. The levels of viral replication, as well as the immune response, in terms of cytokine production and changes in immune system cell populations were evaluated in foetuses and piglets from the infected sows.

2. Results

2.1. Clinical Evaluation of Sows Infected with Pinar del Rio (PdR) vs. Margarita CSFV Strains

In the first experiment, aiming to determine the capacity of CSFV strains of different virulence levels to induce trans-placental infection, two groups of pregnant sows were inoculated with CSFV at 74 days of gestation. Group A (Sows 1 and 2) was infected with the highly virulent CSFV Margarita strain, while Group B (Sows 3 and 4) were inoculated with the low virulence PdR strain. Clinical signs were recorded daily by a trained veterinarian in a blinded manner.

After inoculation, both CSFV Margarita-infected sows (Group A) showed anorexia and apathy between 6 and 11 days post-infection (dpi). Subsequently, Sow 2 started to eat normally, whereas the clinical condition of Sow 1 deteriorated progressively, showing constipation/diarrhoea, some peaks of fever, evident weight loss, and, eventually, weakness of the hindquarters. This animal was euthanised at 17 dpi (91 days of gestation) for animal welfare reasons, while the remaining sows were euthanised at 22 dpi (96 days of gestation). Both Margarita infected sows showed similar lesions at necropsy, consisting of petechiae in the kidneys, stomach, and intestine, and, in the case of Sow 1, also in the urinary bladder. Conversely, Sows 3 and 4, inoculated with the PdR strain, remained healthy throughout the study, and no lesions related to CSFV infection were found at necropsy.

2.2. CSFV RNA Level Detected in Sows after Infection with Margarita or PdR Strains

CSFV RNA was evaluated by reverse transcription-quantitative PCR (RT-qPCR) [18] in serum samples collected weekly and tissue samples collected at necropsy. The RNA load was characterised as high, moderate or low in accordance with the cycle threshold (Ct) value, as described in the materials and methods section. The CSFV RNA load detected in sera oscillated from moderate to low load (Ct value from 28 to 35) regardless of the virulence degree of the strain used to infect the sows. The RNA was detected at 8 dpi in all the animals in Group A and B (infected with Margarita or PdR strains, respectively). However, at 14 dpi, and until the end of the experiment, samples from the two animals in Group B and from Sow 2 (Group A) were negative (Figure 1A). Notably, only Sow 1 infected with the CSFV Margarita strain was positive at 14 dpi and at the time of euthanasia (17 dpi), although with low RNA load (Ct value 34).

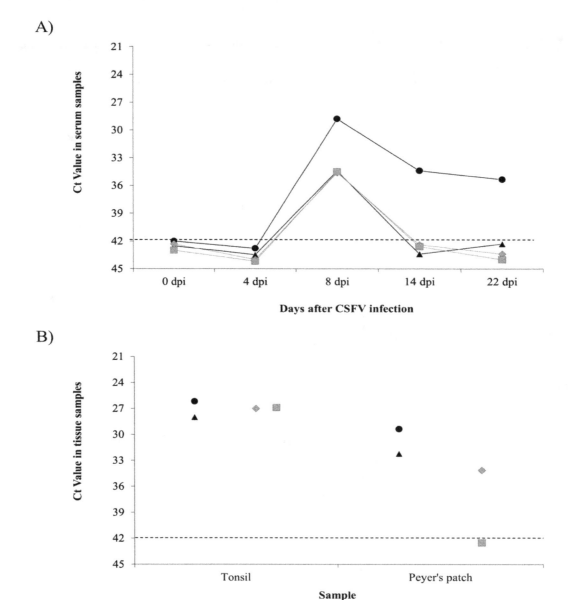

Figure 1. Classical swine fever virus (CSFV) RNA detection by RT-qPCR in sow samples. (**A**) RNA levels detected in sera at different times post-infection. (**B**) RNA levels detected in tissues from sows infected with either the CSFV Margarita (black symbols) or PdR strain (grey symbols). Cycle threshold (Ct) values over 42 (dotted line) were considered as negative. Asterisk indicates the animal that was euthanised at 17 dpi.

In the tissue samples, the CSFV RNA load detected in the tonsils samples was similar in both experimental groups, with Ct value around 27 (moderate RNA load). The viral RNA load in Peyer's patch samples was also similar for both groups, with the exception of Sow 4 (PdR infected), which was negative (Figure 1B).

2.3. The High Virulence CSFV Strain Margarita Elicited Faster and Higher Humoral Response than PdR Strain in the Infected Sows

Specific anti-E2 and neutralising antibodies were evaluated weekly in sera by ELISA and neutralisation peroxidase linked assay (NPLA) [19], respectively. Anti-E2 antibodies were detected in both of the CSFV Margarita-infected sows (Group A) at 14 dpi and at the time of euthanasia. In Group B, infected with the PdR strain, only one animal showed anti-E2 antibodies at 22 dpi (Figure 2A).

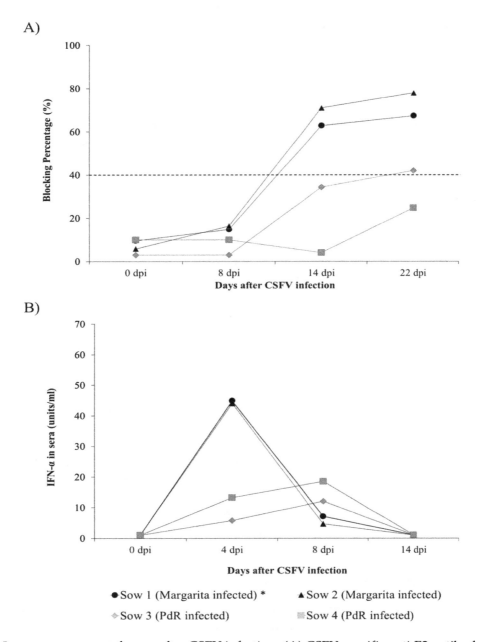

Figure 2. Immune response of sows after CSFV infection. (**A**) CSFV specific anti-E2 antibody response against the E2 glycoprotein detected by ELISA (in blocking %), values above 40% (dotted line) being considered as positive. (**B**) Interferon alpha (IFN-α) response in serum determined by ELISA test from sows infected with either the CSFV Margarita (black symbols) or PdR strain (grey symbols). The IFN-α concentration in sera is expressed as units/mL. Asterisk indicates the animal that was euthanised at 17 dpi.

Similarly, both of the Margarita-infected sows showed neutralising antibody titers by NPLA assay starting at 14 dpi, which increased at 17 and 22 dpi for Sows 1 and 2, respectively. In the case of PdR infected sows, neutralising antibody response was only detected in Sow 3 at 22dpi, while sow 4 did not show neutralising antibodies throughout the whole trial (Table 1).

Table 1. Neutralising antibody response in sows after CSFV infection.

Sow ID		Time after CSFV Infection			
		0 dpi	8 dpi	14 dpi	22 dpi
Margarita	1	0	0	1:640	1:1280 *
infection group	2	0	0	1:320	1:960
PdR infection	3	0	0	0	1:60
group	4	0	0	0	0

* sample taken at 17 dpi.

2.4. IFN-α and IFN-γ Response in Sows Infected with High or Low Virulence CSFV Strains

Interferon alpha (IFN-α) and interferon gamma (IFN-γ) were evaluated by ELISA test in sera from sows at different time-points after infection. IFN-α was detected in the sera of all the sows from Groups A and B at 4 and 8 dpi. Notably, the highest levels were registered in sows from Group A (Sows 1 and 2) at 4 dpi (Figure 2B). For IFN-γ, no detectable levels in sera were found in either experimental group after infection.

2.5. Evaluation of the Foetuses from CSFV Infected Sows at Necropsy

Foetuses from the CSFV Margarita-infected sows showed internal haemorrhages in tonsil, intestine, kidneys, lymph nodes and spleen. Furthermore, four of the foetuses from Sow 1 and three foetuses from Sow 2 had generalised haemorrhagic lesions in the skin (data not shown). Additionally, one mummified foetus was found in both of them. Conversely, foetuses from Sows 3 and 4, inoculated with the PdR low virulence strain, showed no lesions at necropsy.

2.6. Vertical Transmission and CSFV Replication in the Foetuses

Following hysterectomy, serum and tissue samples were collected from all the foetuses, about two weeks before the expected delivery day, in order to determine CSFV transmission from sows to their foetuses. All the foetuses from Group A were RT-qPCR positive with high CSFV RNA load (Ct values between 15.67 and 23) in the majority of sera, tonsil, spleen and thymus samples (see Table 2). In the different organs, the mean Ct value ranged from 17.28 to 20.33 for foetuses from Sows 1 and 2, respectively. By contrast, only 3 out of 13 (23%) foetuses from each of the PdR-infected sows were positive in sera by RT-qPCR, ranging from high to low RNA load (Table 2). However, after analysis by RT-qPCR of tonsil, spleen and thymus samples, the number CSFV positive foetuses increased to 11 out of 13 (Sow 3) and 9 out of 13 (Sow 4), respectively, with high to low CSFV RNA load in the positive tissues.

2.7. Immune Response in the Foetuses from CSFV-Infected Sows

Absence of CSFV specific humoral response was found in sera from all the foetuses in the study. However, IFN-γ levels were detected only in serum sample of five out of the 13 foetuses from the Sow 1 (infected with Margarita strain), in values ranging between 23.2 and 130.9 pg/ml. In addition, detectable levels of IFN-α were also registered in 11 samples in foetuses from both Margarita-infected sows (Table 3). Interestingly, foetuses from sows infected with the low virulence strain (PdR) showed higher levels of IFN-α (between 100 to 200 units/ml). Notably, the positive values were found in the foetuses that were CSFV RNA positive for the four samples analysed or in those that showed the higher CSFV RNA load in the tissue samples (Tables 2 and 3). Finally, detectable levels of soluble CD163 (sCD163) were found in foetal sera samples from both experimental groups, being about 10 times higher the concentration in samples from Group A (Figure 3).

Table 2. Detection of CSFV RNA in foetuses from sows infected with CSFV Margarita or PdR strains.

Margarita Infection Group A	CSFV RT-qPCR (Ct Value)				PdR Infection Group B	CSFV RT-qPCR (Ct Value)			
Foetus ID	Serum	Tonsil	Spleen	Thymus	Foetus ID	Serum	Tonsil	Spleen	Thymus
Foetus from Sow 1					*Foetus from Sow 3*				
1	19.65	18.52	17.91	16.54	1	Undet.	Undet.	34.65	Undet.
2	23.13	20.61	19.56	25.86	2	Undet.	Undet.	Undet.	Undet.
3	20.40	21.96	19.11	15.70	3	Undet.	32.73	29.94	35.45
4	21.35	26.58	18.95	16.85	4	Undet.	Undet.	32.44	Undet.
5	18.48	19.69	17.00	19.18	5	Undet.	Undet.	37.43	Undet.
6	17.65	19.59	16.14	15.92	6	Undet.	35.32	33.82	Undet.
7	18.71	20.53	16.59	16.46	7	22.42	22.75	15.86	17.69
8	23.23	19.92	17.75	15.56	8	Undet.	36.67	Undet.	Undet.
9	18.73	16.13	16.24	14.70	9	Undet.	Undet.	Undet.	Undet.
10	19.55	18.78	16.85	17.31	10	Undet.	36.60	34.56	Undet.
11	20.56	23.52	18.45	17.18	11	24.76	23.18	18.30	21.15
12	17.58	18.05	16.62	16.31	12	32.36	23.37	23.68	24.85
13	17.27	18.61	16.62	16.37	13	Undet.	33.91	31.51	36.33
Mean	**19.72**	**20.33**	**17.49**	**17.28**	**Mean**	**38.50**	**37.19**	**33.28**	**36.33**
Desvest	**2.05**	**2.72**	**1.22**	**2.92**	**Desvest**	**7.16**	**5.88**	**9.89**	**9.02**
Foetus from Sow 2					*Foetus from Sow 4*				
1	20.30	25.16	17.84	20.28	1	Undet.	Undet.	Undet.	Undet.
2	18.68	17.92	17.44	15.79	2	28.26	28.36	18.37	21.79
3	18.50	19.28	17.43	16.95	3	Undet.	35.01	28.32	28.24
4	27.06	28.74	25.01	24.94	4	Undet.	34.59	36.29	Undet.
5	18.94	16.87	17.36	15.70	5	Undet.	Undet.	Undet.	36.54
6	19.51	18.93	17.44	16.78	6	Undet.	Undet.	Undet.	Undet.
7	16.81	18.01	16.93	16.78	7	Undet.	Undet.	Undet.	Undet.
8	16.60	17.25	23.57	17.51	8	Undet.	Undet.	Undet.	36.58
9	18.65	18.36	16.47	16.85	9	Undet.	Undet.	Undet.	Undet.
10	20.67	22.67	17.22	16.97	10	Undet.	Undet.	34.36	Undet.
11	16.91	18.37	17.26	16.92	11	34.54	29.63	26.51	25.84
12	16.94	18.37	18.96	17.66	12	Undet.	36.52	Undet.	Undet.
13	15.67	16.88	16.41	16.26	13	21.52	20.59	18.58	18.32
Mean	**18.75**	**19.30**	**18.46**	**17.43**	**Mean**	**38.87**	**36.88**	**35.16**	**36.70**
Desvest	**2.99**	**3.34**	**2.81**	**2.44**	**Desvest**	**6.69**	**7.01**	**9.21**	**8.55**

Undet: undetectable, negative sample.

Table 3. IFN-α levels in foetal serum.

Margarita Infection Group A		PdR Infection Group B	
Foetus ID	IFN-α	Foetus ID	IFN-α
Foetus from Sow 1		*Foetus from Sow 3*	
1	**48.5**	1	0.0
2	0.0	2	0.0
3	0.0	3	**60.3**
4	**237.7**	4	0.0
5	0.0	5	0.0
6	**18.7**	6	0.0
7	0.0	7	**116.7**
8	0.0	8	0.0
9	0.0	9	0.0
10	**31.3**	10	0.0
11	0.0	11	**102.7**
12	**8.0**	12	**209.6**
13	0.0	13	0.0
Foetus from Sow 2		*Foetus from Sow 4*	
1	0.0	1	0.0
2	**25.5**	2	**227.8**
3	**26.7**	3	**239.5**
4	**49.3**	4	0.0
5	0.0	5	0.0
6	0.0	6	0.0
7	0.0	7	0.0
8	**14.3**	8	0.0
9	0.0	9	0.0
10	**12.2**	10	0.0
11	**43.2**	11	**173.4**
12	0.0	12	0.0
13	0.0	13	**126.9**

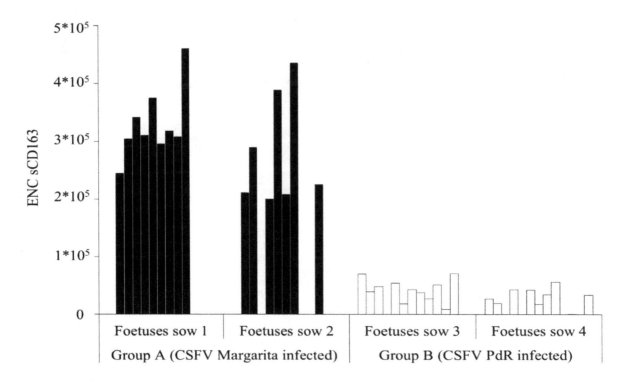

Figure 3. sCD163 levels in foetal sera. Foetuses from sows infected with either the Margarita (black bars) or PdR (white bars) CSFV strains are represented. Results are expressed as the equivalent number of copies of CD163 transfected cells.

2.8. Phenotypical Profile in Foetal PBMCs after CSFV Infection

Samples from whole blood were obtained from three foetuses in each infected group, and peripheral blood mononuclear cells (PBMCs) were isolated. Flow cytometry analysis was performed to study the phenotypical profile in these cells. The PBMCs analysed corresponded with foetuses that showed CSFV RNA levels in serum samples. Additionally, PBMCs of three foetuses from uninfected sows, from the same farm of origin, were also analysed to use as reference, uninfected controls. The $CD4^+$ T-cell subset ranged from 4% to 16% of PBMC from the Margarita infected foetuses (Group A), showing a reduction in two out of three samples analysed with values below 5% (Figure 4). This cell population ranged from 14% to 17% in the three foetal PBMC tested from Group B, while a wider range was detected in the PBMC from naïve samples (from 11% to 38%). By contrast, the $CD8^+$ T-cells were increased in the CSFV infected foetuses, with percentages between 29% and 56% in Group A, and 20% to 27% in Group B (infected with PdR strain), whereas it was always below 15% for the naïve samples (Figure 4).

2.9. Infection with the CSFV Moderately Virulent Strain: Clinical Signs and CSFV Replication in Sows

In the second experiment, in order to evaluate the capacity of a CSFV moderately virulent strain to induce trans-placental infection and congenital viral persistence, two pregnant sows (Sows 5 and 6) were inoculated with the Catalonia 01 (Cat01) strain. As in Experiment 1, the infection was carried out at 74 days of gestation, and a trained veterinarian recorded clinical signs daily.

The Cat01 infected sows did not show any clinical signs after inoculation. However, at 34 dpi (108 days of gestation), Sow 6 went into early labour and gave birth to eight stillbirths and two live piglets. All the stillbirths showed haemorrhagic lesions, whereas the live piglets were very weak and had to be euthanised on the same day for ethical reasons. The sow was also euthanised at this time. Both Cat01 infected sows were CSFV RNA positive in sera, and rectal and nasal swabs at 7dpi. The CSFV RNA load was low in all the samples, with Ct values ranging from 31 to 37. Afterwards, both sows cleared the virus, only Sow 6 was positive in rectal swab at 28 dpi, although at low RNA concentration (Ct 35.59) (data not shown).

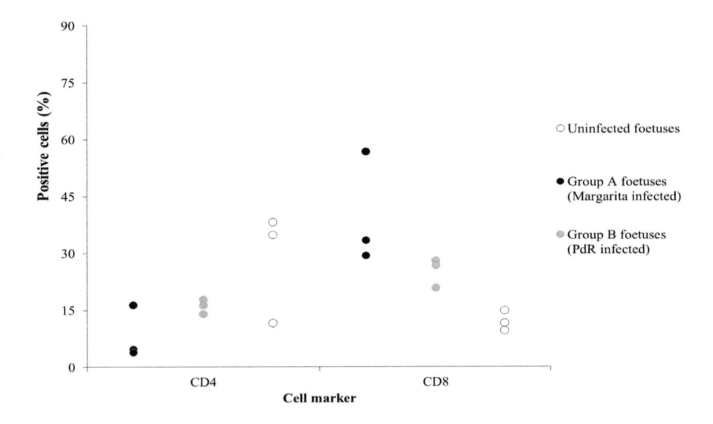

Figure 4. Comparative expression of the CD4+ and CD8+ T-cell subsets in PBMCs from uninfected foetuses (white dots), foetuses infected with the Margarita (black dots), or the PdR (grey dots) CSFV strain.

2.10. Vertical Transmission and Congenital Viral Persistence Generated by the Moderate Virulence CSFV Strain

At 114 days of gestation, Sow 5 gave birth to eight live piglets and six stillbirths, the live animals were active and fed normally from the mother immediately after birth. During the seven days after farrowing, two piglets were found dead in the pen, having being crushed by the sow, whereas no clinical signs were registered in the remaining six animals (Piglets 1 to 6). Piglets 1, 3, and 5 remained clinically healthy during the 32 days of the trial. Meanwhile, the other three piglets (Piglets 2, 4, and 6) developed sporadic fever peaks (below 41 °C) from day 10 until the end of the study. Piglet 6 developed mild polyarthritis from day 10, and Piglets 2 and 4 at days 30 and 23, respectively. Notably, at the time of euthanasia, the piglets weighed around 8.5 kg and continued to show normal feeding behaviour.

On the day of birth, the piglets were positive by RT-qPCR with high CSFV RNA load (Ct values about 23) in the rectal swab samples (Table 4). Despite the absence of CSF specific clinical signs, a high CSFV RNA load (Ct value about 20) was detected in all the serum samples during the study, indicating a permanent viremia in the piglets during the trial (Table 4). In parallel, high and permanent excretion in nasal and rectal swabs was found in all the sampling time points during the 32 days after birth. The Ct values increased in the majority of animals throughout the trial, reaching Ct values around 22 and 24 in nasal and rectal swabs (Table 4).

Table 4. Detection of CSFV RNA in piglets from Sow 5, infected with the CSFV Cat01 strain.

	Day of Birth	7 dpb			15 dpb			23 dpb			27 dpb			32 dpb		
Piglet ID	Rectal Swab	Serum	Nasal Swab	Rectal Swab	Serum	Nasal Swab	Rectal Swab	Serum	Nasal Swab	Rectal Swab	Serum	Nasal Swab	Rectal Swab	Serum	Nasal Swab	Rectal Swab
1	25	17.06	24.77	23.77	16.88	16.87	24.52	16.55	23.03	22.38	16.51	24.70	23.62	17.30	18.80	22.47
2	23.94	16.10	26.09	20.42	16.34	25.76	23.91	16.06	20.82	25.53	15.96	21.16	23.52	17.28	20.59	27.20
3	24.01	16.01	23.15	21.46	16.36	25.88	23.36	16.80	27.16	24.49	17.29	21.66	23.74	19.27	19.25	24.42
4	22.63	16.31	22.30	20.86	16.74	19.26	26.91	17.01	18.02	25.36	16.73	22.20	25.44	16.36	23.53	22.86
5	23.44	15.71	27.94	22.81	16.68	27.00	24.38	16.61	20.42	24.77	16.89	20.41	25.83	17.64	19.30	25.99
6	24.55	15.39	23.20	23.79	25.52	22.65	26.56	16.56	21.28	23.19	16.66	20.57	22.70	16.74	19.86	>22.42
Mean	**23.93**	**16.10**	**24.58**	**22.19**	**18.09**	**22.90**	**24.94**	**16.60**	**21.79**	**24.29**	**16.67**	**21.78**	**24.14**	**17.43**	**20.22**	**24.23**
Desvest	**0.83**	**0.57**	**2.13**	**1.47**	**3.65**	**4.09**	**1.45**	**0.32**	**3.09**	**1.25**	**0.44**	**1.58**	**1.22**	**1.01**	**1.73**	**2.01**

CSFV qRT-PCR (Ct Value)

dpb: days post birth.

2.11. Immune Response Generated by the Moderately CSFV Strain in Sows and Their Litters

After infection, Sow 6 developed CSFV specific humoral response at 14 dpi, while Sow 5 was positive at 21 dpi, with blocking percentage values of 42% and 60%, respectively, which increased throughout the study. Neutralising antibody response appeared at 21 dpi on Sow 5 (titre 1:120), and at 14 dpi in Sow 6 (titre 1:20), and increased, reaching titres of 1:160 in both sows by 28 dpi. Nevertheless, none of the piglets showed an antibody response either by ELISA or NPLA during the 32 days after birth. Interestingly, IFN-α was detected in the sera from 4 piglets at 8 and 15 days post-birth (dpb) (Figure 5A). On the other hand, alterations in the CD4$^+$ and CD8$^+$ T-cell subsets from Cat01-infected piglets were found in the analysed PBMC from persistently infected piglets. While the T-CD4$^+$ population did not exceed 5% in the uninfected, age-matched piglets, these cells ranged from 4% to 16% in persistently infected animals. On the other hand, the CD8$^+$ cell subset was increased (about 50%) in the infected animals, being between 9.6 and 23.5% in the uninfected animals (Figure 5B).

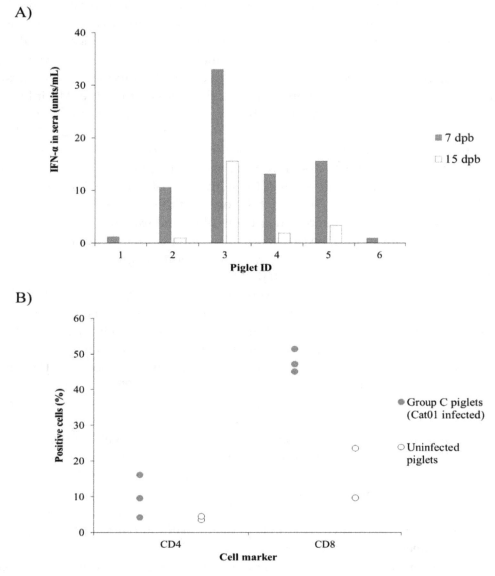

Figure 5. IFN-α levels and phenotypic profile in peripheral blood mononuclear cells (PBMCs) from CSFV congenital persistently infected piglets. (**A**) Concentration of IFN-α in sera expressed as units/mL from CSFV persistently infected piglets at 7 dpb (grey bars) and 15 dpb (white bars). (**B**) Comparative expression of the T-CD4+ and T-CD8+ cell subsets in PBMCs from uninfected piglets (white dots) and piglets infected with the Cat01strain (grey dots).

3. Discussion

CSF congenital persistent infection was described several decades ago; however, some aspects regarding the generation of this form of the disease remain to be elucidated, and the available information is not up to date [4,6]. In the present work, three groups of sows were infected with either the Margarita, Cat01, or PdR CSFV strains. Each of these strains hav been previously characterised as of high, moderate, and low virulence, respectively [20–22]. In accordance with previous studies, the infection was carried out at 74 days of gestation, a time-point in which persistent congenital infection can be generated [4]. The capacity for trans-placental transmission and induction of foetal immune response was compared side by side between the high and low virulence strains (Figures 1 and 2, Tables 1 and 2). In accordance with previous data found in piglets, the highly virulent CSFV Margarita strain induced high serum IFN-α levels in sows over a short period of time [23]. By contrast, the IFN-α response induced by the low virulence PdR strain was lower, although it lasted one week longer. This supports the role of high replication rates for the previously described exacerbated innate immune response in the host after infection with highly virulent CSFV strains. This may explain the differences in pathogenesis between the sows from these two groups, with more severe lesions and an inability to clear the virus in the Margarita-infected sows, compared with the clinically healthy status and low replication of the PdR-infected ones. Trans-placental transmission was more efficient with the highly virulent Margarita strain, and high viral RNA load was detected in sera and tissues from the foetuses in this group. Conversely, a small proportion of the foetuses from the PdR infected sows were viraemic with high viral replication in organs, while the majority of them were either non-infected or only showed low viral RNA in tissues. Despite the immune response developed, mainly in Margarita infected sows, CSFV crossed the trans-placental barrier from the sows to their foetuses (Tables 1 and 2, Figure 2). In agreement with previously described data, the high replication rate found in sows infected with a highly virulent CSFV strain may explain the activation of neutralising antibody response in these animals. However, taking into account that the onset of the antibody response in the sows was after two weeks, it is likely that the generation of trans-placental transmission took place during the first week after infection. Considering the previously described data, in order to avoid trans-placental transmission, it is necessary that effective neutralising antibody response be already present at the moment of infection, with titres of at least 1/320 [24].

Mummifications and haemorrhagic lesions were found in the Margarita infected foetuses. Probably, these animals would have died during the perinatal period. On the contrary, neither mummifications nor macroscopic lesions were observed in the PdR infected foetuses, even in those that showed viremia and high levels of viral replication in organs. It is very well known that sows transmit passive immunity to CSFV to the litters via colostrum [25,26]. These maternally derived antibodies (MDA) protect piglets against disease, including CSF, during their firsts weeks of life [15,25,26]. Considering that, in the case that the piglets had been born, the low immunity generated in the sows after infection with the low virulence PdR strain would result in an inefficient transmission of MDA to these litters. There might be major consequences to this situation since the suboptimal level of MDA would favour the infection of the non-infected piglets by their congenital persistently infected littermates and lead to chronic or postnatal persistent infection [10,11]. Recently, it was reported that the lack of maternal immunity led to a high prevalence of CSFV persistently infected piglets in an endemic scenario [10]. Notably, the CSFV persistently infected piglets have been proven to be refractory to vaccination [10,27]. This complex situation may lead to a vicious circle, which greatly impairs control programs of regions where CSF persistent infections are occurring.

In the case of infection carried out with the moderately virulent CSFV Cat01 strain, early labour in one of the infected sows and mummification and stillbirths in both of them were detected. Interestingly, both Cat01 infected sows developed a CSFV neutralising antibody response. However, the viral trans-placental transmission was not impaired, and all the piglets that were born alive in one of the Cat01 infected litters developed persistent congenital infection. These piglets showed normal weight gain, according to standards [28], despite being infected and excreting high viral load with a lack of

CSFV specific antibody response [1,5,6]. Interestingly, the level of viral replication was comparable, or even higher than those found in the foetuses from sows infected with the high virulence strain (Tables 2 and 4). This finding suggests an immunomodulatory capacity of the moderate virulence CSFV strains in the interaction with the host. Previous data showed the efficacy of this type of CSFV strain to also generate persistent postnatal infection [11,27]. Similar to persistent postnatal infection, low levels of IFN-α were found during congenital viral persistence, despite the high viral replication, pointing towards immunosuppressive regulation. Similar mechanisms might be taking place during the establishment of congenital or postnatal viral persistence. Recently, myeloid-derived suppressor cell populations have been determined to play a relevant role in the generation of CSFV postnatal persistence infection [29]. It cannot be discarded that these cell subsets are playing a role during the establishment of CSFV congenital persistent infection, considering that they have been found in cord blood and during neonatal stages in humans [30,31]. On the other hand, a low CD4/CD8 ratio has been reported as a marker for dysregulation of the immune response [32–35]. An increase in the CD8$^+$ T-cell population, resulting in a low CD4/CD8 ratio, has been reported in CSFV postnatal persistently infected animals [12]. In the present study, an increase in the CD8$^+$ T-cell subset was observed in the PBMC of infected foetuses and piglets from all the experimental groups. This finding may indicate that immunosuppressive mechanisms are also taking place in animals after trans-placental infection by CSFV.

Activation of innate immunity, evidenced by the IFN-α and IFN-γ levels detected in sera, was found in the foetuses and piglets regardless of the infecting strain and the maturity level of the immune system (Table 3 and Figure 5). Type I interferon response activates the innate immunity after viral infection by playing an antiviral and immunomodulatory role. CSFV has the capacity to induce high levels of IFN-α response in pigs, being associated with disease severity and viral replication in the infected animals [36]. The highest IFN-α response was found in the viraemic foetuses or in those that showed higher viral replication in organs from the group infected with the low virulence PdR strain. Notably, the capacity of the PdR strain for high and prolonged IFN-α activation in piglets has been associated with an uninterrupted 36-uridine sequence found in the 3' untranslated region of the CSFV genome [23]. Activation of IFN-α response in ruminant and human foetuses, following infection with bovine viral diarrhoea and Zika virus, respectively, has been described, and it may support the results obtained in this study [37,38]. Thus, the immunotolerance mechanism that was previously associated with the development of CSF congenital persistent form [1,5] is a complex immunologic phenomenon, and further studies may explain this mechanism and its relation with the establishment of viral persistence.

Previous reports have shown that the levels of sCD163 can be increased as a result of tissue damage during acute infection with highly pathogenic viruses, such as the African swine fever virus (ASFV) [39,40]. In addition, increased IFN-γ levels have also been found as part of the cytokine storm phenomenon responsible for the pathogenesis of ASFV [39–41]. In agreement with the haemorrhagic lesions and levels of viral replication found in foetuses infected with the high virulence CSFV Margarita strain, it is likely that the increase of IFN-γ and sCD163 may be associated with the exacerbated immune response in the host after infection, leading to cellular homeostasis imbalance and tissue damage.

Taken together, our results show that the infecting CSFV strain capacity for viral replication influences its efficacy for trans-placental transmission and the establishment of persistent infection. Likewise, the CSFV strain with a moderate virulence degree proved to be very efficient in generating CSFV congenital persistent infection following trans-placental transmission. Our results indicate that trans-placental infection took place very fast before the neutralising antibody response could be generated in sows. Therefore, vaccines against CSFV indicated for pregnant sows must induce fast and strong immunity to guarantee the viral protection of their offspring against this type of infection.

On the other hand, the foetal immune system is able to recognise the virus and generate immune response after trans-placental infection. Further studies are needed to elucidate the mechanisms by which the specific immune response against CSFV is being impaired, following the initial recognition of the pathogen. To the best of our knowledge, this is the first report showing the foetal immune response after CSFV infection.

4. Materials and Methods

4.1. Cells and Viruses

Production of the viral strains was carried out by infecting susceptible cells with viral suspensions in 2% pestivirus-free foetal bovine serum using the porcine kidney cell line PK-15 (ATCC CCL 33, Middlesex, England), cultured in Eagle's minimum essential medium supplemented with 5% foetal calf serum. Following the infection, cells were incubated at 37 °C in 5% CO_2, and after 72 h, the virus was harvested. Peroxidase-linked assay (PLA) [42] was used for viral titration following the statistical methods described by Reed and Muench [43]. The CSFV PdR and the Margarita strains, both belonging to the 1.4 subgenotype [44,45], have been characterised as low and high virulence strains, respectively [20,21]. The Cat01 strain, which belongs to subgenotype 2.3, was selected as a moderate virulence prototype [22].

4.2. Experimental Design

Six pregnant sows (Landrace) of 68 days of gestation, from a commercial farm, were housed in the biosafety level 3 (BSL3) animal facility at CReSA (Barcelona, Spain). The animals were purchased from pestivirus-free farms, and they were also checked for antibodies against CSFV before arriving at the CReSA facilities. Animals were numbered from one to six and distributed in three groups (from A to C), each group in a separate box with standard facilities for pregnant sows. In accordance with the previously established methodology to evaluate the capacity of CSFV for trans-placental transmission, two sows were included in each experimental group [24,46]. After five days of acclimatisation period (74 days of gestation), Sows 1 and 2 (Group A) were inoculated with the CSFV Margarita strain, Sows 3 and 4 (Group B) with the PdR strain and Sows 5 and 6 (Group C) with the Cat01 strain. The viral dose for all the inocula was 10^5 TCID $_{50}$ per animal, and the inoculation was carried out by intramuscular injection in the neck [22,24,47]. After infection, a trained veterinarian recorded clinical signs daily in a blinded manner. Two experiments were carried out, Experiment 1 included Groups A and B, while Experiment 2 included the Group C sows.

In Experiment 1 of the trial, serum and nasal and rectal swab samples were collected on the day of infection and at 4, 8, 14, and 22 dpi, which corresponded with days 74, 78, 82, 88 and 96 of gestation, respectively. At this time, the sows were euthanised, following the accepted procedures accordingly with the European Directive 2010/63/EU. Whole blood in EDTA was obtained in the day of infection and before euthanasia for ex vivo collection of PBMCs. After necropsy, tissue samples from tonsil and Peyer's patch were collected [24]. In parallel, the foetuses from all gilts were obtained, following procedures previously described to avoid foetal distress [24,48]. All foetuses were subjected to an exhaustive necropsy in which the presence of macroscopic lesions in different organs was evaluated [49]. Sera and whole blood samples and tissues (tonsil, spleen, and thymus) were collected from 13 foetuses per each sow.

In Experiment 2, sera samples were collected on the day of infection and at 7, 14, 21, and 28 dpi (days 81, 87, 95, and 102 of pregnancy, respectively). At farrowing, rectal swabs were collected from all piglets. Sows were kept with their litters for 21 days, and, after removal of the sow, piglets were fed an age-appropriate diet (StartRite, Cargill, Spain) until the end of the trial. The handling of the piglets was performed following previously described protocols [11].

Serum and nasal and rectal swabs were collected from piglets at 7, 15, 23, 27, and 32 dpb. At this time, whole blood samples were collected and piglets were euthanised following procedures according to the European Directive, using a pentobarbital overdose of 60–100 mg/kg of weight, administered via the jugular vein. In addition, sows and piglets were euthanised before the end of the trial if they presented clinical signs compatible with severe CSF or exhibited prostration behaviour, in accordance with previous studies [22]. The experiment was approved by the Ethics Committee for Animal Experiments of the Autonomous University of Barcelona (UAB), according to existing Spanish and European regulations.

4.3. Detection of CSFV RNA

The NucleoSpin RNA isolation kit (Macherey-Nagel, Düren, Germany) was used in order to extract RNA from sera and nasal and rectal swab samples, as well as from organ samples, following the protocol provided by the manufacturer. In all cases, a final volume of 50 µL of RNA was extracted from an initial sample volume of 150 µL. The detection of viral RNA was carried out by a previously described RT-qPCR assay [18], validated in our laboratory for the detection of CSFV RNA in sera, nasal, and rectal swabs and tissue samples [11,22]. Samples were considered positive when the Ct values were equal to or less than 42. In addition, using the Ct value, samples were determined to have either high (Ct value below 23), moderate (between 23 and 28), or low (Ct value above 28) CSFV RNA load, as previously described [23,50]. Samples in which fluorescence was undetectable (Undet) were considered negative.

4.4. Determination of E2-Specific and Neutralising Antibodies

CSFV E2-specific antibodies were evaluated in sera from sows, foetuses, and piglets, using a commercial ELISA kit (IDEXX Laboratories, Liebfeld, Switzerland). Positive results were considered when the blocking percentage was ≥40%, following the manufacturer's recommendations. Additionally, neutralising antibodies against the respective infecting strain were determined using an NPLA assay [19]; thus, animals from Groups A, B, and C were evaluated for neutralising antibodies against the Margarita, PdR, and Cat01 strain, respectively. The neutralising antibody titres were expressed as the reciprocal dilution of serum that neutralised 100 TCID of 50% of the culture replicates.

4.5. IFN-α ELISA Test in Serum Samples

IFN-α concentration was determined in sera from foetuses and sows from Groups A and B, as well as piglets from Group C at 7 and 15 dpb, using a previously described in-house ELISA test [11,51]. Briefly, plates were coated overnight with an anti-IFN-α monoclonal antibody (K9 clone, PBL Biomedical Laboratories, Piscataway, New Jersey, USA). After washing, 50 µl of serum samples and serial dilutions of IFN-α recombinant protein (PBL Biomedical Laboratories) were plated by duplicate and incubated for 1 hour at 37 °C. Afterwards, plates were washed, and a biotinylated anti-IFN-α antibody was added (F17 clone, PBL Biomedical Laboratories). Following an incubation of 1 hour at 37 oC, the plates were washed, and streptavidin-HRP was added. Finally, after a 30 minute incubation, 3,3′,5,5′-tetramethylbenzidine (TMB) was used for revealing the technique, using H_2SO_4 1N as a stop solution. Plates were read at 450 nm, and cytokine concentrations (units/ml) were determined using a regression line built with the optical densities of the cytokine standards used in the test.

4.6. ELISA Detection of IFN-γ and sCD163

IFN-γ and sCD163 were analysed in sera from foetuses and sows from Groups A and B. Commercial ELISA test was used for detection of IFN-γ (IFN-γ ELISA Kit, Porcine, Life Technologies), following the manufacturer's instructions and the results were expressed as picograms per millilitre (pg/ml). Finally, a formerly described ELISA using lysates from CD163 transfected CHO cells as standard was used to quantify sCD163 [39,52]. Results were expressed as the equivalent numbers of CD163-transfected CHO cells (ENC).

4.7. PBMCs Collection and Flow Cytometry Assay

PBMCs were obtained from whole blood collected at the time of necropsy from three animals of each group in Experiments 1 and 2 of the trial, previously characterised by RT-qPCR. Cells were separated by density-gradient centrifugation with Histopaque 1077 (Sigma-Aldrich St. Louis, MO, USA), followed by osmotic shock in order to eliminate the remaining red blood cells. The number and viability of the PBMCs were determined by staining with Trypan Blue [21]. Additionally, thymocytes were obtained from three uninfected foetuses, and whole blood samples were also collected from three uninfected foetuses and piglets at the same time of gestation/days after birth as the foetuses from Experiment 1 or the piglets from Experiment 2, respectively.

The phenotypic profile of PBMCs from foetuses and piglets was evaluated by flow cytometry. Single staining was performed using the mAbs to porcine CD4 (74-12-4, IgG2b) Alexa Fluor 647 conjugate (BD Biosciences), and CD8-α (76-2-11, IgG2a) FITC-labelled (BD Biosciences, Franklin Lakes, NJ, USA).

The staining protocols were performed as previously described [11,12]. After staining, cells were filtered and passed in the cytometer (FACSAria IIu, BD Biosciences), with 10,000 cell events being recorded for each sample. The cells were analysed by FACSDiva software, version 6.1.2 and the results were expressed as the percentage of positive cells obtained for each staining, using irrelevant isotype-matched mAbs as staining controls.

Author Contributions: Conceptualization, L.G.; Investigation, J.A.B., S.M.-G., and L.G.; Methodology, L.G., S.M.-G., J.A.B., M.P.-S., I.M., R.R., L.C., and M.D.; Formal Analysis, J.A.B., S.M.-G., and L.G.; Resources, L.G. and R.R.; Writing—Original Draft Preparation, J.A.B., S.M.-G., and L.G.; Writing—Review and Editing, J.A.B., S.M.-G, M.D., and L.G.; Supervision, L.G.; Project Administration, L.G.; Funding Acquisition, L.G. All authors have read and agreed to the published version of the manuscript.

References

1. Blome, S.; Staubach, C.; Henke, J.; Carlson, J.; Beer, M. Classical swine fever—An updated review. *Viruses* **2017**, *9*, 1–24. [CrossRef] [PubMed]
2. Aynaud, J.M.; Corthier, G.; Vannier, P.; Tillon, P.J. Swine fever: In vitro and in vivo properties of low virulent strains isolated in breeding farms having reproductive failures. In *Proceedings of the Agricultural Research Seminar on Hog Cholera. Hog Cholera. Classical Swine Fever and African Swine Fever*; Liess, B., Ed.; Commission of the European Communities, Publication EUR 5904 EN: Brussels, Belgium, 1977; pp. 273–277.
3. Carbrey, E.A.; Stewart, W.C.; Kresse, J.I.; Snyder, M.L. Inapparent Hog Cholera infection following the inoculation of field isolates. In *Proceedings of the Agricultural Research Seminar on Hog Cholera. Hog Cholera. Classical Swine Fever and African Swine Fever*; Lies, B., Ed.; Commission of the European Communities, Publication EUR 5904 EN: Brussels, Belgium, 1977; pp. 214–230.
4. Van Oirschot, J.T.; Terpstra, C. A congenital persistent swine fever infection. I. Clinical and virological observations. *Vet. Microbiol.* **1977**, *2*, 121–132. [CrossRef]
5. Van Oirschot, J.T. Experimental production of congenital persistent swine fever infections. II. Effect on functions of the immune system. *Vet. Microbiol.* **1979**, *4*, 133–147. [CrossRef]
6. Liess, B. Persistent infections of hog cholera: A review. *Prev. Vet. Med.* **1984**, *2*, 109–113. [CrossRef]
7. Vannier, P.; Plateau, E.; Tillon, J.P. Congenital tremor in pigs farrowed from sows given hog cholera virus during pregnancy. *Am. J. Vet. Res.* **1981**, *42*, 135–137.
8. Pérez, L.J.; Díaz de Arce, H.; Perera, C.L.; Rosell, R.; Frías, M.T.; Percedo, M.I.; Tarradas, J.; Dominguez, P.; Núñez, J.I.; Ganges, L. Positive selection pressure on the B/C domains of the E2-gene of classical swine fever virus in endemic areas under C-strain vaccination. *Infect. Genet. Evol.* **2012**, *12*, 1405–1412. [CrossRef]

9. Rios, L.; Coronado, L.; Naranjo-Feliciano, D.; Martínez-Pérez, O.; Perera, C.L.; Hernandez-Alvarez, L.; Díaz De Arce, H.; Núñez, J.I.; Ganges, L.; Pérez, L.J. Deciphering the emergence, genetic diversity and evolution of classical swine fever virus. *Sci. Rep.* **2017**, *7*, 17887. [CrossRef]

10. Coronado, L.; Bohórquez, J.A.; Muñoz-González, S.; Pérez, L.J.; Rosell, R.; Fonseca, O.; Delgado, L.; Perera, C.L.; Frías, M.T.; Ganges, L. Investigation of chronic and persistent classical swine fever infections under field conditions and their impact on vaccine efficacy. *BMC Vet. Res.* **2019**, *15*, 247. [CrossRef]

11. Muñoz-González, S.; Ruggli, N.; Rosell, R.; Pérez, L.J.; Frías-Leuporeau, M.T.; Fraile, L.; Montoya, M.; Córdoba, L.; Domingo, M.; Ehrensperger, F.; et al. Postnatal persistent infection with classical swine fever virus and its immunological implications. *PLoS ONE* **2015**, *10*, e0125692. [CrossRef]

12. Bohórquez, J.A.; Wang, M.; Pérez-Simó, M.; Vidal, E.; Rosell, R.; Ganges, L. Low CD4/CD8 ratio in classical swine fever postnatal persistent infection generated at 3 weeks after birth. *Transbound. Emerg. Dis.* **2019**, *66*, 752–762. [CrossRef]

13. Beer, M.; Goller, K.V.; Staubach, C.; Blome, S. Genetic variability and distribution of Classical swine fever virus. *Anim. Health Res. Rev.* **2015**, *16*, 33–39. [CrossRef] [PubMed]

14. Luo, Y.; Ji, S.; Liu, Y.; Lei, J.-L.; Xia, S.-L.; Wang, Y.; Du, M.-L.; Shao, L.; Meng, X.-Y.; Zhou, M.; et al. Isolation and Characterization of a Moderately Virulent Classical Swine Fever Virus Emerging in China. *Transbound. Emerg. Dis.* **2017**, *64*, 1848–1857. [CrossRef] [PubMed]

15. Henke, J.; Carlson, J.; Zani, L.; Leidenberger, S.; Schwaiger, T.; Schlottau, K.; Teifke, J.P.; Schröder, C.; Beer, M.; Blome, S. Protection against transplacental transmission of moderately virulent classical swine fever virus using live marker vaccine "CP7_E2alf". *Vaccine* **2018**, *36*, 4181–4187. [CrossRef]

16. Postel, A.; Nishi, T.; Kameyama, K.; Meyer, D.; Suckstorff, O.; Fukai, K.; Becher, P. Reemergence of Classical Swine Fever, Japan, 2018. *Emerg. Infect. Dis.* **2019**, *25*, 1228–1231. [CrossRef] [PubMed]

17. Kameyama, K.-I.; Nishi, T.; Yamada, M.; Masujin, K.; Morioka, K.; Kokuho, T.; Fukai, K. Experimental infection of pigs with a classical swine fever virus isolated in Japan for the first time in 26 years. *J. Vet. Med. Sci.* **2019**, *81*, 1277–1284. [CrossRef] [PubMed]

18. Hoffmann, B.; Beer, M.; Schelp, C.; Schirrmeier, H.; Depner, K. Validation of a real-time RT-PCR assay for sensitive and specific detection of classical swine fever. *J. Virol. Methods* **2005**, *130*, 36–44. [CrossRef]

19. Terpstra, C.; Bloemraad, M.; Gielkens, A.L. The neutralizing peroxidase-linked assay for detection of antibody against swine fever virus. *Vet. Microbiol.* **1984**, *9*, 113–120. [CrossRef]

20. Coronado, L.; Liniger, M.; Muñoz-González, S.; Postel, A.; Pérez, L.J.; Pérez-Simó, M.; Perera, C.L.; Frías-Lepoureau, M.T.; Rosell, R.; Grundhoff, A.; et al. Novel poly-uridine insertion in the 3'UTR and E2 amino acid substitutions in a low virulent classical swine fever virus. *Vet. Microbiol.* **2017**, *201*, 103–112. [CrossRef]

21. Ganges, L.; Barrera, M.; Núñez, J.I.; Blanco, I.; Frías, M.T.; Rodríguez, F.; Sobrino, F. A DNA vaccine expressing the E2 protein of classical swine fever virus elicits T cell responses that can prime for rapid antibody production and confer total protection upon viral challenge. *Vaccine* **2005**, *23*, 3741–3752. [CrossRef]

22. Tarradas, J.; de la Torre, M.E.; Rosell, R.; Pérez, L.J.; Pujols, J.; Muñoz, M.; Muñoz, I.; Muñoz, S.; Abad, X.; Domingo, M.; et al. The impact of CSFV on the immune response to control infection. *Virus Res.* **2014**, *185*, 82–91. [CrossRef]

23. Wang, M.; Liniger, M.; Muñoz-González, S.; Bohórquez, J.A.; Hinojosa, Y.; Gerber, M.; López-Soria, S.; Rosell, R.; Ruggli, N.; Ganges, L. A Polyuridine Insertion in the 3' Untranslated Region of Classical Swine Fever Virus Activates Immunity and Reduces Viral Virulence in Piglets. *J. Virol.* **2019**, *94*. [CrossRef]

24. Muñoz-González, S.; Sordo, Y.; Pérez-Simó, M.; Suárez, M.; Canturri, A.; Rodriguez, M.P.; Frías-Lepoureau, M.T.; Domingo, M.; Estrada, M.P.; Ganges, L. Efficacy of E2 glycoprotein fused to porcine CD154 as a novel chimeric subunit vaccine to prevent classical swine fever virus vertical transmission in pregnant sows. *Vet. Microbiol.* **2017**, *205*, 110–116. [CrossRef] [PubMed]

25. Suradhat, S.; Damrongwatanapokin, S.; Thanawongnuwech, R. Factors critical for successful vaccination against classical swine fever in endemic areas. *Vet. Microbiol.* **2007**, *119*, 1–9. [CrossRef] [PubMed]

26. van Oirschot, J.T. Vaccinology of classical swine fever: From lab to field. *Vet. Microbiol.* **2003**, *96*, 367–384. [CrossRef] [PubMed]

27. Muñoz-González, S.; Pérez-Simó, M.; Muñoz, M.; Bohórquez, J.A.; Rosell, R.; Summerfield, A.; Domingo, M.; Ruggli, N.; Ganges, L. Efficacy of a live attenuated vaccine in classical swine fever virus postnatally persistently infected pigs. *Vet. Res.* **2015**, *46*, 78. [CrossRef]

28. Collins, C.L.; Pluske, J.R.; Morrison, R.S.; McDonald, T.N.; Smits, R.J.; Henman, D.J.; Stensland, I.; Dunshea, F.R. Post-weaning and whole-of-life performance of pigs is determined by live weight at weaning and the complexity of the diet fed after weaning. *Anim. Nutr.* **2017**, *3*, 372–379. [CrossRef]

29. Bohórquez, J.A.; Muñoz-González, S.; Pérez-Simó, M.; Revilla, C.; Domínguez, J.; Ganges, L. Identification of an Immunosuppressive Cell Population during Classical Swine Fever Virus Infection and Its Role in Viral Persistence in the Host. *Viruses* **2019**, *11*, 822. [CrossRef]

30. Schwarz, J.; Scheckenbach, V.; Kugel, H.; Spring, B.; Pagel, J.; Härtel, C.; Pauluschke-Fröhlich, J.; Peter, A.; Poets, C.F.; Gille, C.; et al. Granulocytic myeloid-derived suppressor cells (GR-MDSC) accumulate in cord blood of preterm infants and remain elevated during the neonatal period. *Clin. Exp. Immunol.* **2018**, *191*, 328–337. [CrossRef]

31. Rieber, N.; Gille, C.; Köstlin, N.; Schäfer, I.; Spring, B.; Ost, M.; Spieles, H.; Kugel, H.A.; Pfeiffer, M.; Heininger, V.; et al. Neutrophilic myeloid-derived suppressor cells in cord blood modulate innate and adaptive immune responses. *Clin. Exp. Immunol.* **2013**, *174*, 45–52. [CrossRef]

32. Serrano-Villar, S.; Moreno, S.; Fuentes-Ferrer, M.; Sánchez-Marcos, C.; Ávila, M.; Sainz, T.; de Villar, N.G.P.; Fernández-Cruz, A.; Estrada, V. The CD4: CD8 ratio is associated with markers of age-associated disease in virally suppressed HIV-infected patients with immunological recovery. *HIV Med.* **2014**, *15*, 40–49. [CrossRef]

33. Serrano-Villar, S.; Sainz, T.; Lee, S.A.; Hunt, P.W.; Sinclair, E.; Shacklett, B.L.; Ferre, A.L.; Hayes, T.L.; Somsouk, M.; Hsue, P.Y.; et al. HIV-Infected Individuals with Low CD4/CD8 Ratio despite Effective Antiretroviral Therapy Exhibit Altered T Cell Subsets, Heightened CD8+ T Cell Activation, and Increased Risk of Non-AIDS Morbidity and Mortality. *PLoS Pathog.* **2014**, *10*, e1004078. [CrossRef] [PubMed]

34. Dustin, L.B. Innate and Adaptive Immune Responses in Chronic HCV Infection. *Curr. Drug Targets* **2017**, *18*, 826–843. [CrossRef] [PubMed]

35. Gandhi, R.T.; McMahon, D.K.; Bosch, R.J.; Lalama, C.M.; Cyktor, J.C.; Macatangay, B.J.; Rinaldo, C.R.; Riddler, S.A.; Hogg, E.; Godfrey, C.; et al. Levels of HIV-1 persistence on antiretroviral therapy are not associated with markers of inflammation or activation. *PLoS Pathog.* **2017**, *13*, e1006285. [CrossRef] [PubMed]

36. Summerfield, A.; Ruggli, N. Immune responses against classical swine fever virus: Between ignorance and lunacy. *Front. Vet. Sci.* **2015**, *2*, 10. [CrossRef]

37. Smirnova, N.P.; Webb, B.T.; McGill, J.L.; Schaut, R.G.; Bielefeldt-Ohmann, H.; Van Campen, H.; Sacco, R.E.; Hansen, T.R. Induction of interferon-gamma and downstream pathways during establishment of fetal persistent infection with bovine viral diarrhea virus. *Virus Res.* **2014**, *183*, 95–106. [CrossRef]

38. Chen, J.; Liang, Y.; Yi, P.; Xu, L.; Hawkins, H.K.; Rossi, S.L.; Soong, L.; Cai, J.; Menon, R.; Sun, J. Outcomes of Congenital Zika Disease Depend on Timing of Infection and Maternal-Fetal Interferon Action. *Cell Rep.* **2017**, *21*, 1588–1599. [CrossRef]

39. Cabezón, O.; Muñoz-González, S.; Colom-Cadena, A.; Pérez-Simó, M.; Rosell, R.; Lavín, S.; Marco, I.; Fraile, L.; de la Riva, P.M.; Rodríguez, F.; et al. African swine fever virus infection in Classical swine fever subclinically infected wild boars. *BMC Vet. Res.* **2017**, *13*, 227. [CrossRef]

40. Lacasta, A.; Monteagudo, P.L.; Jiménez-Marín, Á.; Accensi, F.; Ballester, M.; Argilaguet, J.; Galindo-Cardiel, I.; Segalés, J.; Salas, M.L.; Domínguez, J.; et al. Live attenuated African swine fever viruses as ideal tools to dissect the mechanisms involved in viral pathogenesis and immune protection. *Vet. Res.* **2015**, *46*, 135. [CrossRef]

41. Alfonso, P.; Rivera, J.; Hernáez, B.; Alonso, C.; Escribano, J.M. Identification of cellular proteins modified in response to African swine fever virus infection by proteomics. *Proteomics* **2004**, *4*, 2037–2046. [CrossRef]

42. Wensvoort, G.; Terpstra, C.; Boonstra, J.; Bloemraad, M.; Zaane, D. Van Production of monoclonal antibodies against swine fever virus and their use in laboratory diagnosis. *Vet. Microbiol.* **1986**, *12*, 101–108. [CrossRef]

43. Reed, L.J.; Muench, H. A simple method of estimating fifty per cent endpoints. *Am. J. Hyg.* **1938**, *27*, 493–497.

44. Díaz De Arce, H.; Núñez, J.I.; Ganges, L.; Barrera, M.; Frías, M.T.; Sobrino, F. Molecular epidemiology of classical swine fever in Cuba. *Virus Res.* **1999**, *64*, 61–67. [CrossRef]

45. Postel, A.; Schmeiser, S.; Perera, C.L.; Pérez Rodríguez, L.J.; Frías-Lepoureau, M.T.; Becher, P. Classical swine fever virus isolates from Cuba form a new subgenotype 1.4. *Vet. Microbiol.* **2013**, *161*, 334–338. [CrossRef] [PubMed]

46. OIE Classical Swine Fever (Infection with Classical Swine Fever Virus). Available online: https://www.oie.int/fileadmin/Home/eng/Health_standards/tahm/3.08.03_CSF.pdf (accessed on 16 February 2020).

47. Leifer, I.; Blome, S.; Blohm, U.; König, P.; Küster, H.; Lange, B.; Beer, M. Characterization of C-strain "Riems" TAV-epitope escape variants obtained through selective antibody pressure in cell culture. *Vet. Res.* **2012**, *43*, 33. [CrossRef] [PubMed]

48. Mellor, D.J.; Diesch, T.J.; Gunn, A.J.; Bennet, L. The importance of "awareness" for understanding fetal pain. *Brain Res. Rev.* **2005**, *49*, 455–471. [CrossRef] [PubMed]

49. Ahrens, U.; Kaden, V.; Drexler, C.; Visser, N. Efficacy of the classical swine fever (CSF) marker vaccine Porcilis Pesti in pregnant sows. *Vet. Microbiol.* **2000**, *77*, 83–97. [CrossRef]

50. Tarradas, J.; Monsó, M.; Fraile, L.; de la Torre, B.G.; Muñoz, M.; Rosell, R.; Riquelme, C.; Pérez, L.J.; Nofrarías, M.; Domingo, M.; et al. A T-cell epitope on NS3 non-structural protein enhances the B and T cell responses elicited by dendrimeric constructions against CSFV in domestic pigs. *Vet. Immunol. Immunopathol.* **2012**, *150*, 36–46. [CrossRef]

51. Tarradas, J.; Argilaguet, J.M.; Rosell, R.; Nofrarías, M.; Crisci, E.; Córdoba, L.; Pérez-Martín, E.; Díaz, I.; Rodríguez, F.; Domingo, M.; et al. Interferon-gamma induction correlates with protection by DNA vaccine expressing E2 glycoprotein against classical swine fever virus infection in domestic pigs. *Vet. Microbiol.* **2010**, *142*, 51–58. [CrossRef]

52. Pérez, C.; Ezquerra, A.; Ortuño, E.; Gómez, N.; García-briones, M.; Martínez de la Riva, P.; Alonso, F.; Revilla, C.; Domínguez, J. Cloning and expression of porcine CD163: Its use for characterization of monoclonal antibodies to porcine CD163 and development of an ELISA to measure soluble CD163 in biological fluids. *Spanish J. Agric. Res.* **2008**, *6*, 59. [CrossRef]

Pathogenicity and Genetic Characterization of Vietnamese Classical Swine Fever Virus: 2014–2018

SeEun Choe [1,†], Van Phan Le [2,†], Jihye Shin [1], Jae-Hoon Kim [3], Ki-Sun Kim [1], Sok Song [1], Ra Mi Cha [1], Gyu-Nam Park [1], Thi Lan Nguyen [2], Bang-Hun Hyun [1], Bong-Kyun Park [1,4] and Dong-Jun An [1,*]

1   Viral Disease Division, Animal and Plant Quarantine Agency, Gimcheon, Gyeongbuk 39660, Korea; ivvi59@korea.kr (S.C.); shinjibong227@gmail.com (J.S.); kisunkim@korea.kr (K.-S.K.); ssoboro@naver.com (S.S.); rami.cha01@korea.kr (R.M.C.); changep0418@gmail.com (G.-N.P.); hyunbh@korea.kr (B.-H.H.); parkx026@korea.kr (B.-K.P.)
2   College of Veterinary Medicine, Vietnam National University of Agriculture, Hanoi 100000, Vietnam; letranphan@gmail.com (V.P.L.); nguyenlan@vnua.edu.vn (T.L.N.)
3   College of Veterinary Medicine and Veterinary Medical Research Institute, Jeju National University, Jeju 63243, Korea; kimjhoon@jejunu.ac.kr
4   College of Veterinary Medicine, Seoul University, Gwanak-ro, Gwanak-gu, Seoul 08826, Korea
*   Correspondence: andj67@korea.kr
†   These authors made an equal contribution to this work.

Abstract: Here, we examined the pathogenicity and genetic differences between classical swine fever viruses (CSFV) isolated on pig farms in North Vietnam from 2014–2018. Twenty CSFV strains from 16 pig farms were classified as genotype 2 (sub-genotypes 2.1b, 2.1c, and 2.2). The main sub-genotype, 2.1c, was classified phylogenetically as belonging to the same cluster as viruses isolated from the Guangdong region in South China. Strain HY58 (sub-genotype 2.1c), isolated from pigs in Vietnam, caused higher mortality (60%) than the Vietnamese ND20 strain (sub-genotype 2.2). The Vietnamese strain of sub-genotype 2.1b was estimated to have moderate virulence; indeed, genetic analysis revealed that it belongs to the same cluster as Korean CSFV sub-genotype 2.1b. Most CSFVs circulating in North Vietnam belong to sub-genotype 2.1c. Geographical proximity means that this genotype might continue to circulate in both North Vietnam and Southern China (Guangdong, Guangxi, and Hunan).

Keywords: CSFV; genotype; virulence; E2 gene; phylogenetic tree

1. Introduction

Classical swine fever virus (CSFV), which belongs to the genus *Pestivirus* within the family *Flaviviridae*, is an enveloped virus containing a single-stranded, positive-sense RNA genome of approximately 12.3 kb [1]. The virus causes a highly contagious disease in pigs, which results in significant economic losses to the pig industry both in Vietnam and worldwide. Depending on the strain, CSFV can cause an acute, subacute, chronic, or asymptomatic disease [2,3]. Highly virulent CSFV results in high morbidity and mortality, whereas low virulent CSFV may cause asymptomatic disease [2,3]. CSFV is categorized into three genotypes (1, 2, and 3), each comprising three to four sub-genotypes (1.1–1.4, 2.1–2.3, and 3.1–3.4) [4]. CSFV strains isolated in China during the 1990s clustered into sub-genotypes 1.1, 2.1, 2.2, and 2.3 [5]; however, the majority of CSFV strains belonged to either sub-genotype 2.1 (49.1%) or 2.2 (36.4%). In Vietnam, some pigs have been vaccinated against CSFV; however, a previous study suggested that antibody responses against the CSF vaccine was significantly reduced in Trypanosoma (T) evansi-infected pigs as compared to uninfected pigs.

This immunosuppression might explain the accounts of poor protection of CSF-vaccinated pigs reported in T. evansi endemic areas of Vietnam [6]. Genetic analysis of the 5' non-translated region (5' NTR) of CSFVs isolated in the Mekong delta area of South Vietnam between 2001 and 2003 showed that the strains clustered into two sub-genotypes: the majority clustered into sub-genotype 2.1, with the remainder clustering into sub-genotype 2.2 [7]. In Thailand, a country neighboring Vietnam, all three sub-genotypes (2.1, 2.2, and 2.3) were isolated throughout the 1980s and early 1990s, but sub-genotype 2.2 was the major isolate from 1996 onwards [8]. CSFVs isolated in the northern provinces of Laos (bordering Vietnam) between 1997 and 1999 belonged to sub-genotype 2.1, whereas most of those isolated in the southern provinces of Laos belonged to subgroup 2.2; CSFVs isolated in central provinces of Laos belonged to sub-genotypes 2.1 and 2.2 [9]. The geographical position of Vietnam makes it particularly vulnerable to CSF outbreaks because pigs come into the country across the borders with Cambodia, Laos, and China.

The objective of the present study was to examine the pathogenicity and phylogenetic genotypes of CSFVs circulating recently in northern Vietnam.

2. Results

2.1. Genotype Analysis and Phylogenetic Tree

The 20 CSFVs identified from samples collected from the 16 backyard pig farms in north Vietnam between 2014 to 2018 were categorized as group 2.1b (one farm), 2.1c (14 farms), and 2.2 (one farms) based on nucleotide sequence analysis of the complete E2 gene (Table 1 and Figures 1 and 2). Three strains (ND2, ND20 and ND21) belonged to sub-genotype 2.2, and an NA5 strain was classified as sub-genotype 2.1b; the 16 remaining strains were sub-genotype 2.1c (Table 1 and Figure 2).

The mean time of the most recent common ancestor (tMRCA) for the Vietnamese strains was estimated to be 1932 (95% highest posterior density (HPD): lower, 1917; upper, 1957), with an effective sample size (ESS) of 729.1967 on the maximum clade credibility (MCC) tree. The clock rate ($\times 10^{-4}$ substitutions/site/year) for Vietnamese strains was 8.49 (95% HPD: lower, 6.4415; upper, 10.589) (Figure 2). The phylogenetic tree suggested that strains belonging to sub-genotype 2.2 circulating in Vietnam are more closely related to strains isolated in European countries (Germany, Austria, the Czech Republic, and Italy) than to strains isolated in Asia (Taiwan, Nepal, and China) (Figure 2). The NA5 strain was on the sub-genotype 2.1b branch of the MCC tree and clustered with seven very similar strains (KSB06N01, YJB08B2, LSG03N46, SW03N8, CW02N13, MBG07N01, and KH2002N1) detected in Korea between 2002 and 2008 (Figure 2).

The 16 Vietnamese CSFV strains (sub-genotype 2.1c) were most similar to CSFV strains GXF29/2013, GDZH.2009, GDHZ.2009, HN.2010, HNLY-11, and GDPY.2008 isolated in the southern regions (Guangdong, Guangxi, and Hunan) of China; phylogenetic analysis placed them in the same cluster (Figure 2). The complete E2 gene sequence of Vietnamese CSFV identified herein was submitted to GenBank under accession numbers KP702206–KP702210, MF977825-MF977830, and MN977260-MN977268.

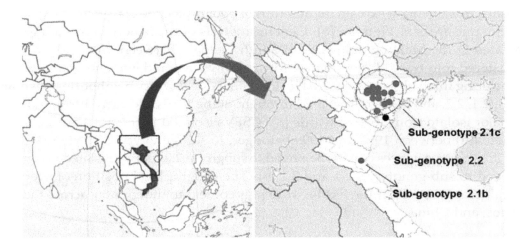

Figure 1. Map showing outbreaks of classical swine fever on pig farms in northern Vietnam. CSFV genotypes are denoted by the red circle (sub-genotype 2.1c), black circle (sub-genotype 2.2), and blue circle (sub-genotype 2.1b).

Table 1. Vietnamese strains of classical swine fever virus examined during the 5-year study.

Date of Collection	Place	Farm Name	Age of Sampled Pig	Strain	CSFV Genotype	Accession Number
June, 2014	[a] Nam Dinh	XTND	60	ND2	2.2	KP702207
June, 2014	[a] Nam Dinh	XTND	60	ND20	2.2	KP702209
June, 2014	[a] Nam Dinh	XTND	60	ND21	2.2	KP702210
June, 2014	[b] Nam Dinh	NDB	90	ND9	2.1c	KP702208
July, 2014	[c] Hai Duong	NGHD	30	HD1	2.1c	KP702206
Jan, 2015	Nghe An	NAN	30	NA5	2.1b	MF977825
June, 2015	Hung Yen	HYen	70	HY58	2.1c	MF977826
Sep, 2015	Hung Yen	HYen	70	HY78	2.1c	MF977827
Feb, 2016	Hung Yen	HYN	50	HY91	2.1c	MF977828
Mar, 2016	Hung Yen	HYY	60	HY92	2.1c	MF977829
Mar, 2016	Bac Giang	BGiang	61	BG47	2.1c	MF977830
Jul, 2017	Hung Yen	HYenI	30	C71	2.1c	MN977260
Aug, 2017	Hung Yen	HYenJ	30	C77	2.1c	MN977261
Aug, 2017	Hung Yen	HYenK	40	C83	2.1c	MN977262
Sep, 2017	Hung Yen	HYenJ	30	C91	2.1c	MN977263
Sep, 2017	Hung Yen	HYenL	60	C94	2.1c	MN977264
Sep, 2017	Hung Yen	HYenM	50	C97	2.1c	MN977265
Oct, 2018	Hung Yen	HYenN	30	P143	2.1c	MN977266
Nov, 2018	Nam Dinh	NDinhO	40	P166	2.1c	MN977267
Dec, 2018	Ha Nam	Ha NamP	40	P192	2.1c	MN977268

[a] Nam Dinh: Xuan Truong-Nam Dinh; [b] Nam Dinh: My Xa-Nam Dinh; [c] Hai Duong: Ninh Giang-Hai Duong.

2.2. Comparison of the Pathogenicity of Different Sub-Genotypes

Four of the five pigs in group 2, which were inoculated with the ND20 strain, survived for 30 days post-infection (dpi) (mortality, 20%); however, the mortality rate in pigs inoculated with the HY58 strain (group 3) was 60% (Table 2). The main clinical signs in pigs inoculated with the ND20 strain were fever, anorexia, and trembling; minor clinical signs included congestion, diarrhea, dehydration, and conjunctivitis. In addition to the clinical signs previously mentioned, pigs inoculated with the HY58 strain showed dehydration and hind leg paralysis (Table 2). The total mean clinical score at 21 dpi for pigs inoculated with ND20 and HY58 strains was 8.4 and 12.4, respectively (Table 3). According to the strain clinical sign scoring system, two Vietnamese strains (sub-genotypes 2.2 and 2.1c) were classified as having moderate virulence. At 7 days post-infection (dpi), the CSFV RNA copy number in the blood of pigs inoculated with the ND20 strain was lower (4.5–5.6 log$_{10}$) than that of pigs inoculated with the HY58 strain (5.6–6.8 log$_{10}$) (Table 2). At 0 to 21 dpi, leukocyte counts in pigs inoculated with the GPE$^-$ strain (control group) were stable (average 18673/ul and 22840/ul, respectively). Pigs inoculated with the ND20 strain showed leukopenia, with leucocyte counts of 9000/ul from 3 to 7 dpi, whereas pigs inoculated with the HY58 strain had leukopenia from 3 to 21 dpi (Figure 3A). Both ND20 and HY58 strain infected pigs showed high rectal temperature (>40 °C) at 5–7 dpi (Figure 3B).

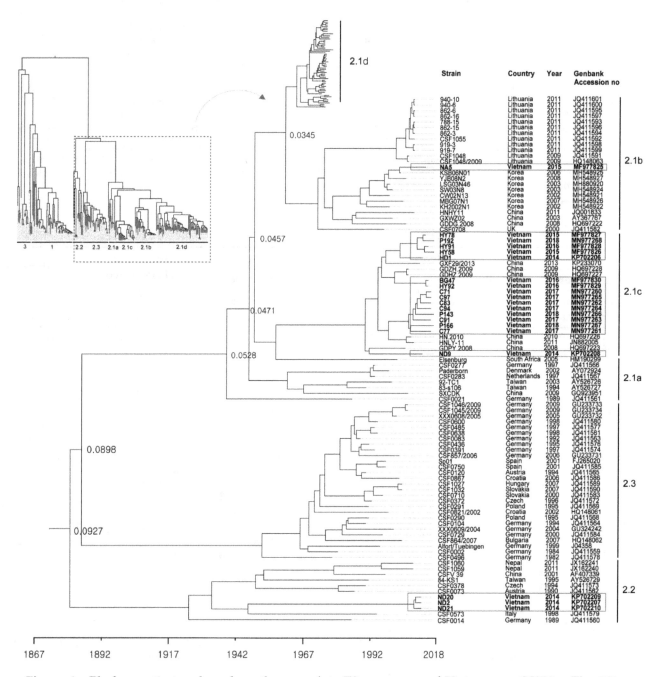

Figure 2. Phylogenetic tree based on the complete E2 sequences of Vietnamese CSFVs. The 171 complete E2 gene sequences, including those of 20 Vietnam strains, were obtained from the NCBI Genbank database. Each dataset was simulated using the following options: generation = 80,000,000; burn-in, 10%; and ESSs > 200. The confidence of the phylogentic analysis is represented by the numbers above the nodes representing branch length (time) based time scale by factor (1.0). Twenty Vietnamese strains are marked by blue boxes.

Table 2. CSFV RNA copy number in blood and clinical signs in pigs infected with CSFV.

Group	Pig No.	SG	[a] Strain	OP	DOP	[b] Clinical Signs	CSFV RNA Copy Number ($\log_{10}$) in Blood (Days of Post-Infection)						
							0	3	5	7	10	14	21
1	11	1.1	GPE⁻	30	alive	None	-	-	-	-	-	-	-
	12	1.1	GPE⁻	30	alive	None	-	-	-	-	-	-	-
2	7	2.2	ND20	30	alive	F, A, Di	-	3.6	5.3	5.6	3.2	3.5	2.7
	8	2.2	ND20	30	alive	F, A, T, Co	-	2.7	4.1	5.3	3.8	3.1	2.4
	9	2.2	ND20	30	alive	F, A, T, Di	-	3.0	5.5	5.1	3.3	4.2	1.8
	16	2.2	ND20	30	28	F, A, Di, T, C	-	3.4	5.8	5.4	4.5	2.5	2.9
	34	2.2	ND20	30	alive	F, A, T, C	-	2.5	4.9	4.5	2.7	2.6	1.7
3	21	2.1c	HY58	30	alive	F, A, De, T	-	3.2	5.7	5.9	5.2	3.5	3.7
	24	2.1c	HY58	30	22	F, A, Di, De, C, T	-	2.7	6.4	6.1	4.3	4.2	3.5
	29	2.1c	HY58	30	23	F, A, De, C, HP	-	2.9	6.1	6.8	5.7	5.3	3.7
	31	2.1c	HY58	30	alive	F, A, De, T, Co	-	3.3	4.7	5.6	5.8	4.2	2.6
	38	2.1c	HY58	30	25	F, A, Di, T, Co, HP	-	3.6	5.4	6.7	4.9	4.8	3.5

[a] Strain: an inoculation of virus ($4 \times 10^{5.0}$ TCID$_{50}$/mL/dose) was administered via the oral and intramuscular routes (half of the dose via each of these routes). SG: sub-genotype; OP: observation period (days); DOP: day of death during observation period. [b] Clinical signs were F (fever), A (anorexia), Di (diarrhea), De (dehydration), T (tremble), C (congestion), Co (conjunctivitis), and HP (hind leg paralysis).

Table 3. Clinical score of pigs infected with CSFV.

Parameter	Mean Clinical Sore (21 dpi)										Total Mean Clinical Score	Virulent
	*Li	BT	BS	Br	Wa	Sk	Ey	Ap	De	Le		
ND20 strain	0.8	0.2	0.5	0.8	0.8	0.9	1.0	1.5	0.5	1.4	8.4	moderate
HY58 strain	1.4	1.0	1.2	1.2	1.2	1.0	1.0	1.6	0.8	2.0	12.4	moderate

*Li: liveliness; BT: body tension; BS: body shape; Br: breathing; Wa: walking; Sk: skin; Ey: eyes; Ap: appetite; De: defecation; Le: leftovers in feeding trough.

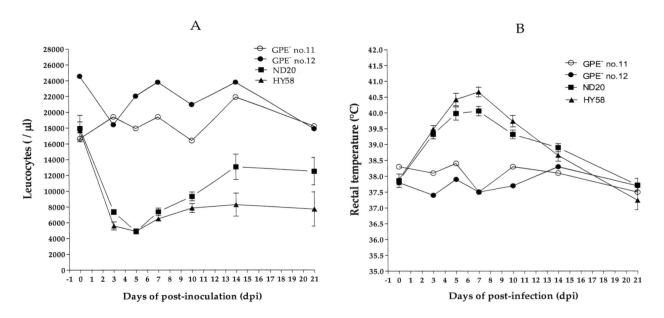

Figure 3. Leukocyte counts and rectal temperature of pigs inoculated with CSFV. Vietnamese strains inoculated group showed leukopenia and a high temperature. GPE⁻ vaccine control group was shown individually and other Vietnam CSFV groups shown as mean standard ± deviation. White blood cell count (**A**) and rectal temperature (**B**) were measured for 21 days post-infection.

2.3. Tissue Lesion Finding between Sub-Genotype 2.2 and 2.1c

Pigs inoculated with the CSFV ND20 strain (sub-genotype 2.2) showed histopathologic lesions in various organs. Multifocal hemorrhage or nonspecific mild bronchopneumonia was observed in the lungs. Mild to moderate infiltration of macrophages and reticular cells around lymphoid follicles and lymphoid depletion in follicles were observed in the tonsils. Dilated tonsillar crypts contained cellular debris, keratin, and neutrophils. In addition, the proliferation of reticular cells and macrophages and atrophy of lymphoid follicles were confirmed in the lymph nodes (Figure 4B). The liver showed signs of multifocal pericholangitis, characterized by mild-to-moderate infiltration in the portal triad by lymphocytes and macrophages. Mild chronic interstitial nephritis and multifocal infiltration by lymphocytes and plasma cells was observed in the kidney. Perivascular cuffing (PVC), characterized by mild-to-moderate infiltration of the perivascular space (Virchow Robin space), was observed in the brain parenchyma, arachnoid space, and glial nodules (Figure 4E). However, there were no specific CSFV-associated lesions in the heart, spleen, ileum, or urinary bladder. CSFV HY58 strain (sub-genotype 2.1c) inoculated pigs showed more pathologic lesions in various organs compared to ND 20 group. The tonsils showed moderate infiltration of reticular cells and macrophages around lymphoid follicles, and severe lymphoid depletion in the follicles. In addition, cystic-dilated tonsillar crypts were also plugged with degenerated cellular debris, inflammatory cells, and keratin. Typical peripheral hemorrhage, proliferation of macrophages, and severe lymphoid depletion were observed in the lymph nodes (Figure 4C). Atrophy of the splenic white pulp and histiocytic infiltration were observed, along with non-suppurative interstitial nephritis and pericholangitis in the kidney and liver. Moderate-to-severe lesions typical of viral non-suppurative encephalitis, characterized by severe PVC, formation of glial nodules, and neuronophagia, were observed throughout the brain parenchyma (Figure 4F). However, no specific lesions were observed in the heart, ileum, or urinary bladder. There were no pathognomonic lesions or very mild histopathologic changes in the internal organs from pigs inoculated with the GPE⁻ strain (Figure 4A,D). Occasionally very mild atrophy of white pulp in spleen and mild interstitial nephritis were detected from the GPE⁻ strain inoculated group.

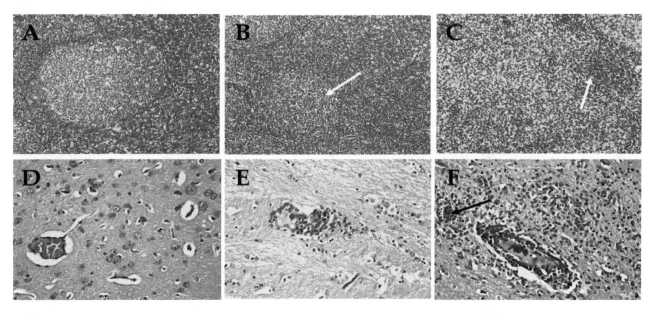

Figure 4. Histopathologic lesions in organs of pigs infected with GPE⁻ strain (**A,D**), Vietnamese CSFV ND20 strain (**B,E**) and HY58 strain (**C,F**). Nearly normal (A), mild (B, arrow), and severe (C, arrow) atrophy of follicle in lymph nodes of pigs (H&E stain; magnification × 200). Note focal hemorrhage and infiltration of macrophages (C). Normal brain parenchyma (D), mild perivascular cuffing (E), and severe PVC and glial nodule (F, arrow) in the brains of pigs (H&E stain; magnification × 400).

2.4. Immunohistochemical Staining for Sub-Genotypes 2.2 and 2.1c

In pigs inoculated with the ND20 strain (sub-genotype 2.2), immunohistochemical (IHC) analysis revealed specific CSFV antigens in 6 organs (lung, heart, spleen, tonsil, lymph nodes, and bladder) from animal (no. 16) dead at 28 dpi and in 3 organs (lymph nodes and ileum) from animal (no. 34) survived at 30 dpi (Tables 2 and 4). However, most CSFV antigens were detected in lymphoid tissues such as tonsil, lymph node, and spleen (Figure 5A–C). In addition, CSFV antigens by the IHC analysis of pigs inoculated with the HY58 strain (sub-genotype 2.1c) were detected in all organs including CNS from animal (no. 29) dead at 23 dpi and in 5 organs (lung, tonsil, lymph nodes, ileum, and bladder) from animal (no. 31) survived at 30 dpi (Tables 2 and 4 and Figure 5D–F). CSFV antigens were demonstrated not only in lymphoid tissues but also in other parenchyma including liver, urinary bladder, and brain. Histopathologically, CSFV antigens of pigs (no. 29 and no. 31) were observed in the cytoplasm of bronchial and bronchiolar epithelial cells in the lungs (Table 2 and Figure 5E), but focal deposits were observed in cardiac muscle cells in the heart of pig (no. 29) infected with the HY58 strain (Tables 2 and 4). In the brain of pig (no. 29) inoculated with the HY58 strain, viral antigens were observed within infiltrating lymphocytes in PVC lesions (Tables 2 and 3). QRT-PCR analysis of various organs from pigs inoculated with the ND20 strain detected a CSFV RNA copy number of 2.5 to 6.4 log $_{10}$ (Table 4). CSF RNA copy number in all organs of pigs inoculated with the HY58 strain was higher (2.1–6.6 log $_{10}$) than that in pigs infected with the ND20 strain (Table 4). The mean percentage ± SEM for CSF-positive organs of pigs infected with the ND20 strain and HY58 strain was 38.00% ± 9.638% and 72.00% ± 7.424%, respectively, the difference between two means was 34.00% ± 12.17% (Figure 6).

Table 4. The qRT-PCR and immunohistochemical staining results for various pig organs.

*G	Strain	Pig No.	CSF RNA Copy Number (log 10)/Foci Score									
			Lung	Heart	Liver	Spleen	Tonsil	LN	SI	Ki	Bl	CNS
1	GPE⁻	11	-	-	-	-	-	-	-	-	-	-
		12	-	-	-	-	-	-	-	-	-	-
2	ND20	7	-	-	-	3.3/*	4.5/*	-	-	4.3/*	3.1/*	-
		8	-	-	-	-	3.7/*	3.8/*	-	2.5/*	-	-
		9	-	-	-	4.1/*	4.9/*	3.1/*	-	-	-	-
		16	3.3/+	4.1/+	-	5.2/+	6.4/+++	6.2/++	-	3.7/-	3.8/+	-
		34	-	-	-	-	3.6/-	5.4/+	4.5/+	-	-	-
3	HY58	21	-	2.1/*	-	5.2/*	5.7/*	4.2/*	3.4/*	-	-	-
		24	4.4/*	-	-	4.1/*	5.9/*	4.6/*	-	3.8/*	4.8/*	-
		29	5.1/++	4.2/+	4.6/+	5.5/+	6.6/++	6.1/++	5.3/++	3.5/+	5.2/++	5.8/++
		31	4.7/+	-	-	3.7/-	6.2/++	5.9/+	4.8+	3.6/-	4.7/+	-
		38	3.5/*	-	3.4/*	4.8/*	5.2/*	-	3.9/*	4.6/*	3.1/*	4.5/*

*G: group. +: 1–3 foci/section, ++: 4–10 foci/section, +++: >10 foci/section. LN: lymph node; SI: small intestine; Ki: kidney; Bl: bladder; CNS: central nervous system. *: not tested.

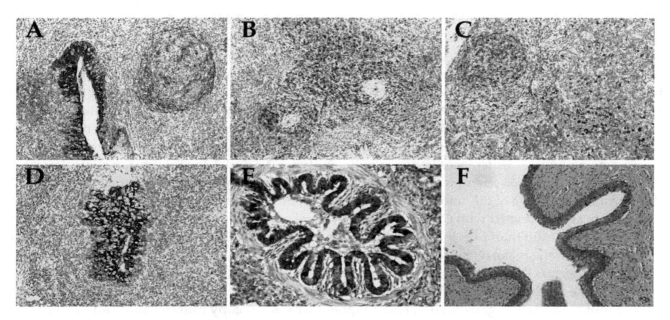

Figure 5. Immunohistochemical results in organs of pigs infected with the Vietnamese CSFV ND20 strain (**A–C**) and the HY58 strain (**D–F**). CSFV antigens were observed in the cryptal epithelium of the tonsils (A), infiltrated lymphocytes or macrophages of the spleen (B) and lymph nodes (C) of pigs with the ND20 strain (IHC; magnification × 200). Note CSFV antigens in the epithelial cells in the crypts of tonsil (D, IHC; × 200), the bronchiolar epithelium of the lung (E, IHC; × 400), and transitional epithelium of the urinary bladder (F, IHC; × 200) of pigs with the HY58 strain.

Pig oragns

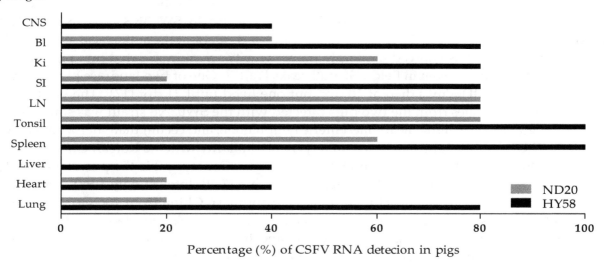

Percentage (%) of CSFV RNA detecion in pigs

Figure 6. Ratio of CSFV-positive antigen detection in organs. CSFV RNA detection percentage from each organs of pigs (n = 5) infected with the Vietnamese CSF ND20 strain (light bar) and HY58 strain (black bar) by the qRT-PCR. CNS: central nervous system; BI: bladder; Ki: kidney; SI: small intestine; LN: lymph node.

3. Discussion

The most common clinical signs of CSF worldwide over the last 30–40 years have changed from acute to subacute, chronic, or asymptomatic disease [10,11]. In general, highly virulent CSFV strains (e.g., ALD, Brescia/IVI, and Eystrup) have high rates of morbidity and mortality when infecting domestic pigs and wild boar, regardless of age [12]. However, CSFV strains with moderate-to-low virulence may cause low or moderate morbidity and low mortality, and the rates can vary according to age, weight, and breed. Highly virulent CSFV strains spread rapidly throughout the body and are shed via all types of secretion [13]. By contrast, excretion of low virulent strains occurs only via the oronasal route because these strains are restricted to specific target organs [13]. Previous studies suggest that this difference in secretion pattern between highly virulent strains and low virulent strains is due to virus tropism [3,13]. Genetic analysis of recent genotypes 2 and 3 suggests that they are less virulent than the old genotype 1. A phylodynamic study suggests that genotype 2 has emerged via an antigenic avoidance phenomenon because live attenuated CSF vaccines were based on genotype 1 [14]. Overall, we found that Vietnamese CSFV genotype 2 had moderate pathogenicity; however, there were some pathogenic differences between sub-genotypes 2.2 and 2.1c. Total mean clinical score of sub-genotype 2.1c (HY58 strain) was slightly higher than sub-genotype 2.2 (ND20 strain), even though they are all in the range of the "moderate" score. The overall histopathologic lesions (including lymph node and brain) associated with CSFV in this study were more frequent and severe in pigs inoculated with the HY58 strain than pigs inoculated with the ND20 strain. The antigenic distributions by the IHC staining analysis, correlated with histopathologic lesions, were also more wide and intense in the internal organs (lymphoid tissues, liver, urinary bladder, and brain) with the HY58 strain than those with the ND20 strain. The HY58 strain belonging to sub-genotype 2.1c caused higher mortality, caused more lesions in organs/tissues, had a higher CSFV RNA copy number, induced higher rectal temperatures, and caused more severe leukopenia than the ND20 strain (sub-genotype 2.2). Although the HY58 strain caused 60% mortality in 30-day-old pigs within 30 days after inoculation, we expect it to be less pathogenic in heavier and/or older pigs. Comparative genetic analysis between the ND20 (sub-genotype 2.2) and HY58 (sub-genotype 2.1c) strains isolated from Vietnam revealed sequence identities of 86.7% for the N^{pro} gene, 87.9% for the E^{rns} gene, 88.3% for the E1 gene, 86.1% for the E2 gene, 88.9% for the NS4B gene, and 86.1% for the NS5A gene [15]. The NA5 strain detected in the Nghe An region in north Vietnam in 2015 belonged to sub-genotype 2.1b, as did CSFV strains circulating among Korean domestic pigs from 2002 to 2009 [16]. The NA5 strain showed high sequence similarity with seven Korean CSFV strains (KSB06N01, YJB08B2, LSG03N46, SW03N8, CW02N13, MBG07N01, and KH2002N1): 96.7–99.5% at the nucleotide level and 97.3–99.5% at the amino acid level. The Korean sub-genotype 2.1b strains showed moderate pathogenicity when inoculated into pigs and did not show high pathogenicity, even in field CSF outbreaks [16,17]. One of two landrace pigs infected with strain SW03 ($10^{6.0}$TCID$_{50}$/mL) died at 18 dpi, but one lived until 21 dpi [17]. The viral RNA copy number in organs/tissues from the two pigs infected with the SW03N8 strain was somewhat lower ($10^{1.08-4.82}$ log$_{10}$) in tonsil, lung, heart, mesenteric lymph node, and cecum than that with the YC11WB strain [17]. Therefore, we think that based on its genetic similarity with the Korean CSFV sub-genotype 2.1b, the Vietnamese NA5 strain has moderate virulence. Genotype 2 is the prevalent genotype in countries (Cambodia, Laos, and Thailand) around Vietnam [7–9]. Interestingly, CSFV strains detected in the Guangdong, Guangxi, and Hunan regions in southern China from 2008 to 2013 are closely related to Vietnamese CSFV genotype 2.1c; indeed, genetic analysis revealed that they belonged to the same cluster. Therefore, it may be that direct and indirect transmission of CSFV occurred via livestock movements or livestock vehicle movements between the two countries. The phylogenetic tree suggests that sub-genotype 2.2 strains circulating in Vietnam are more closely related to strains isolated from European countries (Germany, Austria, the Czech Republic, and Italy) than to strains isolated in Asia (Taiwan, Nepal, and China). Here, we show that the complete E2 nucleotide sequence of strain ND20 is more similar to that of strains isolated from European countries (CSF0378, CSF0573, CSF0073, and CSF0014) (96.3–97.6%) than to that of strain 84-KS1 (96.1%) isolated from Taiwan [18], or to that of strain CSF1059 (94.1%) isolated from Nepal [19]. The finding that the Vietnamese strains within subgroup 2.2 are similar to strains isolated in Europe is interesting because it is unclear how they entered Vietnam; further genetic analyses of strains from neighboring countries (e.g., Cambodia, Laos, and China) may clarify this.

   In conclusion, sub-genotype 2.1c is the major genotype of CSFV in northern Vietnam, which is a geographically important location. Sub-genotype 2.1c, which is prevalent in northern Vietnam, has characteristics similar to those of strains isolated in the Guangdong, Guangxi, and Hunan regions in Southern China, suggesting that mutual exchange between the two regions will continue. The pathogenicity of genotype 2 in Vietnam is moderate, although that of sub-genotypes 2.1c is slightly higher than that of sub-genotype 2.2. Further genetic and pathogenic analyses of Vietnamese CSFV strains will help us to understand their characteristics, thereby enabling improved control strategies and policies for control of CSF in Vietnam.

4. Materials and Methods

4.1. Samples, RT-PCR, Phylogenetic Tree, and Virus Isolation

Blood samples from pigs (30–90 days old) with suspected CSF were collected from 16 pig farms from June 2014 to December 2018. Samples were collected from farms in Xuan Truong-Nam Dinh, Hi Duong, Nghe An, Hung Yen, Bac Giang, My Xa-Nam Dinh, and Ninh Giang-Hai Duong (Table 1 and Figure 1). None of the pigs on the 16 pig farms were vaccinated. Total RNA was extracted from blood using a micro column-based QIAamp Viral RNA Mini kit (Qiagen, USA) to identify CSFV. The RT-PCR conditions and specific primers used to amplify the complete E2 gene have been reported previously [4]. The complete E2 gene sequences of CSFVs (including the Vietnam strains examined in this study) were obtained from the NCBI GenBank database and aligned using the CLUSTAL X alignment program. Next, a BEAST input file was generated using BEAUti within BEAST package v1.8.1 [20]. Rates of nucleotide substitution per site per year and the tMRCA were estimated using a Bayesian MCMC approach. The exponential clock and expansion growth population model in the BEAST program was used to obtain the best-fit evolutionary model and the MCC tree was visualized using Figtree 1.4 [21]. For virus isolation, CSFV-positive blood samples were inoculated to porcine kidney 15 (PK-15) cell (grown to 80% confluence in 6-well plates) using alpha-minimum essential medium (GIBCO Cat. No. 12571-063) with L-glutamine (GIBCO Cat. No. 25030-081), sodium pyruvate (GIBCO Cat. No. 11360-070), and antibiotic-antimycotic solution (GIBCO Cat. No. 15240-062). The six-well plate (PK-15 cells) were inoculated for 3–5 days at 37 °C and the virus was identified by immunochemical staining using the CSFV monoclonal antibody 3B6 (Median Diagnostics Co., South Korea).

4.2. Animal Experiments

After virus inoculation, pigs were monitored to confirm the pathogenicity of two isolated sub-genotypes (2.2 and 2.1c). ND20 strain (sub-genotype 2.2) and HY58 strain (sub-genotype 2.1c) were each inoculated into pigs (30 days old) via two simultaneous administration (2 mL orally and 2 mL intramuscularly) ($10^{5.0}$ $TCID_{50}$/mL). GPE^- strain, a CSFV vaccine strain used in Japan, was inoculated via the same route and dose as a control. Pigs were divided into group 1 (n = 2, GPE^- strain), group 2 (n = 5, ND20 strain), and group 3 (n = 5, HY58 strain), and observed for 30 days. To detect CSFV RNA copies and to check for leukopenia (leucocyte counts below 9000/μL), blood samples were collected at 0, 3, 5, 7, 10, 14, and 21 dpi. During the course of the experiment, pigs were monitored daily for clinical signs (anorexia, diarrhea, dehydration, tremble, congestion, conjunctivitis, and hind leg paralysis). The clinical score was determined by ten parameters following previous procedure [22]. Briefly, ten parameters (liveliness, body tension, body shape, breathing, walking, skin, eyes, appetite, defecation, and leftovers in feeding trough) were graded according to the following scoring system: 0, normal; 1, slightly altered; 2, showing distinct clinical signs; and 3, showing severe CSF clinical signs. Virus strains were classified as highly virulent (total clinical score: >15), moderately virulent (5–15), low virulent (<5), or avirulent (0) [22]. Rectal temperature was checked at the time of blood collection. Pigs were necropsied and ten organs (lung, heart, liver, spleen, tonsil, lymph node, intestinal, kidney, bladder, and central nervous system) were examined to detect histopathologic lesions and the presence of CSFV antigens. Collected tissues were processed routinely for histopathologic examination and stained with hematoxylin and eosin (H&E). Mortality was calculated over the 30-day observation period.

4.3. Immunohistochemical Assay and qRT-PCR

IHC staining was performed as described previously [23,24]. CSF antigens derived from the ND20, HY58, and GPE⁻ strains were detected using DAB and the EnVision™ peroxidase-conjugated polymer reagent (DAKO, Denmark). The results were scored according to the strength of straining as follows: +: 1–3 foci/section, ++: 4–10 foci/section, +++: >10 foci/section. The CSF RNA copy number within the organs of pigs was measured using quantitative real-time PCR (qRT-PCR) and calculated as log 10/g. The AnyQ CSFV qRT-PCR (Median Diagnostic Co. Cat No. NS-CSF-31, Korea) system and TaqMan probes targeting the 5'-UTR region with high specificity were used. The reaction conditions for qRT-PCR have been reported previously [24]. IHC staining was performed on the pigs showing most severe or mild clinical signs of each group. Whereas, qRT-PCR was performed on all pigs of each group.

Author Contributions: Conceptualization, S.C., V.P.L., and D.-J.A.; methodology, K.-S.K., J.-H.K., S.S., R.M.C., J.S., G.-N.P., and T.L.N.; writing/review and editing, B.-H.H., B.-K.P., and D.-J.A. All authors have read and agreed to the published version of the manuscript.

References

1. Meyers, G.; Ruemenapf, T.; Thiel, H.J. Molecular cloning and nucleotide sequence of the genome of hog cholera virus. *Virology.* **1989**, *171*, 555–567. [CrossRef]
2. Moenning, V.; Floegel-Niesmann, G.; Greiser, W. Clinical signs and epidemiology of classical swine fever: A review of new knowledge. *Vet. J.* **2003**, *165*, 11–20. [CrossRef]
3. Brown, V.R.; Bevins, S.N. A review of classical swine fever virus and routes of introduction into the United States and the potential for virus establishment. *Front. Vet. Sci.* **2018**, *5*, 31. [CrossRef]
4. Paton, D.J.; Mcgoldrick, A.; Greiserwilke, A.; Parchariyanon, A.; Song, J.Y.; Liou, P.P.; Stadejek, T.; Lowings, J.P.; Bjorklund, H.; Belak, S. Genetic typing of classical swine fever virus. *Vet. Microbiol.* **2000**, *73*, 137–157. [CrossRef]
5. Tu, C.; Lu, Z.; Li, H.; Yu, X.; Liu, X.; Li, Y.; Zhang, H.; Yin, Z. Phylogenetic comparison of classical swine fever virus in China. *Virus Res.* **2001**, *81*, 29–37. [CrossRef]
6. Holland, W.G.; Do, T.T.; Huong, N.T.; Dung, N.T.; Thanh, N.G.; Vercruysse, J.; Goddeeris, B.M. The effect of Trypanosoma evansi infection on pig performance and vaccination against classical swine fever. *Vet. Parasitol.* **2003**, *111*, 115–123. [CrossRef]
7. Kamakawa, A.; Ho, T.V.; Yamada, S. Epidemiological survey of viral diseases of pigs in the Mekong delta of Vietnam between 1999 and 2003. *Vet. Microbiol.* **2006**, *118*, 47–56. [CrossRef]
8. Parchariyanon, S.; Inui, K.; Damrongwatanapokin, S.; Pinyochon, W.; Lowings, P.; Paton, D. Sequence analysis of E2 glycoprotein genes of classical swine fever viruses: Identification of a novel genogroup in Thailand. *Dtsch. Tierarztl. Wochenschr.* **2000**, *107*, 236–238.
9. Blacksell, S.D.; Khounsy, S.; Boyle, D.B.; Gleeson, L.J.; Westbury, H.A.; Mackenzie, J.S. Genetic typing of classical swine fever viruses from Lao PDR by analysis of the 5' non-coding region. *Virus Genes* **2005**, *31*, 349–355. [CrossRef]
10. Wensvoort, G.; Terpstra, C. Swine fever: A changing clinical picture. *Tijdschr Diergeneeskd.* **1985**, *110*, 263–269.
11. Koenen, F.; Van Caenegem, G.; Vermeersch, J.P.; Vandenheede, J.; Deluyker, H. Epidemiological characteristic of an outbreak of classical swine fever in an area of high pig density. *Vet. Rec.* **1996**, *12*, 367–371. [CrossRef]
12. Mayer, D.; Thayer, T.M.; Hofmann, M.A.; Tratschin, J.D. Establishment and characterization of two cDNA-derived strains of classical swine fever virus, one highly virulent and one avirulent. *Viurs Res.* **2003**, *98*, 105–116. [CrossRef]
13. Weesendrop, E.; Stegeman, A.; Loeffen, W. Dynamics of virus excretion via different routes in pigs experimentally infected with classical swine fever virus strain of high, moderated, or low virulence. *Vet. Microbiol.* **2009**, *133*, 9–22. [CrossRef]
14. Yoo, S.J.; Kwon, T.; Kang, K.; Kim, H.; Kang, S.D.; Richt, J.A.; Lyoo, Y.S. Genetic evolution of classical swine fever virus under immune environments conditioned by genotype 1-based modified live virus vaccine. *Transbound Emerg. Dis.* **2018**, *65*, 735–745. [CrossRef]

15. Kim, K.S.; Le, V.P.; Choe, S.; Cha, R.M.; Shin, J.; Cho, I.S.; Hung, N.P.; Thach, P.N.; Hang, V.T.T.; An, D.J. Complete genome sequences of classical swine fever virus subgenotype 2.1 and 2.2 strains isolated from Vietnamese pigs. *Microbiol. Resour. Announc.* **2019**, *8*, e01634-18. [CrossRef]

16. An, D.J.; Lim, S.I.; Choe, S.; Kim, K.S.; Cha, R.M.; Cho, I.S.; Song, J.Y.; Hyun, B.H.; Park, B.K. Evolutionary dynamics of classical swine fever virus in South Korea: 1987–2017. *Vet. Microbiol.* **2018**, *225*, 79–88. [CrossRef]

17. Lim, S.I.; Kim, Y.K.; Lim, J.A.; Han, S.H.; Hyun, H.S.; Kim, K.S.; Hyun, B.H.; Kim, J.J.; Cho, I.S.; Song, J.Y.; et al. Antigenic characterization of classical swine fever virus YC11WB isolates from wild boar. *J. Vet. Sci.* **2017**, *18*, 201–207. [CrossRef]

18. Postel, A.; Jha, V.C.; Schmeiser, S.; Becher, P. First molecular identification and characterization of classical swine fever virus isolates from Nepal. *Arch. Virol.* **2013**, *158*, 207–210. [CrossRef]

19. Pan, C.H.; Jong, M.H.; Huang, T.S.; Liu, H.F.; Lin, S.Y.; Lai, S.S. Phylogenetic analysis of classical swine fever virus in Taiwan. *Arch. Virol.* **2005**, *150*, 1101–1119. [CrossRef]

20. Drummond, A.J.; Suchard, M.A.; Xie, D.; Rambaut, A. Bayesian phylogenetics with BEAUti and the BEAST 1.7. *Mol. Bio. Evol.* **2012**, *29*, 1969–1973. [CrossRef]

21. Rambaut, A. FigFree. Tree Figure dra3wing Tool. 2012. Available online: https://www.semanticscholar.org/paper/Transatlantic-disjunction-in-fleshy-fungi.-II.-The-Petersen-Borovi%C4%8Dka/f8aeaf51c17f62a3c281961756b0c01b408340ba/figure/2 (accessed on 27 February 2020).

22. Mittelholzer, C.; Moser, C.; Tratschin, J.; Hofmann, M.A. Analysis of classical swine fever virus replication kinetics allows differentiation of highly virulent from avirulent strains. *Vet. Microbiol.* **2000**, *74*, 293–308. [CrossRef]

23. Choe, S.; Kim, J.H.; Kim, K.S.; Song, S.; Kang, W.C.; Kim, H.J.; Park, G.N.; Cha, R.M.; Cho, I.S.; Hyun, B.H.; et al. Impact of a Live Attenuated Classical Swine Fever Virus Introduced to Jeju Island, a CSF-Free Area. *Pathogens* **2019**, *20*, 8. [CrossRef]

24. Choe, S.; Kim, J.H.; Kim, K.S.; Song, S.; Cha, R.M.; Kang, W.C.; Kim, H.J.; Park, G.N.; Shin, J.; Jo, H.N.; et al. Adverse Effects of Classical Swine Fever Virus LOM Vaccine and Jeju LOM Strains in Pregnant Sows and Specific Pathogen-Free Pigs. *Pathogens* **2019**, *23*, 9. [CrossRef]

Classical Swine Fever Virus Biology, Clinicopathology, Diagnosis, Vaccines and a Meta-Analysis of Prevalence

Yashpal Singh Malik [1,*], Sudipta Bhat [1], O. R. Vinodh Kumar [2], Ajay Kumar Yadav [3], Shubhankar Sircar [1], Mohd Ikram Ansari [1], Dilip Kumar Sarma [4], Tridib Kumar Rajkhowa [5], Souvik Ghosh [6] and Kuldeep Dhama [7,*]

[1] Division of Biological Standardization, ICAR-Indian Veterinary Research Institute, Izatnagar, Bareilly, Uttar Pradesh 243001, India; sudiptabhat1991@gmail.com (S.B.); shubhankar.sircar@gmail.com (S.S.); mohd.ikram.ansari@gmail.com (M.I.A.)

[2] Division of Epidemiology, ICAR-Indian Veterinary Research Institute, Izatnagar, Bareilly, Uttar Pradesh 243122, India; vinodhkumar.rajendran@gmail.com

[3] Animal Health, ICAR-National Research Centre on Pig (ICAR-NRCP), Guwahati, Assam 781015, India; dr.ajayyadav07@gmail.com

[4] Department of Veterinary Microbiology, Assam Agricultural University, Khanapara, Guwahati 781022, India; dksarma1956@gmail.com

[5] College of Veterinary Sciences & Animal Husbandry, Central Agricultural University, Selesih, Aizawl, Mizoram 796001, India; tridibraj09@gmail.com

[6] Department of Biomedical Sciences, One Health Center for Zoonoses and Tropical Veterinary Medicine, Basseterre, St. Kitts PO Box 334, West Indies; sghosh@rossvet.edu.kn

[7] Division of Pathology, ICAR-Indian Veterinary Research Institute, Izatnagar, Bareilly, Uttar Pradesh 243122, India

[*] Correspondence: malikyps@gmail.com (Y.S.M.); kdhama@rediffmail.com (K.D.);

Abstract: Classical swine fever (CSF) is an economically significant, multi-systemic, highly contagious viral disease of swine world over. The disease is notifiable to the World Organization for Animal Health (OIE) due to its enormous consequences on porcine health and the pig industry. In India, the pig population is 9.06 million and contributes around 1.7% of the total livestock population. The pig industry is not well organized and is mostly concentrated in the eastern and northeastern states of the country (~40% of the country's population). Since the first suspected CSF outbreak in India during 1944, a large number of outbreaks have been reported across the country, and CSF has acquired an endemic status. As of date, there is a scarcity of comprehensive information on CSF from India. Therefore, in this review, we undertook a systematic review to compile and evaluate the prevalence and genetic diversity of the CSF virus situation in the porcine population from India, targeting particular virus genes sequence analysis, published reports on prevalence, pathology, and updates on indigenous diagnostics and vaccines. The CSF virus (CSFV) is genetically diverse, and at least three phylogenetic groups are circulating throughout the world. In India, though genotype 1.1 predominates, recently published reports point toward increasing evidence of co-circulation of sub-genotype 2.2 followed by 2.1. Sequence identities and phylogenetic analysis of Indian CSFV reveal high genetic divergence among circulating strains. In the meta-analysis random-effects model, the estimated overall CSF prevalence was 35.4%, encompassing data from both antigen and antibody tests, and region-wise sub-group analysis indicated variable incidence from 25% in the southern to nearly 40% in the central zone, eastern, and northeastern regions. A country-wide immunization approach, along with other control measures, has been implemented to reduce the disease incidence and eliminate the virus in time to come.

Keywords: classical swine fever virus; CSFV; swine; genome; phylogeny; diversity; immunobiology; diagnosis; vaccines; publication bias; prevalence; meta-analysis; India

---

1. Introduction

Classical swine fever (CSF), also known as hog cholera or more commonly swine fever, is a systemic, extremely contagious, and notifiable disease of viral origin affecting domestic and wild pigs [1]. The causative agent, the classical swine fever virus (CSFV), belongs to the genus *Pestivirus* in the family *Flaviviridae*. This genus also contains Bovine viral diarrhea virus (BVDV-1, 2), Border disease virus, Bungowannah virus, and HoBi-like virus. The disease was first reported in the year 1833 from the state of Ohio in the United States, and thereafter, the virus was identified in 1904 [2]. The incubation period in CSF disease varies between 3 and 10 days, and the course of the disease is influenced by the virulence of the virus and the age of the animals. CSF is characterized by several clinicopathological signs such as high fever (>40 °C), conjunctivitis, respiratory signs, constipation and/or diarrhea, skin hemorrhages, lethargy, and neurological symptoms like convulsions, clumsy movements, and staggering gait of infected animals. The disease in pregnant sows manifests abortions, stillbirths, mummified fetuses, and malformations [3]. CSF can cause high mortalities and morbidities in porcine populations, inflicting devastating economic losses and severely impacting the socio-economic conditions of pig farmers. The disease spreads by direct contact between pigs or through contaminated feed (swill feeding) and water, fomites, farm equipment, transport vehicle, and visitors. Moreover, the disease can also spread through infected boar semen, artificial insemination, and/or coitus. A characteristic feature of CSFV in infected pigs is noticeable immuno-suppression, including the depletion/reduction of B-lymphocytes and T-lymphocytes [4].

Disease outbreaks at regular intervals in endemic geographical regions, as well as preventive and vaccination costs to combat the virus, have great economic consequences, as the disease impacts pig breeding, national and international trade of pigs, and pork production. Because the disease has a tremendous impact on the pig industry, which ultimately affects the economy of both developed and developing countries, CSF is notifiable to the OIE, the World Organization for Animal Health [5]. Along with informing the higher authorities, there must be some standard procedures on culling methods of infected pig herds and biosecurity measures for the non-infected herds. The prohibition of trading of any pork meat products from the CSF endemic country to the disease-free region is an essential part of the strategy of control. The only effective measure to control/eradicate the disease is by way of following the vaccination strategy with cell-culture-adapted live attenuated vaccine. To control the disease, strict biosecurity guidelines and vaccination strategies have been adopted by many CSF endemic countries as part of control programs. The systematic/disciplined implementation of the vaccines, along with the coordinated control measures, could result in the eradication/elimination of the disease from both domestic and wild boar (natural reservoir) population. The CSF vaccine's manufacturing relies on the procedures outlined in the OIE Manual of Diagnostic Tests and Vaccines for Terrestrial Animals, ensuring the production of safe and effective vaccines [6]. The Chinese (C) strain of the CSFV is a conventionally and frequently used strain for the manufacture of the vaccine globally. The C-strain-based vaccines are acclaimed highly safe and effective against the disease [7]. Recently, an indigenous CSFV isolate cell culture-based vaccine has also been developed in India. The CSF is endemic in the country, and wide variations in its prevalence are noted since its first report in 1944.

In India, the pig population is 9.06 million and shares about 1.7% of the cumulative livestock data as per the recent livestock census (20th national livestock census). Here, the pig population is mostly concentrated in the northeastern (NE) states. The average number of pigs per household is around 4.03, indicating that most of the piggery sector is maintained under a backyard condition. The number of organized farms maintaining pigs in India is less than 5000, with 100 to 2000 pigs per farm. The recent 20th Livestock Census revealed that 90.27% of the pig population is in rural India and 9.73% of pig population is reared in urban settings. The first CSF case in India was reported during 1944 in northern parts, Uttar Pradesh [8], trailed by outbreaks in West Bengal (eastern parts), and Andhra Pradesh (southern parts) during 1951 and 1959, respectively. Subsequently, a report on CSF appeared from central parts of the country, Maharashtra [9].

In this review, we intend to provide a systematic review of the prevalence and genetic diversity of the CSF virus situation in the porcine population in India, targeting complete virus genome sequence analysis, published reports on prevalence, pathology, and updates on indigenous diagnostics and vaccines from an Indian perspective.

2. CSFV Genome and Classification

The CSFV is a member of the genus *Pestivirus* in the family *Flaviviridae* [5]. Recently, pestivirus species are renamed and classified as Pestivirus A to K, like Bovine viral diarrhea virus (BVDV)-1 named as Pestivirus A, BVDV-2 as Pestivirus B, CSFV as Pestivirus C, and so on [10].

The CSFV genome comprises a single-stranded positive-sense RNA, of nearly 12.3 kb in length [11]. The genomic RNA is infectious because it is a positive sense and possesses a single open reading frame (ORF) with a flanked non-translated region at both the ends of the genome (5'-UTR and 3'-UTR). The ORF encodes a single polyprotein, and further downstream, processing of this polyprotein by viral and cellular enzymes generates four structural (C, E^{rns}, E1, and E2) and eight/nine non-structural (N^{pro}, p7, NS2-3, NS2, NS3, NS4A, NS4B, NS5A, and NS5B) proteins [12,13].

3. Phylogenetic and Sequence Analysis of Indian CSFV Isolates

Three genomic locations (3'end of the NS5B polymerase gene (RdRp), 5' untranslated region (5'UTR), and E2 glycoprotein genes) are recognized to classify CSFV isolates as well as to know genetic relatedness and phylogenetic tree placements. As of now, CSFV strains are categorized in three genotypes and 3–4 subgenotypes [14,15]: (i) Genotype 1: four subgenotypes (1.1/1.2/1.3/1.4), (ii) Genotype 2: three subgenotypes (2.1/2.2/2.3), and (iii) genotype 3: four subgenotypes (3.1/3.2/3.3/3.4) [15,16]. Genotype 1 mainly contains historical strains of the virus that were retrieved globally and that contained the in-use live-attenuated vaccine strains. Genotype 2 CSFVs have been spreading since the 1980s with increasing prevalence and epidemic infections all over the world, along with two subgenotypes, namely CSFV 2.1 and 2.2, where subgenotype 2.1 is further split into 2.1a and 2.1b [17–20]. Due to the high genetic diversity among genotype 2, a few reports further suggest splitting of subgenotype 2.1 into 2.1a–2.1j [18,21]. The CSFV strains of genotype 3 are primarily found in different European and Asian (Thailand, Taiwan, Japan, Korea) regions [17]. However, all these genotypes have been reported in Asian countries [15,17].

3.1. CSFV Complete Genome Based Phylogenetic Analysis and Percent Similarity

We performed the phylogenetic and sequence distance analysis on 53 CSFV complete genome sequences retrieved from different Asian countries, including 14 whole-genome sequences of CSFV from India and representatives of other genotypes/subgenotypes from other countries. These sequences were retrieved from NCBI GenBank (https://www.ncbi.nlm.nih.gov/genbank/) and aligned using ClustalW in MEGA 6.0 software (Phoenix, AZ, USA) (available online: http://www.megasoftware.net/). Phylogenetic analysis was completed following the Maximum Likelihood method (1000 bootstrap replicates) [21]. The pair-wise similarity among the nucleotide sequences was calculated, and for aligning the sequences by the ClustalW program in high-speed Multiple Alignment using Fast Fourier Transform (MAFFT) online software program from the EBI website was used (https://www.ebi.ac.uk/Tools/msa/mafft/) [22].

In the phylogenetic analysis of complete genomes of the representative CSFV isolates of major genotypes, two major clades were identified, one containing genotype 1 (1.1) and the other containing genotype 2 (2.1 and 2.2) (Figure 1). Genetic divergence among the circulating Indian CSFV strains was observed, which belongs to the subgenotype 1.1, and the results are evident in their phylogenetic clustering pattern. Indian CSFV 1.1 strains were distributed in different branches inside the 1.1 clade, among which two strains (Accession no. EU857642 and MK405703) formed separate branching near Chinese isolates whereas four strains (Accession no. KM262189, MN128600, MH734359, and KC503764) from India clustered separately near a Thailand isolate. One Indian strain (Accession no. KY860615) clustered alongside South Korean strains. In subgenotype 2.2, all the Indian CSFV strains appeared distributed in several branches inside the same clade. One of the Indian CSFV strains from the state of Haryana (Accession no. MK405702) appeared to be independent inside the clade 2.2. A single strain of subgenotype 2.1 from India seemed to be divergent and appeared distantly from isolates of other countries. Apart from genotypes circulating in India, the other reported genotypes worldwide (1.2, 1.3, 1.4, 2.3, 3.2, and 3.4) constituted their respective independent clades. It is significant to note that the data set does not include two underrepresented genotypes (3.1 and 3.3) where searching of the previous literature could not reveal any accession number associated with these two subgenotypes.

Previous CSFV detection and genotyping reports from India revealed the historical prevalence of subgenotype 1.1 along with current increasing evidence and co-circulation of subgenotype 2.2 followed by 2.1 [20]. Genotype 1 contains highly virulent strains and vaccine strains, whereas genotype 2 and 3 refer to the comparatively moderately virulent strains [15]. Therefore, the changing pattern may be because of vaccine pressure [19]. The emergence of CSFV genotype 2 has already been documented in other countries like Europe, China, and Taiwan [14,17,23]. Although in India, to date, genotype 1.1 is most prevalent , analysis of genotype 2.2 has been done from a limited state only [24–27]. Therefore, the hypothesis of switching of prevalent genotypes needs further studies [26,27]. The analysis of archived sequences of Indian origin CSFV, partial or complete genome, also indicates the maximum prevalence of genotype 1.1. Notably, the phylogenetic patterns retrieved targeting the full-length (1119 bp) E2 gene of all CSFV isolates from India are similar to the whole genome-based phylogeny, suggesting that either the whole CSFV genome or E2 gene-targeted phylogeny can be used for typing and analysis of the circulating virus genotypes/subgenotypes.

As there are many Indian sequences available for CSFV 1.1 and 2.2, we have calculated the nucleotide (nt) similarity within the Indian strains (Table 1). Whole genome-based nucleotide similarity within Indian 1.1 strains was found to be between 92.075% and 96.38%, whereas it was between 83.425 and 84.99% within the whole genome of Indian 2.2 strains. The nucleotide identity of a single isolate of subgenotype 2.1 from India was 90.84%, 91.33%, 90.13%, 91.83% and 90.88% with South Korean, Mongolian, Vietnamese, Taiwanese and Japanese isolates, respectively. Whereas it ranged between 90.65% and 91.35% with Chinese isolates of 2.1 specificity.

3.2. Sequence Percent Homology Similarity Index of Other CSFV Gene Targets

The sequence percentage similarity of E2 and NS5B genes and 5'UTR between Indian isolates of subgenotype 1.1, 2.1, and 2.2 is given in Table 1. The percentage similarity between Indian isolates of subgenotype 1.1 is 89.2%–99.8% based on the E2 gene, 92%–99.8% based on NS5B gene, and 93.9%–98.2% based on the 5'UTR (Table 1). The higher similarity (90.7%–99.8% at nucleotide levels) of the CSFV 1.1 strains to the South Korean strain is notable as of the geographic distance, and it could possibly be due to the uses of the bovine kidney adapted CSFV vaccine imported from Korea. However, these assumptions need further detailed investigations.

Whereas, Indian 2.2 subgenotype showed similarity between 95.9% and 98.4% for E2 gene, 92.6% and 99.6% for NS5B gene, and 91% and 97.4% for 5' UTR. As there was only a single isolate present for 2.1 subgenotype from India, its nucleotide percentage similarity was assessed with other countries 2.1 subgenotype isolates based on E2 and NS5B genes and 5'UTR. The Indian CSFV subgenotype 2.1 has shown highest similarity range of 84.2%-86.5% with Chinese CSFV strains, 89.3%–89.9% with Taiwanese, and 88.7%–95% with Chinese strains for E2 and NS5B genes, and 5'UTR, respectively.

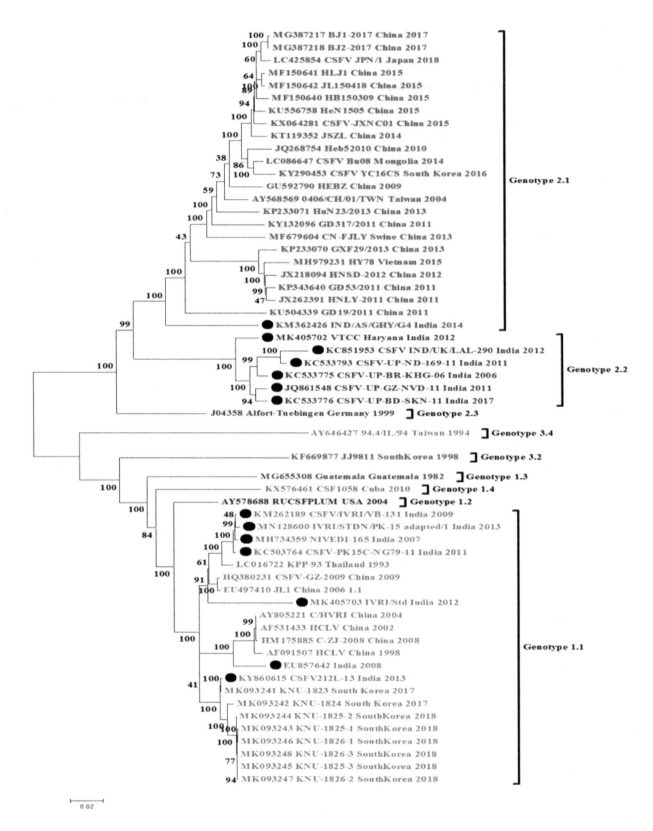

Figure 1. Phylogenetic analysis of Asian classical swine fever virus (CSFV) strains based on the complete genome. The different genotypes used in the current study are depicted in different color codes, and Indian CSFV strains are designated in solid black dots. Phylogenetic analysis was achieved following the Maximum Likelihood method (1000 bootstrap replicates) based on the General Time Reversible model in MEGA 6 software (v 6.06, Phoenix, AZ, USA).

Table 1. Nucleotide percent similarity based on whole genome, E2, NS5B genes, and 5′UTR of Indian CSFV strains with isolates from different Asian countries.

CSFV Genotype	Gene/Target	Country	Nt Similarity (%) India
CSFV 1.1	Whole Genome	India	92.07–96.38
		China	94.8–98.16
		South Korea	93.15–99.88
	E2	India	89.2–99.8
		China	90.1–97.5
		South Korea	90.7–99.8
	NS5B	India	92–99.8
		China	92.1–97.6
		South Korea	93.1–99.1
	5′ UTR	India	93.9–98.2
		China	91–96.8
		South Korea	91.6–98.4
CSFV 2.2	Whole Genome	India	83.42–84.99
	E2	India	95.9–98.4
	NS5B	India	92.6–99.6
	5′ UTR	India	91–97.4
CSFV 2.1	Whole Genome	South Korea	90.84
		China	90.65–91.35
		Mongolia	91.33
		Vietnam	90.13
		Taiwan	91.83
		Japan	90.88
	E2	South Korea	84.2–85.4
		China	84.2–86.5
		Mongolia	84.4–85.7
		Vietnam	83.7—84.8
		Taiwan	85.1–86.3
		Japan	84.3–85.6
	NS5B	South Korea	88.9–89.1
		China	88.5–89.7
		Mongolia	89–89.3
		Vietnam	87.9–88.1
		Taiwan	89.3–89.9
		Japan	88.7–89.2
	5′ UTR	South Korea	90–93.4
		China	88.7–95
		Mongolia	89.4–92.6
		Vietnam	89.4–91.8
		Taiwan	90.8–94.2
		Japan	62–63.1

4. Meta-Analysis of CSF Prevalence in India

The current meta-analysis study of CSF presents more comprehensive data compared to previous studies from India [26,27]. Additionally, CSF meta-analysis in the present study compared different diagnostic test-wise prevalence and identified the outlier and influential studies [28,29]). The basic idea to employ meta-analysis was to comprehend the scattered information on CSF disease prevalence in India over the time interval of nearly two decades. We performed a published article search to recognize all peer-reviewed articles documenting the prevalence of CSF in India using electronic databases like PubMed, ScienceDirect, Scopus, Indianjournals.com, J-Gate @Consortium of e-Resources in Agriculture (CeRA), Google Scholar, Springer, and handpicked publications (2001–2018). The keywords used for the search were CSF, India, swine, prevalence, pig, and epidemiology. All the articles on CSF prevalence in India were collected, and the Quality criteria were developed using MOOSE (Meta-analysis of Observation Studies in Epidemiology) and PRISMA (Preferred Reporting Items for Systematic Reviews) protocol. Screening at title and abstract level followed by full-text screening, data extraction, and quality assessment, were also carried out before starting the review of full papers.

All the individual studies were reviewed and screened manually by two investigators independently using both inclusion and exclusion criteria, and the third investigator resolved the discrepancy between the two investigators. The PRISMA protocol is depicted in Figure 2. The included publication was extracted into the author's name, article title, year of publication, sample size, number of positives, study area, study year, and diagnosis method used. From the 323 papers screened (from 1980 to 2018), 23 (from 2011–2019) publications were incorporated in the systematic review and meta-analysis. The proportion for CSF prevalence was carried out using 23 studies with 79 strata level data with a total sample size of 14,123. The publication year was classified into two intervals: 2011–2015 and 2016–2019. The states which reported the prevalence of CSF were categorized into the following six regions: (i) Northern region—Jammu and Kashmir, Punjab, Uttar Pradesh, Uttarakhand; (ii) Eastern region—West Bengal, Odisha, Bihar, Jharkhand; (iii) Northeast Region—Assam, Tripura, Meghalaya, Nagaland; (iv) Western region—Rajasthan, Gujarat, Maharashtra, (v) Central region—Madhya Pradesh, Chhattisgarh; and (vi) Southern region—Kerala, Tamil Nadu, undivided Andhra Pradesh, Karnataka. The studies included in the analysis used diagnostic techniques such as AGID, ELISA, I-ELISA, S-ELISA, and RT–PCR. The details of the included studies are given in Supplementary Materials.

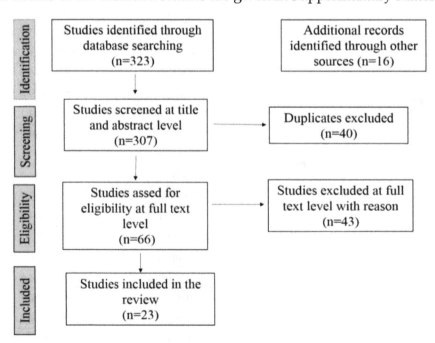

Figure 2. Schematic diagram showing the PRISMA (Preferred Reporting Items for Systematic Reviews) chart for the studies from India on classical swine fever (CSF) prevalence.

Summary reports on CSF prevalence were performed by using descriptive statistics. Between-study heterogeneity was assessed graphically by visual inspection of the Baujat plot [28] and quantified by Higgin's I^2 and Cochran's Q method. The meta-analysis was completed through a random effect (RE) model using the inverse-variance model [29,30]. The pooled estimate was measured and described as prevalence, with point and 95% confidence intervals (CI). Forest plots were employed to identify the prevalence in each study and the collectively estimated prevalence. Publication bias was assessed graphically by visual inspection of the funnel plot, and the Egger method [31,32]. A set of case deletion diagnostics such as studentized residuals, the difference in fits values (DFFITS), Cook's distances, COVRATIO, and leave-one-out estimates, for the amount of heterogeneity as well as the test statistic for heterogeneity, were used to identify the influential studies [33]. The sensitivity analysis was carried out with and without the exclusion of influential studies to verify the robustness of the study design, sample size, study conclusions, and the effect of missing data. Subgroup analysis was conducted to identify the stratified prevalence in different regions, study period, diagnostic tests, and species Table 2). The R statistical platform (R Foundation for Statistical Computing, Vienna, Austria version 3.5.1 with "meta" package (version 4.9-2) and "metafor" package (version 2.0-0) was employed for statistical analyses.

Table 2. Details of the sub-group analysis for seroprevalence of CSF in India.

S. No	Variables		Samples Tested	Positive Samples	Pooled Estimate (RE) (95% CI)	Pooled Estimate (FE) (95% CI)	p-Value	I^2 Value	Tau Square
1.	Geographic region	Northern India	2569	272	30% (14%–50%)	8% (7%–9%)	<0.01	99%	0.05
		Western India	332	145	37% (8%–73%)	39% (34%–45%)	<0.01	98%	0.22
		Central India	593	302	42% (24%–61%)	51% (47%–55%)	<0.01	94%	0.04
		Southern India	3661	883	25% (18%–33%)	22% (21%–23%)	<0.01	95%	0.03
		Eastern India	54	28	41% (10%–75%)	52% (37%–66%)	<0.01	80%	0.09
		North Eastern India	6064	2678	40% (29%–51%)	43% (41%–44%)	<0.01	98%	0.07
		India	1207	786	72% (54%–87%)	65% (63%–68%)	<0.01	95%	0.01
2.	Serological test	ELISA	9224	3200	30% (22%–38%)	31% (30%–32%)	0.00	98%	0.08
		RT–PCR	1988	423	33% (8%–64%)	17% (15%–18%)	< 0.01	99%	0.10
		S-ELISA	357	27	52% (0%–100%)	4% (2%–7%)	< 0.01	97%	0.63
		AGID	196	136	60% (18%–95%)	71% (64%–77%)	<0.01	97%	0.09
		I-ELISA	2605	1253	61% (42%–78%)	48% (46%–50%)	<0.01	99%	0.07
		IIP	110	65	59% (50%–68%)	59% (50%–68%)	NA	NA	NA
3.	Study period	2011-15	9019	2356	36% (28%–43%)	21% (20%–22%)	0.00	98%	0.07
		2016-19	5461	2738	35% (24%–47%)	50% (48%–51%)	<0.01	98%	0.06

From the 323 publications screened (from 1980 to 2019), 23 papers (2011–2019) were incorporated in the systematic review and meta-analysis. The other publication before 2011 reported mainly outbreaks and ambiguous samples and diagnostic tests. Hence, most of such studies were excluded from the analysis. From 23 papers, 79 strata level data were extracted. For example, the survey by NIVEDI (2008) was obtained into four strata levels representing different regions where the study was performed.

A meta-analysis of these studies showed significant variability/heterogeneity (Q = 8869.91) between the studies, and the between-study variance (Tau square) was as 0.08. The RE model revealed better symmetry than the fixed effect (FE) model and indicated that the RE model is a better one. Sub-group analysis showed a significant heterogeneity (I^2 indices > 90%, p-values < 0.01) was noticed for all subgroups. In funnel plot identified publication bias (Figure 3) and due to significant publication bias ($p = 0.41$), the RE model results were considered. The Baujat plot showed that the studies that contributed to overall heterogeneity were two, and no study was identified as an influential study.

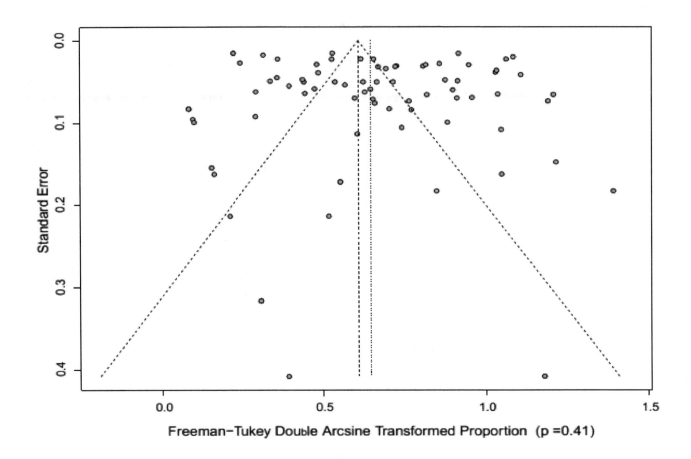

Figure 3. Funnel plot of the included articles for analysis demonstrates potential publication bias.

The pooled prevalence for CSF in an RE model was 35% (95% CI: 28%–43%). The sub-group analysis of diagnostic tests showed that the CSF seroprevalence with ELISA was 30% (95% CI: 22%–38%), i-ELISA 61% (95% CI: 42%–78%), s-ELISA 52% (95% CI: 0–100%), AGID 60% (95% CI: 18%–95%), RT–PCR 33% (95% CI: 8%–64%). The region-wise sub-group analysis showed CSF prevalence in the central zone (42%), East zone (41%), Northeast zone (40%), North zone (30%), southern zone (25%), and West (37%) (Figure 4; Supplementary data S1–S4).

The disease causes severe economic losses to pig farmers, and despite its devastating impact and recurrent outbreaks, CSF continued to be misconstrued and neglected for decades in India. The prevalence of CSF has been reported in most of the states of India [20]. In this meta-analysis, we included more data compared to the other previous studies carried out on CSF in India [26,27]. Compared to earlier studies on CSF meta-analysis in India, the present study compared the different diagnostic test-wise prevalence and identified the outlier and influential studies [28,29]. In this analysis, the prevalence estimate by a sandwich and indirect ELISA is comparatively higher than RT–PCR. The probable reason may be due to the higher false positives. In most of the studies, ELISA is often used to estimate the prevalence of CSF as it is convenient and has higher sensitivity and specificity. Serological assays provide better and quick information about CSF prevalence in the large pig population. Furthermore, serological tests are more realistic in serosurvey and extended epidemiological investigations provided assay targeted should not cross-react with other pestiviruses. The available antigen ELISA is quick but has low sensitivity [34]. As of now, the nucleic acid-based RT–PCR assay remains the method of choice due to high sensitivity for detecting virus at an early stage of infections. The possible limitations of this meta-analytic study could be that most of the studies did not clearly mention the diagnostic methodology and sampling procedures. The potential bias in the prevalence of CSF estimate might be due to low reporting and use of highly accurate RT–PCR based assays, though they are expensive.

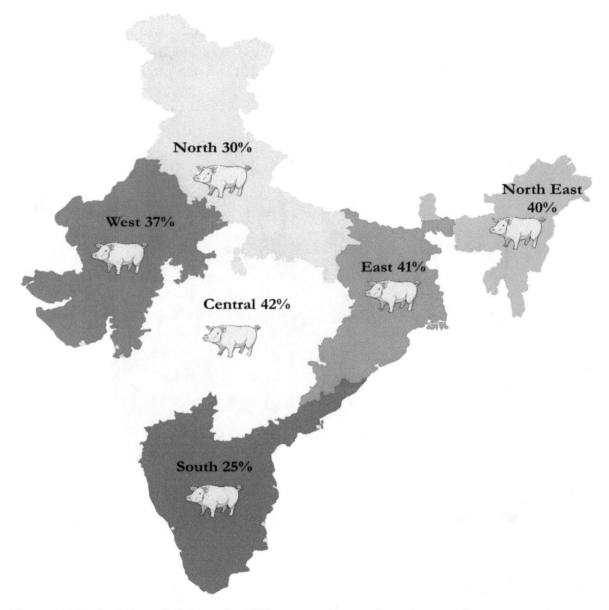

Figure 4. The depiction of region-wise CSF percentage prevalence in central, eastern, northeastern, northern, southern, western, and central zones of India.

5. Clinical Disease and Pathology on the CSF Outbreaks in India

CSFV is a known disease of domestic, feral, and wild suids [35]. The infection setup in vulnerable populations through the oro-nasal route and spreads via direct or indirect contact with clinically infected pigs and consuming virus-contaminated feed. Reports also support the vertical transmission of infection from sow to the offspring. The incubation period varies 3–10 days after infection. Depending on the CSFV strain, viral load, and host factors (age, breed, and immune status), CSFV infection classically takes either of the acute, chronic, or prenatal forms [36]. The clinical form of CSF has been extensively studied and presented in previous reports [36–43].

The pathological findings of CSF rely upon the clinical progression of the disease. During CSF field case investigations, we noticed a wide spectrum of clinical–pathological changes (Figure 5). In the acute course of CSF, pathology often reveals erythematous lesion in the skin of the ear, ventral surface of the abdomen, perianal region, tail, and extremities (Figure 5A). Lymph nodes (particularly mesenteric lymph nodes, inguinal lymph nodes) appear swollen with hemorrhages (Figure 5D). Serosal and mucosal surfaces of several organs such as the heart, kidneys, lungs, urinary bladder, and intestine show petechial hemorrhages. Non-collapsing, oedematous lungs with petechial to echymotic hemorrhages are frequently observed. Splenic infarctions at the edges are considered pathognomic for CSF (Figure 5B) [41]. Petecheation on the cortical surface presents a turkey egg appearance to the kidneys. Hemorrhagic enteritis (Figure 5C) and non-purulent encephalitis are also frequently observed in the acute clinical form of CSF.

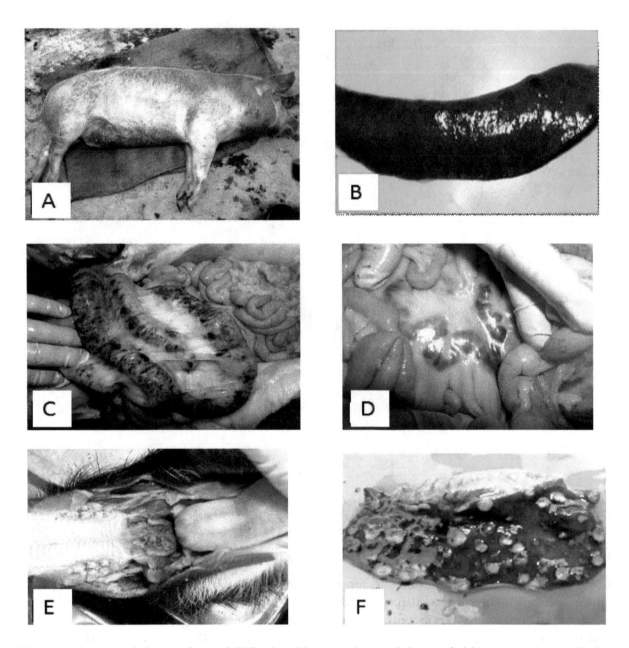

Figure 5. Acute and chronic form of CSF related lesions observed during field investigations in India. (**A**), Hemorrhages in skin, acute CSF form; (**B**), infarction in spleen, acute CSF form; (**C**), Hemorrhagic enteritis, acute CSF form; (**D**), hemorrhagic mesenteric lymph nodes, acute CSF form; (**E**), necrotic tonsillitis, chronic CSF form; and (**F**), Button ulcers in colon, chronic CSF form.

The long course of the diseases in the chronic form of CSF leads to wasting in affected pigs. The acute inflammatory lesions of the initial stage of the disease are later transformed into necrotic and ulcerative lesions. Necrotic and ulcerative tonsillitis and enteritis (small intestine, colon, and ileocecal valve) are frequently observed (Figure 5E,F). The red infarction at the edges of the spleen may transform into necrotic and ulcerative lesions with the progression of the disease. Importantly, these pathological lesions vary among animals based on the host factors like age, breed and immune status, and the CSFV strain virulence [41].

Histopathological lesions of acute CSF include hemorrhagic interstitial pneumonia, hemorrhagic lymphadenitis with depletion of lymphocytes, and hemorrhagic enteritis. The alveoli and bronchiolar air spaces are often filled with sero-fibrinous exudates, necrotic debris, desquamated epithelial cells with thickened alveolar wall due to edema, congestion, hemorrhages, and mononuclear infiltration. Severe congestion and hemorrhages with depletion of lymphocytes occur in spleen and lymph nodes. Moderate to severe hemorrhages are frequently observed in the cortex and corticomedullary junction of kidneys with tubular degeneration. Similar changes but with the predominance of necrotic and ulcerative lesions were observed in chronic cases [41].

6. CSF Laboratory Diagnosis in India

In routine, the provisional diagnosis of CSF disease is done looking at the clinical signs and pathological changes. The laboratory confirmation of the disease is crucial to differentially diagnose it with other infectious diseases of swine [44–46]. Sampling a greater number of animals is advisable as this disease may progress in a chronic form [47,48]. Virus isolation in the cell culture system and subsequent characterization remains the method of choice and a gold standard as well. The virus isolation is attempted in homologous primary cells (pig kidney) or in preferred cell lines (PK-15, RK-13, SK6, PS, and swine testicular epithelioid cells). Being non-cytopathic, the CSFV growth in the cell culture system is verified by detection using several immunological techniques like immunofluorescence (FAT) or peroxidase linked assay (PLA) using staining with poly- or monoclonal antibodies.

6.1. Serological Methods of Diagnosis of CSF

In India, primarily serological methods are applied for surveillance epidemiological investigations. The commonly used immunological tests for detection of the virus antigen in tissue samples are ELISA (Enzyme-Linked Immunosorbent Assay) and FAT (Fluorescent Antibody Test). The antibodies in the serum samples can be detected by ELISA and VNT (virus neutralization test). Blocking ELISA with the whole virus antigen, indirect ELISA (i-ELISA), neutralization peroxidase linked assay (NPLA), complex trapping blocking ELISA, and immuno-chromatographic strip/lateral flow assays (LFA), etc. have become available in the past for the anti-CSFV antibody detection [44–46]. Nonetheless, these assays fail to differentiate the infected from vaccinated animals.

In India, E^{rns} and E2 proteins-based ELISAs are available for the serodiagnosis of CSFV. A double antibody-based sandwich ELISA was standardized for the detection of CSFV antigen in clinical samples [44]. Assessment of the sandwich ELISA and dot-ELISA in CSFV antigen detection in tissues of naturally infected pigs and slaughtered pigs showed 86% and 80% of the samples from diseased pigs and 20% and 14% of the samples from pigs slaughtered for human consumption positivity by the tests, respectively, and statistical analysis also showed excellent agreement between these tests [45]. A comparative evaluation of antibody-based serological assays and nucleic acid-based assays for detecting CSFV in India showed 58% to 65% positivity by sandwich ELISA and direct FAT, respectively, and 76% positivity by nested RT–PCR [46].

Recently, in India, a recombinant Newcastle disease virus (NDV) viral expression vector was developed expressing the CSFV E2 and E^{rns} proteins and inducing production of CSFV-neutralizing antibodies on pig inoculation. Its diagnostic potential was assessed in an indirect ELISA measuring antibody titers in serum samples [47]. In another study, Bhattacharya et al. [48], employing a lentivirus-based gene delivery system, constructed a stable PK-15 cell line expressing E^{rns} (PK-E^{rns}) for using it to develop an ELISA detecting E^{rns}-specific antibodies in pig sera helping in differentiation of infection from vaccinated animals. Notably, a study from the northeastern region of India reported detection of CSFV in bovine samples after screening 134 cattle serum samples using a commercial antigen capture ELISA, where 10 samples were found positive for CSFV antigen by ELISA [49].

6.2. Molecular Methods of Diagnosis of CSF

In the current era, molecular tools are considered the backbone of disease diagnosis, genotyping, and analysis of virulence of the virus [50]. Among the several molecular tools available, real-time PCR (quantitative-PCR or qPCR) appears as the method with the highest sensitivity for the CSFV detection [51,52] and has been adopted as a test of choice for confirmatory diagnosis of the disease. Using the real-time PCR assay, CSFV was detected in tissues from 1120 slaughtered pigs in India, providing baseline prevalence data on CSF infection [40]. For CSFV RNA detection in infected tissue, a fluorescence-based in-situ hybridization (FISH) based method has been reported. The FISH assay uses a biotinylated DNA probe targeting the E2/NS2 gene of CSFV. This technique helped in demonstrating CSFV nucleic acids in the lymphoid tissues, such as spleen and lymph nodes [53]. The RT–PCR assays have been employed to detect CSFV RNA in formalin-fixed tissues, making it useful where the supply of fresh biological samples is difficult [54].

Immunochromatographic strip assay using a poly- or monoclonal colloidal gold conjugation system is being in use as a rapid pen-side test for the detection of CSF virus antigen [55]. Further, immunomagnetic bead-based assay use in the detection of CSFV antigen has been reported [56]. Another useful assay is the RT-loop-mediated isothermal amplification (RT-LAMP), which is a highly rapid 100-fold more sensitive than conventional gel-based RT–PCR while detecting CSFV. Further, it was highly specific and could differentiate other viruses like BVDV, porcine reproductive and respiratory syndrome virus (PRRSV), swine influenza virus (SIV), porcine parvovirus (PPV), porcine circovirus (PCV), and pseudorabies virus (PRV). Several advantages, like low-cost input (devoid of any specific instrument) and quick results, makes it an excellent assay for CSFV surveillance in the field. The development of qPCR and multiplex qPCR for the diagnosis of CSFV and simultaneous detection of CSFV has also been reported [57,58].

6.3. Compelete Genome Sequencing of Indian CSFV Isolates

Recently, different research groups from India have provided a complete genome sequence of local isolates from India using either next-generation sequencing methodology or conventional RT–PCR method. In a study, targeting the overlapping fragments of CSFV in RT–PCR, the complete genome of a lapinized CSFV vaccine strain was retrieved. The genetic analysis showed 92.6%–98.6% similarities at the nucleotide level with other CSFV strains, and it was typed as subgroup 1.1. The 5'-UTR had more than 97.0% similarity with several CSFV vaccine strains from China [59]. Subsequently, the first whole genome of a CSFV subgroup 2.2 (CSFV/IND/UK/LAL-290) was reported from the Uttarakhand state of India recovered from a backyard pig [60]. At the same time, a complete genome from a CSFV field isolate of subgenotype 1.1 was reported from India [61]. Subsequently, a complete genome from CSFV subgroup 2.1 that caused local outbreak in the northeastern state, Assam, India was sequenced. The isolate exhibited high genetic divergence [62]. Another CSFV genotype 1.1 isolate adapted in a porcine kidney cell line was deciphered with some T insertions in 3' UTR [63]. The same group successively provided a complete genome sequence of CSFV strain (CSFV-UP-BR-KHG-06), genotype 2.2 [64].

7. CSF Virus Vaccines in India

Keeping the prioritization for the CSF control in the country, the Ministry of Fisheries, Animal Husbandry and Dairying, Govt. of India has initiated the Classical Swine Fever Control Programme (CSF-CP) in the year 2014–2015 to control the CSF in pigs by mass vaccination using the live attenuated vaccines. There are two major activities in this control program: (i) strengthening of laboratories, including consumables for laboratories; and (ii) vaccination in identified villages including vaccination cost, on a 90:10 allocation basis between centre and the northeastern states. The variation in quality, safety, efficacy, and potency of CSF live vaccines are major hindrances in the success of vaccination programs, and it is, therefore, a significant step to perform thorough quality control of vaccines from different suppliers regularly/batch-wise.

The CSF vaccines are to be produced following the standard operating procedures listed in the OIE Manual of Diagnostic Tests and Vaccines for Terrestrial Animals to ensure a high level of efficacy and safety [6]. The systematic prophylactic vaccination and a stamping-out policy is followed usually to restrain CSF in endemic countries. In India, CSF is endemic, and for its control, a mass vaccination approach is adopted. The lapinized vaccine using the Weybridge strain of the virus, which belongs to the sub-genogroup 1.1, has been used since 1964 [2,7]. The lapinized vaccines are produced mostly by the Institute of Veterinary Biologicals located in different states of the country to meet the local demand of the vaccines. A few of the Institute of Veterinary Biologicals have lately shifted to producing local CSFV strain based cell culture attenuated live vaccines [65]. The systematic vaccination using a live-attenuated vaccine appears to be the best way forward for elimination/eradication of the CSF, including vaccination of the reservoir hosts like wild boars [66].

The present domestic pig population of India is 9.06 million, as per the 20th livestock census of the government of India. The vaccination coverage of all the domestic pigs twice in a year requires about 20 million doses per annum, and only 1.2 million doses are produced per year by the lapinized vaccine. The reason behind this is that only 50 doses of vaccines are produced from a single rabbit spleen. To meet out the demand and overcome the constraints in producing a large quantity of the lapinized vaccine, attempts are underway to produce a cell-culture-based vaccine using either the lapinized vaccine strain or the local CSFV isolates. There are reports on developing effective cell-culture-based live attenuated vaccines against CSFV (using foreign strain, Weybridge) by the Indian Veterinary Research Institute (IVRI), the premier veterinary institute of the country. The vaccine was reported to be safe, potent, and provides immunity for a period of one year [63]. A commercial Bovine Kidney cell culture adapted vaccine for CSFV (Himmvac Hog Cholera (T/C) Vaccine) is also available from KBNP Inc. Korea through Panav Bio-Tech, India.

On 3 February 2020, IVRI released a new safe, potent live-attenuated CSFV cell culture vaccine using indigenous strain (Press Information Bureau, 2020). The vaccine would be the best choice for use in the CSF Control Programme (CSF-CP) already launched by DAHD, Govt. of India. There is a huge demand for transfer of this vaccine technology from various state governments and private manufacturers, and the vaccine has huge export potential, especially to Asian countries. Due to a very high titer of vaccine virus, this vaccine would be the most economical CSF vaccine, costing around less than Rs 2/- per dose, compared to Rs 15-25/- of lapinized CSF vaccine and Rs. 30/dose (approx.) for an imported Korean vaccine being used in the country. Besides, the new vaccine gives immunity for two years as compared to 3 to 6 month's protection under the vaccines currently being used. The vaccine is safe, potent, does not revert to virulence, and provides protective immunity from 14-day post-vaccination (DPV) of the vaccination until 2 years, studied so far. The yield of this vaccine is 1000 times more than the existing CSF vaccine. The evaluation of different parameters along with the protective humoral immune response of pigs vaccinated with a live attenuated cell culture vaccine has been reported from the state of Assam, India. The vaccine was reported to be safe, elicited better and stable immune response after booster doses, and maternally derived antibodies persist up to 42 days in newborn piglets when pregnant pigs are vaccinated at one month of gestation [66].

8. Conclusions and Prospects

CSF is one of the dreaded diseases affecting mostly pigs and wild boars worldwide, causing a severe impact on the global economy. In India, the disease is endemic and mainly present in the northeastern states of the country and pig-populated states. The genotypes 1.1, 2.1, and 2.2 are circulating all over India, with the highest prevalence of genotype 1.1. Recently, increases in prevalence of 2.1 and 2.2 are also reported but need exhaustive epidemiological studies before deriving the conclusion. In India, several socio-economic impacts pose challenges to researchers for the development of potent vaccines against CSFV. Backyard pig farming and highly mobile pig products are the major factors regarding the epidemiology of CSFV in India. The key factors of the CSFV control program should include better diagnostic facilities, potent and effective vaccination, and stamping out along with control of animal movements and biosecurity. Regarding diagnostics, there is a need for rapid and cost-effective point-of-care assay to screen the disease at the farmer's level. Along with CSFV infection, secondary infections are widespread, which sometimes overshade the disease manifestation. The multiplex assay will be better in these situations to detect concurrent infections. To avoid the occasionally observed cross-reaction with pestiviruses, more reliable and accurate CSFV-specific screening assays must be employed for confirmation. Although many ELISAs are available detecting CSFV specifically, the definitive confirmation must use serum neutralization test. Regarding vaccination strategy, the marker vaccines should be chosen for effective vaccination, which can differentiate infected and vaccinated animals. Finally, the culling of infected animals and the adoption of animal identification systems to trace the disease transmission pathway will be helpful in disease control. To eradicate the disease in near future, there is a need for increasing awareness about CSFV, mainly in the poor population who are mostly engaged with pig rearing.

Supplementary Materials:
Data S1, Forest plot showing the prevalence of CSF in India; Data S2, Forest plot showing the diagnostic test wise prevalence of CSF in India; Data S3, Forest plot showing the region wise prevalence of CSF in India; Data S4, Forest plot showing the yearwise prevalence of CSF in India.

Author Contributions: All the authors substantially contributed to the conception, compilation of data, checking and approving the final version of the manuscript, and agree to be accountable for its contents. All authors have read and agreed to the published version of the manuscript.

Acknowledgments: All the authors acknowledge and thank their respective Institutes and Universities. Y.S.M. acknowledges the Education Division, ICAR, GoI for National Fellowship.

References

1.   Everett, H.; Crooke, H.; Gurrala, R.; Dwarka, R.; Kim, J.; Botha, B.; Lubisi, A.; Pardini, A.; Gers, S.; Vosloo, W.; et al. Experimental infection of common warthogs (Phacochoerus africanus) and bushpigs (Potamochoerus larvatus) with classical swine fever virus. I: Susceptibility and transmission. *Transbound. Emerg. Dis.* **2011**, *58*, 128–134. [CrossRef] [PubMed]

2.   Dong, X.N.; Chen, Y.H. Marker vaccine strategies and candidate CSFV marker vaccines. *Vaccine* **2007**, *25*, 205–230. [CrossRef] [PubMed]

3.   Dewulf, J.; Laevens, H.; Koenen, F.; Mintiens, K.; De Kruif, A. An experimental infection with classical swine fever virus in pregnant sows: Transmission of the virus, course of the disease, antibody response and effect on gestation. *J. Vet. Med. B.* **2001**, *48*, 583–591. [CrossRef] [PubMed]

4.   Li, M.; Wang, Y.F.; Wang, Y.; Gao, H.; Li, N.; Sun, Y.; Liang, B.B.; Qiu, H.J. Immune responses induced by a BacMam virus expressing the E2 protein of ckoopokkokkokjjjlassical swine fever virus in mice. *Immunol. Lett.* **2009**, *125*, 145–150. [CrossRef]

5.   Edward, S.; Fukusho, A.; Lefevre, P.C.; Lipowski, A.; Pejsak, Z.; Roehe, P.; Westergaard, J. Classical swine fever: The global situation. *Vet. Microbiol.* **2000**, *73*, 103–119. [CrossRef]

6.   Manual of Diagnostic Tests and Vaccines for Terrestrial Animals. 2016. Available online: http://www.oie.int/fileadmin/Home/eng/Health_standards/tahm/2.08.03_CSF.pdf (accessed on 1 February 2017).

7.   Xia, H.; Wahlberg, N.; Qiu, H.J.; Widén, F.; Belák, S.; Liu, L. Lack of phylogenetic evidence that the Shimen strain is the parental strain of the lapinized Chinese strain (C-strain) vaccine against classical swine fever. *Arch. Virol.* **2011**, *156*, 1041–1044. [CrossRef]

8.   Krishnamurthy, D.; Adlakha, S.C. A preliminary report on the swine fever epidemic in Uttar Pradesh. *Indian Vet. J.* **1962**, *39*, 406–419.

9.   Sapre, S.N.; Moghe, R.G.; Bhagwat, S.V.; Choudhary, P.G.; Purohit, B.L. Observations on swine fever in Maharashtra. *Indian Vet. J.* **1962**, *39*, 527–529.

10. Smith, D.B.; Meyers, G.; Bukh, J.; Gould, E.A.; Monath, T.; Muerhoff, A.S.; Pletnev, A.; Rico-Hesse, R.; Stapleton, J.T.; Simmonds, P.; et al. Proposed revision to the taxonomy of the genus Pestivirus, family Flaviviridae. *J. Gen. Virol.* **2017**, *98*, 2106–2112. [CrossRef]

11. Rümenapf, T.; Unger, G.; Strauss, J.H.; Thiel, H.J. Processing of the envelope glycoproteins of pestiviruses. *J. Virol.* **1993**, *67*, 3288–3294. [CrossRef]

12. Lowings, P.; Ibata, G.; Needham, J.; Paton, D. Classical swine fever virus diversity and evolution. *J. Gen. Virol.* **1996**, *77*, 1311–1321. [CrossRef] [PubMed]

13. Zhang, H.; Wang, Y.H.; Cao, H.W.; Cui, Y.D.; Hua, Z. Phylogenetic analysis of E2 genes of classical swine fever virus in China. *Israel J. Vet. Med.* **2010**, *65*, 151–155.

14. Paton, D.J.; McGoldrick, A.; Greiser-Wilke, I.; Parchariyanon, S.; Song, J.Y.; Liou, P.P.; Belak, S. Genetic typing of classical swine fever virus. *Vet. Microbiol.* **2000**, *73*, 137–157. [CrossRef]

15. Chander, V.; Nandi, S.; Ravishankar, C.; Upmanyu, V.; Verma, R. Classical swine fever in pigs: Recent developments and future perspectives. *Anim. Health. Res. Rev.* **2014**, *15*, 87–101. [CrossRef] [PubMed]

16. Zhou, B. Classical swine fever in China-an update Minireview. *Front. Vet. Sci.* **2019**, *6*, 187. [CrossRef] [PubMed]

17. Deng, M.C.; Huang, C.C.; Huang, T.S.; Chang, C.Y.; Lin, Y.J.; Chien, M.S.; Jong, M.H. Phylogenetic analysis of classical swine fever virus isolated from Taiwan. *Vet. Microbiol.* **2005**, *106*, 187–193. [CrossRef]

18. Gong, W.; Wu, J.; Lu, Z.; Zhang, L.; Qin, S.; Chen, F.; Peng, Z.; Wang, Q.; Ma, L.; Bai, A.; et al. Genetic diversity of subgenotype 2.1 isolates of classical swine fever virus. *Infect. Genet. Evol.* **2016**, *41*, 218–226. [CrossRef]

19. Sarma, D.K.; Mishra, N.; Vilcek, S.; Rajukumar, K.; Behera, S.P.; Nema, R.K.; Dubey, P.; Dubey, S.C. Phylogenetic analysis of recent classical swine fever virus (CSFV) isolates from Assam, India. *Comp. Immunol. Microbiol. Infect. Dis.* **2011**, *34*, 11–15. [CrossRef]

20. Singh, V.K.; Rajak, K.K.; Kumar, A.; Yadav, S.K. Classical swine fever in India: Current status and future perspective. *Trop. Anim. Health Prod.* **2018**, *50*, 1181–1191. [CrossRef]

21. Tamura, K.; Stecher, G.; Peterson, D.; Filipski, A.; Kumar, S. MEGA6: Molecular evolutionary genetics analysis version 6.0. *Mol. Biol. Evol.* **2013**, *30*, 2725–2729. [CrossRef]

22. Madeira, F.; Park, Y.M.; Lee, J.; Buso, N.; Gur, T.; Madhusoodanan, N.; Basutkar, P.; Tivey, A.R.; Potter, S.C.; Finn, R.D.; et al. The EMBL-EBI search and sequence analysis tools APIs in 2019. *Nucleic Acids Res.* **2019**, *2*, W636–W641. [CrossRef] [PubMed]

23. Tu, C.; Lu, Z.; Li, H.; Yu, X.; Liu, X.; Li, Y.; Zang, H.; Yin, Z. Phylogenetic comparison of classical swine fever virus in China. *Virus Res.* **2011**, *81*, 29–37. [CrossRef]

24. Patil, S.S.; Hemadri, D.; Shankar, B.P.; Raghavendra, A.G.; Veeresh, H.; Sindhoora, B.; Chandan, S.; Gagendragad, M.R.; Sreekala, K.; Prabhudas, K. Genetic typing of recent classical swine fever isolates from India. *Vet. Microbiol.* **2010**, *141*, 367–373. [CrossRef] [PubMed]

25. Shivaraj, D.B.; Patil, S.S.; Rathnamma, D.; Hemadri, D.; Isloor, S.; Geetha, S.; Manjunathareddy, G.B.; Gajendragad, M.R.; Rahman, H. Genetic clustering of recent classical swine fever virus isolates from Karnataka, India revealed the emergence of subtype 2.2 replacing subtype 1.1. *VirusDisease* **2015**, *26*, 170–179. [CrossRef]

26. Patil, S.S.; Suresh, K.P.; Saha, S.; Prajapati, A.; Hemadri, D.; Roy, P. Meta-analysis of classical swine fever prevalence in pigs in India: A 5-year study. *Vet. World* **2018**, *11*, 297–303. [CrossRef]

27. Barman, N.N.; Patil, S.S.; Kurli, R.; Deka, P.; Bora, D.P.; Deka, G.; Ranjitha, K.M.; Shivaranjini, C.; Roy, P.; Suresh, K.P. Meta-analysis of the prevalence of livestock diseases in North Eastern Region of India. *Vet. World* **2020**, *13*, 80–91. [CrossRef] [PubMed]

28. Baujat, B.; Mahe, C.; Pignon, J.P.; Hill, C. A Graphical Method for Exploring Heterogeneity in Meta-Analyses: Application to a Meta-Analysis of 65 Trials. *Stat. Med.* **2002**, *21*, 2641–2652. [CrossRef] [PubMed]

29. DerSimonian, R.; Laird, N. Meta-analysis in clinical trials. *Controll. Clin. Trials* **1986**, *7*, 177–188. [CrossRef]

30. Harris, R.J.; Deeks, J.J.; Altman, D.G.; Bradburn, M.J.; Harbord, R.M.; Sterne, J.A. Metan: Fixed-and random-effects meta-analysis. *Stata J.* **2008**, *8*, 3–28. [CrossRef]

31. Egger, M.; Smith, G.D.; Schneide, M.; Minder, C. Bias in meta-analysis detected by a simple, graphical test. *BMJ* **1997**, *315*, 629–634. [CrossRef]

32. Deeks, J.J.; Higgins, J.; Altman, D.G. Analysing data and undertaking meta-analyses. In *Cochrane Handbook for Systematic Reviews of Interventions: Cochrane Book Series*; Wiley: Hoboken, New Jersey, USA, 2008; pp. 243–296. [CrossRef]

33. Viechtbauer, W.; Cheung, M.W.L. Outlier and influence diagnostics for meta-analysis. *Res. Synth. Methods* **2010**, *1*, 112–125. [CrossRef] [PubMed]

34. Dewulf, J.; Koenen, F.; Mintiens, K.; Denis, P.; Ribbens, S.; de Kruif, A. Analytical performance of several classical swine fever laboratory diagnostic techniques on live animals for detection of infection. *J. Virol. Meth* **2004**, *119*, 137–143. [CrossRef] [PubMed]

35. Blome, S.; Gabriel, C.; Staubach, C.; Leifer, I.; Strebelow, G.; Beer, M. Genetic differentiation of infected from vaccinated animals after implementation of an emergency vaccination strategy against classical swine fever in wild boar. *Vet. Microbiol.* **2011**, *153*, 373–376. [CrossRef] [PubMed]

36. Moennig, V.; Floegel, N.G.; Greiser-Wilke, I. Clinical signs and epidemiology of classical swine fever: A review of new knowledge. *Vet. J.* **2003**, *165*, 11–20. [CrossRef]

37. Dahle, J.; Liess, B. A review on classical swine fever infections in pigs: Epizootiology, clinical disease and pathology. *Comp. Immunol. Microbiol. Infect Dis.* **1992**, *15*, 203–211. [CrossRef]

38. Muñoz-González, S.; Ruggli, N.; Rosell, R.; Pérez, L.J.; Frías-Leuporeau, M.T.; Fraile, L.; Montoya, M.; Cordoba, L.; Domingo, M.; Ehrensperger, F.; et al. Postnatal persistent infection with classical swine fever virus and its immunological implications. *PLoS ONE* **2015**, *10*, e0125692. [CrossRef]

39. Blome, S.; Staubach, C.; Henke, J.; Carlson, J.; Beer, M. Classical Swine Fever—An Updated Review. *Viruses* **2017**, *9*, 86. [CrossRef]

40. Rout, M.; Saikumar, G. Virus load in pigs affected with different clinical forms of classical swine fever. *Transbound. Emerg. Dis.* **2012**, *59*, 128–133. [CrossRef]

41. Rajkhowa, T.K.; Hauhnar, L.; Lalrohlua, I.; Jagan, M.G. Emergence of 2.1 subgenotype of classical swine fever virus in pig population of India in 2011. *Vet. Q.* **2014**, *34*, 224–228. [CrossRef] [PubMed]

42. Teifke, J.P.; Lange, E.; Klopfleisch, R.; Kaden, V. Nictitating membrane as a potentially useful postmortem diagnostic specimen for classical swine fever. *J. Vet Diagn. Investig.* **2005**, *17*, 341–345. [CrossRef]

43. Van Oirschot, J. Hog cholera. In *Infectious Diseases of Livestock*, 2nd ed.; Coetzer, J.A.W., Tustin, R.C., Eds.; Oxford University Press: Oxford, UK, 2004; pp. 975–986.

44. Sarma, D.K.; Sarma, P.C. ELISA for detection of hog cholera virus antigen. *Ind. J. Anim. Sci.* **1995**, *65*, 650–651.

45. Sarma, D.K.; Meshram, D.J. Comparison of sandwich and dot ELISA for detection of CSF virus antigen in pigs. *Indian Vet. J.* **2008**, *85*, 915–918.

46. Barman, N.N.; Gupt, R.S.; Singh, N.K.; Tiwari, A.K.; Singh, R.K.; Das, S.K. Comparative evaluation of molecular and antibody based technique for detection of classical swine fever virus infecting pigs of NE region, India. *Indian J. Anim. Sci.* **2009**, *79*, 974–977.

47. Kumar, R.; Kumar, V.; Kekungu, P.; Barman, N.N.; Kumar, S. Evaluation of surface glycoproteins of classical swine fever virus as immunogens and reagents for serological diagnosis of infections in pigs: A recombinant Newcastle disease virus approach. *Arch. Virol.* **2019**, *164*, 3007–3017. [CrossRef]

48. Bhattacharya, S.; Saini, M.; Bisht, D.; Rana, M.; Bachan, R.; Gogoi, S.M.; Buragohain, B.M.; Barman, N.N.; Gupta, P.K. Lentiviral-mediated delivery of classical swine fever virus Erns gene into porcine kidney-15 cells for production of recombinant ELISA diagnostic antigen. *Mol. Biol. Rep.* **2019**, *46*, 3865–3876. [CrossRef] [PubMed]

49. Chakraborty, A.K.; Karam, A.; Mukherjee, P.; Barkalita, L.; Borah, P.; Das, S.; Sanjukta, R.; Puro, K.; Ghatak, S.; Shakuntala, I.; et al. Detection of classical swine fever virus E2 gene in cattle serum samples from cattle herds of Meghalaya. *VirusDisease* **2018**, *29*, 89–95. [CrossRef]

50. Moennig, V.; Becher, P. Pestivirus control programs: How far have we come and where are we going? *Anim. Health Res. Rev.* **2015**, *16*, 83–87. [CrossRef]

51. Depner, K.; Hoffmann, B.; Beer, M. Evaluation of real-time RT-PCR assay for the routine intra vitam diagnosis of classical swine fever. *Vet. Microbiol.* **2007**, *121*, 338–343. [CrossRef]

52. Le Dimna, M.; Vrancken, R.; Koenen, F.; Bougeard, S.; Mesplede, A.; Hutet, E.; Kuntz-Simon, G.; Le Potier, M.F. Validation of two commercial real-time RT-PCR kits for rapid and specific diagnosis of classical swine fever virus. *J. Virol. Methods* **2008**, *147*, 136–142. [CrossRef]

53. Nagarajan, K.; Saikumar, G. Fluorescent in-situ hybridization technique for the detection and localization of classical swine fever virus in infected tissues. *Veterinarski Arhiv* **2012**, *82*, 495–504.

54. Singh, V.K.; Kumar, G.S.; Paliwal, O.P. Detection of classical swine fever virus in archival formalin-fixed tissues by reverse transcription-polymerase chain reaction. *Res. Vet. Sci.* **2005**, *79*, 81–84. [CrossRef] [PubMed]

55.   Zhang, C.; Huang, Y.; Zheng, H.; Fang, Y.; Fande, K.; Shen, H.; He, Q.; Huang, Y.; Wen, F. Study on colloidal gold strip in detecting classical swine fever virus. *Fujian J. Anim. Husb. Vet. Med.* **2007**, *6*, 3–5.

56.   Conlan, J.V.; Khounsy, S.; Blacksell, S.D.; Morrissy, C.J.; Wilks, C.R.; Gleeson, L.J. Development and evaluation of a rapid immunomagnetic bead assay for the detection of classical swine fever virus antigen. *Trop. Anim. Health Prod.* **2009**, *41*, 913–920. [CrossRef] [PubMed]

57.   Huang, Y.L.; Pang, V.F.; Pan, C.H.; Chen, T.H.; Jong, M.H.; Huang, T.S.; Jeng, C.R. Development of a reverse transcription multiplex real time PCR for the detection and genotyping of classical swine fever virus. *J. Virol. Methods* **2013**, *160*, 111–118. [CrossRef]

58.   Haines, F.J.; Hofmann, M.A.; King, D.P.; Drew, T.W.; Crooke, H.R. Development and validation of a multiplex real time RT-PCR assay for the simultaneous detection of classical and African swine fever viruses. *PLoS ONE* **2013**, *8*, e71019. [CrossRef] [PubMed]

59.   Gupta, P.K.; Saini, M.; Dahiya, S.S.; Patel, C.L.; Sonwane, A.A.; Rai, D.V.; Pandey, K.D. Molecular characterization of lapinized classical Swine Fever vaccine strain by full-length genome sequencing and analysis. *Anim. Biotechnol.* **2011**, *22*, 111–117. [CrossRef]

60.   Kumar, R.; Rajak, K.K.; Chandra, T.; Thapliyal, A.; Muthuchelvan, D.; Sudhakar, S.B.; Sharma, K.; Saxena, A.; Raut, S.D.; Singh, V.K.; et al. Whole-genome sequence of a classical Swine Fever virus isolated from the uttarakhand state of India. *Genome Announc.* **2014**, *2*, e00371-14. [CrossRef]

61.   Kamboj, A.; Patel, C.L.; Chaturvedi, V.K.; Saini, M.; Gupta, P.K. Complete genome sequence of an Indian field isolate of classical Swine Fever virus belonging to subgenotype 1.1. *Genome Announc.* **2014**, *2*, e00886-14. [CrossRef]

62.   Ahuja, A.; Bhattacharjee, U.; Chakraborty, A.K.; Karam, A.; Ghatak, S.; Puro, K.; Das, S.; Shakuntala, I.; Srivastava, N.; Ngachan, S.V.; et al. Complete genome sequence of classical swine fever virus subgenogroup 2.1 from Assam, India. *Genome Announc* **2015**, *3*, e01437-14. [CrossRef]

63.   Tomar, N.; Sharma, V.; John, J.K.; Sethi, M.; Ray, P.K.; Arya, R.S.; Das, T.; Saikumar, G. Complete Genome Sequence of a Field Isolate of Classical Swine Fever Virus Belonging to Subgenotype 2.2 from India. *Genome Announc.* **2018**, *6*, e00288-18. [CrossRef]

64.   Tomar, N.; Gupta, A.; Arya, R.S.; Somvanshi, R.; Sharma, V.; Saikumar, G. Genome sequence of classical Swine Fever virus genotype 1.1 with a genetic marker of attenuation detected in a continuous porcine cell line. *Genome Announc.* **2015**, *3*, e00375-15. [CrossRef] [PubMed]

65.   Bardhan, D.; Singh, R.K.; Dhar, P.; Kumar, S. Potential role of technology in increasing productivity and income at National level: A case of cell-culture vaccine against classical swine fever. *Agric. Econ. Res. Rev.* **2017**, *30*, 161–170. [CrossRef]

66.   Nath, M.K.; Sarma, D.K.; Das, B.C.; Deka, P.; Kalita, D.; Dutta, J.B.; Mahato, G.; Sarma, S.; Roychoudhury, P. Evaluation of specific humoral immune response in pigs vaccinated with cell culture adapted classical swine fever vaccine. *Vet. World* **2016**, *9*, 308–312. [CrossRef] [PubMed]

Impact of a Live Attenuated Classical Swine Fever Virus Introduced to Jeju Island, a CSF-Free Area

SeEun Choe [1], Jae-Hoon Kim [2], Ki-Sun Kim [1], Sok Song [1], Wan-Choul Kang [3], Hyeon-Ju Kim [3], Gyu-Nam Park [1], Ra Mi Cha [1], In-Soo Cho [1], Bang-Hun Hyun [1], Bong-Kyun Park [1,4] and Dong-Jun An [1,*]

[1] Viral Disease Division, Animal and Plant Quarantine Agency (APQA), Gimcheon, Gyeongbuk 39660, Korea; ivvi59@korea.kr (S.C.); kisunkim@korea.kr (K.-S.K.); ssoboro@naver.com (S.S.); changep0418@gmail.com (G.-N.P.); rami.cha01@korea.kr (R.M.C.); chois38@korea.kr (I.-S.C.); hyunbh@korea.kr (B.-H.H.); park026@korea.kr (B.-K.P.)
[2] College of Veterinary Medicine and Veterinary Medicine Institute, Jeju National University, Jeju Island 63243, Korea; kimjhoon@jejunu.ac.kr
[3] Jeju Special Self-Governing Provincial Veterinary Research Institute, Jeju Island 63344, Korea; kwc1041@korea.kr (W.-C.K.); bluemouse@korea.kr (H.-J.K.)
[4] Colleage of Veterinary Medicine, Seoul University, Gwanak-ro, Gwanak-gu, Seoul 08826, Korea
* Correspondence: andj67@korea.kr

Abstract: Here, we examine the effects of LOM(Low virulence of Miyagi) strains isolated from pigs (Jeju LOM strains) of Jeju Island, where vaccination with a live attenuated classical swine fever (CSF) LOM vaccine strain was stopped. The circulation of the Jeju LOM strains was mainly caused by a commercial swine erysipelas (*Erysipelothrix rhusiopathiae*) vaccine mixed with a LOM vaccine strain, which was inoculated into pregnant sows of 20 pig farms in 2014. The Jeju LOM strain was transmitted to 91 pig farms from 2015 to 2018. A histopathogenic investigation was performed for 25 farms among 111 farms affected by the Jeju LOM strain and revealed pigs infected with the Jeju LOM strain in combination with other pathogens, which resulted in the abortion of fetuses and mortality in suckling piglets. Histopathologic examination and immunohistochemical staining identified CSF-like lesions. Our results also confirm that the main transmission factor for the Jeju LOM strain circulation is the vehicles entering/exiting farms and slaughterhouses. Probability estimates of transmission between cohabiting pigs and pigs harboring the Jeju LOM strain JJ16LOM-YJK08 revealed that immunocompromised pigs showed horizontal transmission (r = 1.22). In a full genome analysis, we did not find genetic mutation on the site that is known to relate to pathogenicity between Jeju LOM strains (2014–2018) and the commercial LOM vaccine strain. However, we were not able to determine whether the Jeju LOM strain (2014–2018) is genetically the same virus as those of the commercial LOM vaccine due to several genetic variations in structure and non-structure proteins. Therefore, further studies are needed to evaluate the pathogenicity of the Jeju LOM strain in pregnant sow and SPF pigs and to clarify the characteristics of Jeju LOM and commercial LOM vaccine strains.

Keywords: classical swine fever virus (CSFV); LOM vaccine strain; Jeju LOM strain; omega value; transmission

1. Introduction

Classical swine fever virus (CSFV), a member of the genus *Pestivirus* within the family *Flaviviridae*, comprises a single positive-stranded RNA genome of approximately 12.3 kb, which encodes a polyprotein of 3898 amino acids [1]. The viral genome comprises a 5′ untranslated region (5′ UTR), an N-terminal protease (N^{pro}), a capsid (C) protein, envelope (E) proteins (E^{rns}, E1, E2, p7), non-structural

(NS) proteins (NS2, NS3, NS4A, NS4B, NS5A, NS5B), and a 3' UTR [2]. CSFV is categorized into three genotypes, 1, 2, and 3, each of which can be subdivided into three subgenotypes (1.1–1.3, 2.1–2.3, and 3.1–3.4) [3]. Classical swine fever (CSF) is a highly contagious multisystemic hemorrhagic viral disease of domestic pigs and wild boar, which can manifest as acute, subacute, chronic, or late onset disease [4]. Vaccination is used to prevent and/or reduce the number of outbreaks of CSF and, together with other control measures, was an important factor in eradicating CSF from Holland in 1985 and from the Rivas region of Nicaragua [5]. Historically, CSF vaccines have been based on attenuated strains, i.e., lapinized Chinese and tissue culture-adapted strains. Modified live vaccines (MLVs) based on several attenuated virus strains (e.g., C-strain, Thiverval, PAV-250, GPE-, and K-strains) are used most widely. The advantages and disadvantages of MLV vaccination during an outbreak have been described in previous studies [5]. Briefly, the advantages include ease of use, low cost, and an induction of life-long immunity by a single dose. However, in the 1980s and early 1990s (the time when a lapinized Chinese strain was used in Mexico), vaccinated pigs occasionally exhibited adverse reactions; some even died [5]. The CSF vaccine virus multiplies in actively replicating cells such as fetal cells and reticuloendothelial cells; some reports show that animals vaccinated with a Chinese strain virus had more respiratory infections due to a concurrent *Pasteurella multocida* infection [6]. In addition, the CSF vaccine virus may induce embryonic death and myoclonia congenita when administered to pregnant sows [5]. When herds that include pregnant sows are vaccinated for the first time, there can be a fall in sow fertility in the 6 weeks following vaccination, after which it returns to normal; therefore, researchers concluded that vaccination reduces herd productivity [5]. The OIE requirements for the safety of MLVs in young animals states that vaccination should not induce a high body temperature or leukopenia and should not allow horizontal transmission. For pregnant sows, safe MLV vaccination requires no transplacental transmission and no evidence of reversion-to-virulence after passage in piglets. The CSF MLV (LOM vaccine strain) used to vaccinate pigs in South Korea since 1974 has caused abortion in some pregnant sows [7], and prolonged virus shedding by immunosuppressed pigs after vaccination [8].

The South Korean government maintained a CSF (LOM) vaccine policy to control the disease on the mainland; however, vaccination on Jeju Island (located at the southern end of Korea) was stopped in 2000 (Jeju Island declared itself a "CSF-free region"). However, pig farms of Jeju Island have suffered continuous outbreaks of the LOM vaccine strain via various routes from the mainland, raising suspicion about the safety and reversion-to-pathogenicity of commercial LOM vaccine strains. Five outbreaks of the LOM vaccine strain infection of pigs have occurred over 19 years. The first (from 2004 to 2007) occurred through feed contaminated with the commercial LOM vaccine strain present in an animal plasma protein supplement [9]. The second was caused by the delivery of incorrect vaccine material from the mainland; in 2010, one farm accidently inoculated pigs with a vaccine mixed with the LOM vaccine strain. The third and fourth occurred on one farm (2012) and two farms (2013); the route of LOM vaccine strain exposure was not revealed, but feed contaminated with the LOM vaccine strain, or an unintentional injection of an incorrect CSF (LOM) vaccine from the mainland was suspected. In the fifth case (in 2014), pregnant sows on 20 pig farms were inoculated with a commercial swine erysipelas vaccine mixed with the LOM vaccine strain. Vaccination was stopped immediately, but a total of 111 pig farms (20 in 2014, 22 in 2015, 32 in 2016, 26 in 2017, and 11 in 2018) were exposed to the Jeju LOM strains (LOM strains isolated from Jeju pigs). Farm-to-farm transmission patterns showed mainly between high-density pig farms in the Hanlim region (located in northwestern Jeju) from 2015 to 2018 and the Daejeong region (located in southwestern Jeju) from 2016 to 2018.

Here, we investigated pig-to-pig and/or farm-to-farm transmissions, and the possibility of reversion-to-pathogenicity by comparing genetic mutations in the Jeju LOM strain viruses.

2. Results

2.1. Histopathological Analysis to Detect Infection by CSFV (Jeju LOM) Alone or Co-Infection with CSFV (Jeju LOM) and Other Pathogens

Overall, 122 samples (from 100 piglets and 22 fetuses) obtained from 25 pig farms were tested; all were positive for CSFV (Jeju LOM). The Jeju LOM strain was identified in 103 of 122 samples (81 piglets and 22 fetuses). Antigens derived from the Jeju LOM strain were detected in tissue samples from 51 suckling piglets, 14 piglets were infected with Jeju LOM alone, and the remaining 37 were co-infected with Jeju LOM plus enteric pathogens (six with *Clostridium* spp, six with *E. coli*, three with PEDV, and four with rotavirus), respiratory pathogens (three with PRRSV), or *Streptococcus* (n = 7), and *Staphylococcus* spp. (n = 2) (Table 1). Samples from the 37 suckling piglets co-infected with the Jeju LOM strain and other pathogens showed evidence of interior visceral hemorrhage (18 of the kidney, 12 of the exo-endocardium, and nine of the lung), and 14 had non-purulent brain lesions (perivascular cuffing, gliosis, and neuronophagia). Fourteen piglets infected with the Jeju LOM strain only showed interior visceral hemorrhage (eight of the kidney, six of the exo-endocardium, and three of the lung), and six had non-purulent brain lesions (perivascular cuffing, gliosis, and neuronophagia). Seven of the 14 suckling piglets identified to have CSF-like specific histopathologic lesions (Figure 1). Pathogenic lesions in weaning pigs included broncho-interstitial pneumonia or fibrinous lobor pneumonia (n = 16), lung hemorrhage (n = 10), kidney hemorrhage (n = 9), peripheral lymph node hemorrhage (n = 11), exo-endocardium hemorrhage (n = 5), and non-suppurative encephalitis of brain and spinal cord (n = 5) (Table 1). Co-infection of 22 fetuses with other pathogens (i.e., PPV, ADV, EMCV, JEV, PRRSV, and PCV2) was not confirmed, and no specific pathogenic lesions were observed in their organs. Organ tissue immunohistochemistry (IHC) staining detected Jeju LOM strains in 25 of 48 suckling pigs; 17 were cases of co-infection and eight were single infections. The following organs harbored the Jeju LOM strain: tonsil (40%), spleen (22.9%), lymph node (15%), lung (14.6%), small intestine (4.3%), kidney (4.2%), and liver (2.1%) (Table 2). IHC staining of pathogenic tissues from weaning pigs detected the Jeju LOM strain in internal organs (28.6%; 6/21): lymph nodes (20%), spleen (16.7%), lung (15.0%), and tonsil (5%) (Table 2). However, no virus was detected in other internal organs (heart, liver, intestine, spinal, and brain). One of the 22 fetuses showed an infection of the kidney alone (Table 2).

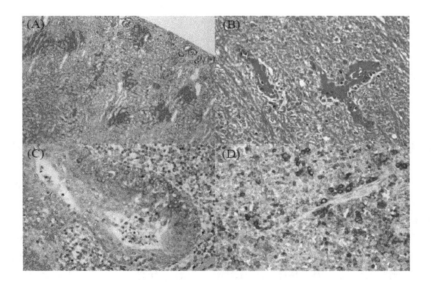

Figure 1. Immunohistochemistry (IHC) staining to detect histopathogenic lesions. Severe multifocal hemorrhages in the renal cortex of a suckling piglet (hematoxylin & eosin (HE); mag ×100) (**A**). Perivascular cuffing in the white matter of the cerebellum of a suckling piglet (HE; mag ×400) (**B**). Brown-stained viral antigens in the cryptal epithelium of the tonsil (IHC; mag ×400) (**C**). Brown-stained viral antigens in macrophages infiltrating the spleen (IHC; mag ×400) (**D**).

Table 1. Classical swine fever virus (CSFV; the Jeju LOM strain) and other pathogens detected in pigs (2014–2018).

Infection Pattern with CSFV (Jeju LOM Strain)	Pathogens (or Diseases)	2014	2015	2016	2017	2018
Suckling piglets — Co-infection with other pathogens	Porcine epidemic diarrhea (PED)			1	2	2
	Rotavirus enteritis				2	1
	Rota viral enteritis + *Strep* or *Staphylo* pneumonia					2
	Colibacillosis			1	4	
	Clostridium difficile associated disease	2				
	Clostridium enteritis (+ exudative epidermitis)				1	
	Porcine reproductive and respiratory syndrome (PRRS)				2(1)	
	PRRS + *Pasteurella* pneumonia		2			
	Streptococcal infection (abscess etc.)			1	3	3
	Staphylococcal infection			1	2	
	Viral encephalitis suspect or bacterial meningitis			1		2
Suckling piglets — Infection (only Jeju LOM)				3	6	5
Weaning piglets — Co-infection with other pathogens	PRRS			1		
	PRRS + *Streptococcal* pneumonia			1		
	PRRS + PCV-2 + APP			1		
	Actinobacillus pleuropneumoniae (APP)			1	2	
	APP + PCV-2				1	
	PCV-2 (+ *Salmonellosis/Staphylo*)					3
	Pasteurella (or *E. coli*) pneumonia			1	1	
	Streptococcal infection					
	Rotavirus enteritis					4
	Salmonellosis (Colibacillosis)				2(1)	2
Total		2	2	14	28(2)	24

Table 2. Immunohistochemical analysis of CSFV (Jeju LOM strain) in the internal organs of pigs.

Infection Pattern with CSFV (Jeju LOM Strain)		Internal Organs (No. of Positive Pigs/No. Tested)									Total
		Tonsil	Lymph Node	Spleen	Lung	Heart	Kidney	Liver	GI Tract	CNS	
Suckling piglets	Co-infection	11/24	3/30	8/34	4/29	0/32	2/34	1/34	2/33	0/26	17/34
	Infection (only Jeju LOM)	3/11	3/10	3/14	2/12	0/13	0/14	0/13	0/13	0/12	8/14
	Subtotal	14/35	6/40	11/48	6/41	0/45	2/48	1/47	2/46	0/38	25/48
Weaning pigs	Co-infection	1/20	4/20	3/18	3/20	0/20	0/20	0/19	0/21	0/15	6/21
Aborted fetuses	Infection (only Jeju LOM)	NT	NT	0/8	0/8	0/8	1/8	0/8	NT	0/8	1/8

GI: Gastrointestinal, CNS: Central Nervous System.

2.2. Detection of Antibodies on Pig Farms Exposed to the Jeju LOM Strain

The average anti-CSF (Jeju LOM) antibody-positive rates on seven pig farms in the Jeju region was as follows: $87.1\% \pm 4.2\%$ of sows, $77.8\% \pm 8.6\%$ of suckling piglets, $24.2\% \pm 14.1\%$ of weaning pigs, $21.4\% \pm 11.2\%$ of growing pigs, and $38.5\% \pm 13.7\%$ of finishing pigs (Table 3). There were significant differences ($p < 0.05$) in the average anti-CSF (Jeju LOM) antibody-positive rates between sows and weaning pigs/growing pigs, and between suckling piglets and growing pigs, respectively. Serum neutralizing antibody ($\log_2$) titers in pigs on antibody-positive farms were 9.42 ± 0.25 ($\log_2$) in sows, 7.04 ± 0.54 ($\log_2$) in suckling pigs, 7.2 ± 1.04 ($\log_2$) in weaning pigs, 5.52 ± 0.12 ($\log_2$) in growing pigs, and 7.44 ± 0.74 ($\log_2$) in finishing pigs (Table 3). There were significant differences in the average anti-CSF (Jeju LOM) neutralizing antibody titers between sows and growing pigs ($p < 0.05$).

Table 3. CSF (Jeju LOM) seropositive rates and anti-CSFV (Jeju LOM) antibody titers in pigs of seven farms on Jeju Island.

Pig Farm	Antibody Positive Ratio (%) against CSFV (Jeju LOM Strain)					Average Antibody Titers (Log 2) for CSFV (Jeju LOM Strain)				
	Sow	Piglet (10–20 days)	Pig (40–60 days)	Pig (90–120 days)	Pig (150–180 days)	Sow	Piglet (10–20 days)	Pig (40–60 days)	Pig (90–120 days)	Pig (150–180 days)
A	80	40	30	0	0	9.5	7.0	9.1	-	-
B	90	95	100	80	0	10.0	10.0	7.1	5.2	-
C	100	100	40	40	90	8.1	6.1	5.5	5.5	8.0
D	100	90	0	10	70	9.1	6.3	-	5.6	8.5
E	90	95	0	0	40	9.5	6.2	-	-	8.9
F	80	65	0	0	10	9.6	6.0	-	-	7.1
G	70	60	0	20	60	10.2	7.7	-	5.8	4.7

2.3. Farm-Slaughterhouse-Farm Transmission

Of the 242 samples collected from vehicles at a slaughterhouse in Jeju, 151 (62.4%) were positive for Jeju LOM antigens by qRT-PCR. The detailed results regarding infected sites were as follows: 66.2% (47/71) driver foot floor, 38% (27/71) vehicle wheels, 71.6% (53/74) pig-holding compartment, and 92.3% (24/26) "other". Among the virus-positive samples, 92 positive samples had an estimated $TCID_{50}$/mL of $10^{3.0-3.9}$, and 11 samples had an estimated $TCID_{50}$/mL of $10^{4.0-4.9}$. One sample had a $TCID_{50}$/mL $> 10^{5.0}$ (Table 4). A peroxidase-link immunosorbent assay (PLA) virus viability test revealed strong staining of 13 samples (4 driver foot floor, 2 vehicle wheels, and 7 pig-holding compartment) and weak staining of 32 samples; 129 samples were unconfirmed due to cellular contamination by bacteria (Table 4).

Table 4. Contamination by the Jeju LOM strain via exposure during transport to or at a slaughterhouse.

qRT-PCR			Immuno Histo Chemistry (IHC) Staining			
Ct Value (Range)	Jeju LOM Strain * $TCID_{50}$ (Log 10)	Sample no.	Negative Samples	Weak Positive Samples	Strong Positive Samples	** No Test
>40	<1.0	91	43			48
36.1–39.9	1.0–2.0	26	9	1		16
30.5–36.0	2.0–3.0	21	4	8		9
26.7–30.4	3.0–4.0	92	12	22	3	55
24.4–26.6	4.0–5.0	11		1	9	1
<24.3	>5.0	1			1	

* $TCID_{50}$: Tissue culture infective dose 50. ** No test: samples were inoculated PK-15 cells but IHC was not performed due to contamination by bacteria.

2.4. Pig-to-Pig Transmission and Reproduction Rate (R)

Six pigs were inoculated with the Jeju LOM strain JJ16LOM-YJK08 and, after 24 h, were placed in a pen with six non-inoculated pigs. For Group 1, we used pigs (unhealthy) with PRRSV or PCV2, and Group 2 used pigs (healthy) without specific wasting diseases. In Group 1, two non-inoculated pigs were positive for anti-CSF (Jeju LOM) antibodies on Day 21 and Day 28. However, no non-inoculated pigs in Group 2 had detectable anti-CSF (Jeju LOM) antibodies on Day 45 (Table 5). The transmission possibility estimate for group 1 was R0 = 1.22 (95% confidence interval (CI), 0.980–1.765), whereas that for Group 2 was R0 = 0.00 (95% CI, not applicable) (Table 5).

Table 5. Estimated transmission probability between non-inoculated pigs and pigs inoculated with the Jeju LOM strain.

Group	Number of Pigs Inoculated with the Jeju LOM Strain	Non-Inoculated Pigs Exposed to Jeju LOM Virus Inoculated Pigs (1 DPI [a])	Pigs Detected with Jeju LOM Strain Antigens and/or Antibodies in Non-Inoculated Pigs (45 DPI)	Transmission Probability Estimate	
				R0 [b]	95% CI [c]
1	6	6	2	1.22	0.980–1.765
2	6	6	0	0.00	NA [d]

R0 calculated as $-\ln((1 - AR)/S0)/(AR - (1 - S0))$, CI calculated as $AR \pm 1.96\sqrt{AR \times (1 - AR)/n}$. [a] DPI, days post-infection. [b] R0: reproduction number; [c] CI: confidence interval; [d] NA: not applicable.

2.5. Comparison of LOM Strain Genome Sequences

The amino acid sequences of four commercial LOM vaccine strains were compared with those of five Jeju LOM strains (2004–2007), and three unique amino acid changes in the E1 (V-577-A/M) and NS4B (M-2378L and V-2383A) proteins were detected (Supplemental Table S1). Comparison of the Jeju LOM strain JJ04LOM-Tamra01 (2004) with the four other Jeju LOM strains (2005–2007) revealed six amino acid changes: E^{rns} (D-386-N, R-480-G), E2 (L-1065-S), NS3 (K-1165-R), NS4B (A-2352-V), and NS5A (N-2816-T) (Supplemental Table S1). Comparison of the four commercial LOM vaccine strains with 12 Jeju LOM strains (2014–2018) identified unique changes in the N^{pro} (K-57-R, L-143-Q), E^{rns} (Y-351-H, R-476-S), E1 (I-651-T), NS3 (V-1381-I, H-1584-N, K-2006-I), NS4B (M-2348-I, T-2371-I, I-2398-M, and V-2483-A), NS5A (A-2978-T), and NS5B (N-3409-S and S-3786-N) proteins (Supplemental Table S2).

2.6. Root-to-Top Divergence and Positive Selection Analyses

Application of the heuristic residual mean squared method to all strains (the commercial LOM vaccine and Jeju LOM strains) using the TempEst program revealed a slope of 3.93×10^{-5} (rate), an X-intercept (TMRCA) of 1797.24, a correlation coefficient of 0.1272, an R squared value of 1.6173×10^{-2}, and a residual mean squared value of 6.9076×10^{-6}. Root-to-top divergence for Jeju LOM strain JJ07LOM-JSG02 was >0.0130. Mainly, the Jeju LOM strains isolated from the field showed a high divergence value of between 0.0070 and 0.0130 (Figure 2). However, seven LOM vaccine strains (excluding 88LOM-Suri) and two Jeju LOM strains (JJ14LOM-WSH01 and JJ17LOM-LHH10) showed a low divergence value (0.0040–0.0060) (Figure 2). The omega value (*dN/dS*) for the commercial LOM vaccine strains and the Jeju LOM strains isolated from the field (2004–2007 and 2014–2018) showed high homology with respect to the E^{rns}, E1, E2, NS2, NS3, NS4A, NS4B, NS5A, and NS5B proteins (Figure 3A). However, the omega value for the C and P7 proteins of commercial LOM vaccine strains was a little higher (0.34224 and 0.43781, respectively) than that of the five Jeju LOM strains isolated in 2004 to 2007. The omega values for the C, E1, and E2 structural proteins of the Jeju LOM strains isolated in the field in 2014 to 2018 were higher than for the NS proteins (Figure 3A). Jeju LOM strains isolated from pigs from 2004 to 2007 were 98.8% to 99.2% identical at the nucleotide level and 99.2% to 99.4% identical at the amino acid level, with an omega value of 0.14088. Jeju LOM strains isolated from 2014 to 2018 showed 98.2% to 99.4% identity at the nucleotide level and 99.1% to 99.6% identity at the amino acid level, with an omega value of 0.16196 (Supplemental Table S3). The Bayes empirical Bayes (BEB) analysis of Jeju LOM strains isolated from 2004 to 2007 showed the possible inclusion mutation sites at 237, 259, 577, and 2467 aa positions, but a BEB analysis of Jeju LOM strains from 2014 to 2018 showed mutations at 173, 176, 386, 564, 1337, 2676, 2988, and 3605 aa positions. A native empirical Bayers (NEB) analysis performed with Jeju LOM strains (2014–2018) revealed the mutation site of the 564 aa position (*p* > 99%; Supplemental Table S3).

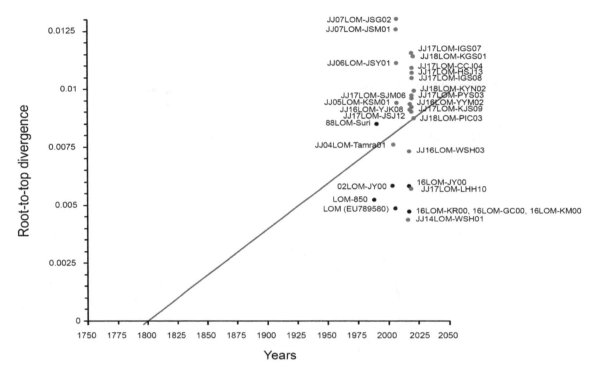

Figure 2. Root-to-top divergence analysis of Jeju LOM strains and commercial LOM vaccine strains. Complete genomes of 29 strains (8 commercial LOM vaccines and 21 Jeju LOM strains) were analyzed using the TempEst v1.5.1 program. The commercial LOM vaccine strains are marked with a black rectangle and the Jeju LOM strains are marked with a red rectangle. The heuristic residual mean squared method used to analyze all strains revealed the following: slope (rate), 3.93×10^{-5}; X-intercept (TMRCA), 1797.24; correlation coefficient, 0.1272; R squared value, 1.6173×10^{-2}; and residual mean squared value, 6.9076×10^{-6}.

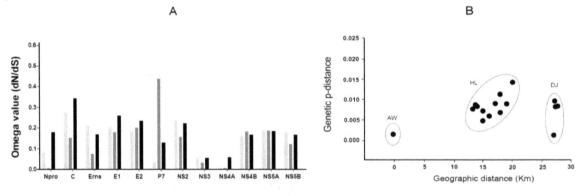

Figure 3. Omega values (dN/dS), genetic p-distances, and geographic distances for Jeju LOM strains. The dN/dS value for each of the structure proteins (N^{Pro}, C, E^{rns}, E1, E2, p7) and non-structural proteins (NS2, NS3, NS4A, NS4B, NS5A, NS5B) was calculated and compared among 8 commercial LOM vaccine strains, 5 Jeju LOM strains (2004–2007), and 16 Jeju LOM strains (2014–2018) (**A**). Light gray denotes the commercial LOM vaccine strain, dark gray denotes the Jeju LOM strains (2004–2007), and black denotes Jeju LOM strains (2014–2018) (A). Jeju LOM strains (2014–2018) from the Aeweal (AW), Hanlim (HL), and Daejeong (DJ) regions show genetic p-distances of 0.0018 (one strain), 0.0045–0.0139 (11 strains) and 0.0011–0.0086 (4 strains), respectively (**B**).

2.7. Geographic Distance and MCC Tree Analysis

A correlation between geographic distance and genetic p-distance of the Jeju LOM strains contaminating the commercial LOM vaccine strain 16LOM-KM00 from 2014 to 2018 was confirmed, as shown in Figure 3B. Jeju LOM strain JJ14LOM-WSH01, isolated at a pig farm in the Aeweal region in 2014, showed a genetic p-distance from commercial LOM vaccine strain 16LOM-KM00 of 0.0018.

Eleven Jeju LOM strains (Hanlim region: geographic distance, 13.5–20.1 km) and four Jeju LOM strains (Daejeong region: geographic distance, 27.4–28.1 km) isolated from pig farms showed a genetic p-distance of 0.0045–0.0139 and 0.0011–0.0086, respectively (Figures 3B and 4). Among genotypes 1, 2, and 3 in the beast tree constructed after global analysis of the complete E2 protein of CSFV, all LOM strains (including the Jeju LOM strains) belonged to independent groups within subgenotype 1.1 (Figure 5). From the mid-1980s, LOM strains were divided into two clusters: a lower cluster comprising commercial LOM vaccine strains and an upper cluster comprising mainly Jeju LOM strains isolated from pigs (Figure 5). In the above cluster, Jeju LOM strains isolated from pigs on Jeju Island were divided according to the year of isolation (2004–2007 and 2014–2018; Figure 5). The mean tMRCA for the LOM strains was 41.466, with an ESS (effective sample size) of 2340.2436 and a 95% highest posterior density (HPD) interval of 39.018–44.3142. The clock rate for LOM strains was 5.215×10^{-4}, with a 95% HPD interval of 4.1721×10^{-4}–6.159×10^{-4}.

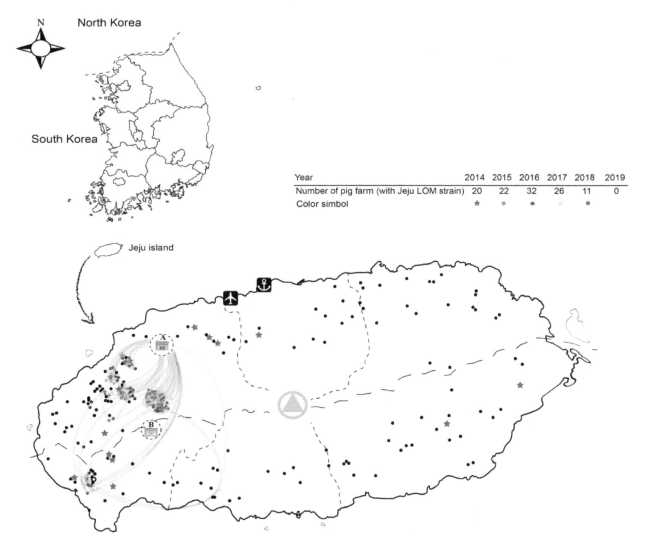

Year	2014	2015	2016	2017	2018	2019
Number of pig farm (with Jeju LOM strain)	20	22	32	26	11	0
Color simbol	★	●	●	▵	●	

Figure 4. Map of Jeju Island showing locations of the pig farms harboring the Jeju LOM strains (2014–2018). Pig farms harboring Jeju LOM strains (2014–2018) are marked with a red star (2014), an orange rectangle (2015), a purple rectangle (2016), a light green rectangle (2017), or a deep green rectangle (2018). Black rectangles denote pig farms without Jeju LOM strains. An old slaughterhouse (**A**) and a new slaughterhouse (**B**) built at the end of 2018 are located in the upper and middle left, respectively. The light brown and light purple curved lines denote the estimated routes by which Jeju LOM strains entered the pig farms.

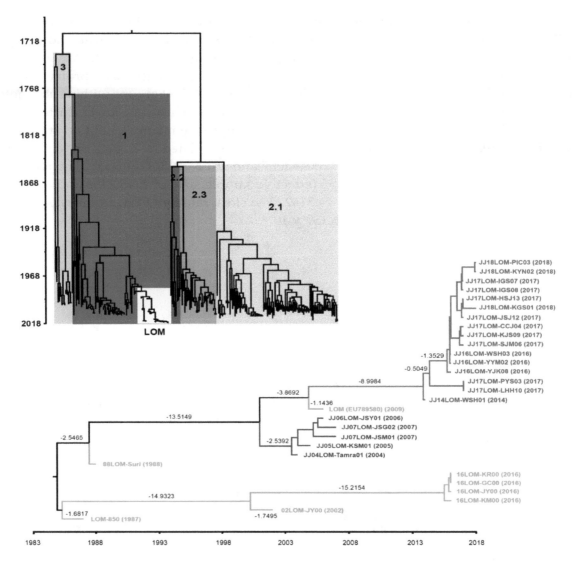

Figure 5. A maximum clade credibility tree based on complete E2 sequences of CSFVs. Rates of nucleotide substitution per site and per year, and the most recent common ancestor (tMRCA), were estimated using a Bayesian MCMC approach. Each dataset was simulated with the following options: generation = 100,000,000, burn-in of 10%, and ESSs > 200. The confidence of the phylogentic analysis is present to numbers representing branch length (time) above the nodes. The yellow block comprises LOM strains within Genotype 1. The light green line denotes 8 commercial LOM vaccine strains. The blue line denotes 5 Jeju LOM strains (2004–2007) and the red line denotes 16 Jeju LOM strains (2014–2018).

3. Discussion

The main characteristics of the LOM strain are attenuated; however, inoculation into pregnant sows lacking anti-CSF antibodies triggers abortion [7]. In addition, LOM vaccination of immunocompetent pigs leads to an antigen release period of more than 4 weeks, which results in the worsening of lesions if an animal is co-infected with other pathogens [8]. A previous study tested the effect of a live attenuated BVDV vaccine on pig-to-pig transmission and found that the R value was <1 [10]. Here, we found that transmission of the Jeju LOM strain differed significantly depending on the health status of the pig (Group 1 (unhealthy): r = 1.22; and Group 2 (healthy): r = 0). This is because, as for other wasting diseases, the period of virus release from infected pigs is prolonged and the amount of virus shed in the feces increases [8]. A commercial LOM vaccine strain showed 10% of the average transmission rate from inoculated pigs to cohabiting non-inoculated pigs [11]. Although a small number of pigs were used for the transmission experiment in this study, the transmission characteristics of the Jeju LOM strain were revealed to be similar to the commercial LOM vaccine. In a previous study, after oral inoculation of the LOM vaccine strain of $2 \times 10^{4.0} TCID_{50}/mL$, the LOM vaccine virus was detected in blood and feces in the 9 days post-inoculation [9]. We also detected 11 samples of live Jeju LOM viruses with more than $10^{4.0} TCID_{50}/mL$ in the slaughterhouse experiment, which support the possibility of farm-slaughterhouse-farm transmission.

From 2004 to 2005, LOM-infected pigs in Jeju showed varying symptoms. The clinical symptoms showed both the similarities and differences from those associated with CSF [10]. Similarities to more current Jeju LOM strain infections (2014–2018) included skin ulcers, ulceration of the tonsil, petechial hemorrhage in the kidney, button ulceration of the ileocecal region, infarction of the spleen, and pneumonia. Differences in histologic findings were a weakness in endothelial cell lesions of organs such as the spleen, lymph nodes, and brain. These lesions seem to be more related with PRRS not CSF. In addition, meningitis was observed in the central nervous system, CSF did not show meningitis, and lymphoid organs showed little increase in volume other than lymphocytic atrophy. The Jeju LOM strain that was prevalent from 2004 to 2007 was not related to CSF pathogenicity [10]. IHC (2004–2005) was Jeju LOM virus positive in 52.1% (25/48) of suckling piglets and 28.6% (6/21) of weaned pigs [10]. Our Jeju LOM antigen results (2014–2018) were lower than the results of the Jeju LOM antigen (2004–2005) test (58.3%) from a previous report [10]. Jeju LOM strains (2014–2018) were also suspected to have caused CSF-like lesions in 7 young piglets (average age of 10 days), which was proved by histopathological findings and IHC analysis. It may be deduced that some CSF lesions in suckling piglets, as well as abortion during pregnancy, are associated with LOM strains. However, in this case, it is unlikely that persistent infection will continue to circulate the virus among pigs.

Some experts suggest that Jeju LOM strains detected on Jeju pig farms from 2014 to 2018 have recovered pathogenicity and that it is now different from that of the commercial LOM vaccine strain on the current market. However, gene analysis of Jeju LOM strains revealed no evidence for restoration of pathogenicity. Previous studies have identified differences in pathogenic regions between the ALD and GPE strains as E2 (T830A), NS4B (V2475A, A2563V), and N^{pro} (N136D) [12,13]. Other studies revealed that Shimen's pathogenicity-related gene locus is within E2 (T745I, M979K) [14] and E2 (N850S) [15]. Our analysis of the amino acid sequences of the commercial LOM vaccine strain and the Jeju LOM strains detected in Jeju pigs revealed no changes at these sites. In addition, although there are differences in pathogenicity linked to changes in N-linked glycosylation sites on the E2 protein of CSF, there was no change of N-linked glycosylation sites in the Jeju LOM strains [16]. A study comparing the complete nucleotide and amino acid sequences of the ALD and GPE strains revealed 98.2% and 98.8% identity, respectively [17]. Although the Jeju LOM strain (2014–2018) harbors several amino acid mutations, it is difficult to interpret this as conferring recovery of pathogenicity or additional attenuation. There was no significant difference in the gene mutation rate among Jeju LOM strains, nor was there a significant difference in omega values. Therefore, Jeju LOM strains (2014–2018) from Jeju cannot be considered a pathogenically-reversed LOM strain, which is virulent in pigs but shows a safety profile characteristic of the commercial LOM vaccine strain described in previous study [7]. More precisely, the presence of Jeju LOM strains with recovered pathogenicity should be evaluated in animals (i.e., pregnancy sows and SPF pigs).

In conclusion, the CSF-like histopathogenic lesions of Jeju pigs revealed to be more related to other viral pathogens rather than the Jeju LOM strains (2014–2018), despite the presence of the Jeju LOM strain in organs of piglets. We also confirmed that the pig-to-pig transmission of the Jeju LOM strain and farm-to-farm transmission may have been caused by vehicles visiting the slaughterhouse. Although we found some genetic differences between the Jeju LOM strains (2014–2018) and commercial LOM vaccine strains, more pathogenesis studies may be needed using animals such as pregnant sows and SPF pigs.

4. Materials and Methods

4.1. Detection of Histopathologic Lesions and Immunohistochemical Straining Analysis

From 2014 to 2018, tests in this study performed by the diagnostic services of a veterinary medicine college in Jeju national university to detect animal infectious disease identified 122 samples (100 piglets and 22 fetuses) from 25 pig farms that were positive for CSFV by RT-PCR, histopathology, and IHC. The amplification targets for RT-PCR were CSFV [9], porcine circovirus type 2 (PCV2) [18], porcine reproductive and respiratory syndrome virus (PRRSV), swine influenza virus (SIV), cytomegalovirus (PCMV), *Salmonella* spp, *Streptococcus* spp, *Actinobacillus, pleuropneumoniae,* and *Haemophilus parasuis.* Histopathologic lesions specific to CSFV were examined by staining tissues with hematoxylin and eosin. The following were examined: skin (hemorrhage and endothelial damage), lymph nodes (peripheral hemorrhage, lymphoid depletion, and reticular cell hyperplasia), kidney and bladder (hemorrhage, swelling and peripheral hemorrhage), spleen (hemorrhagic infarction, endothelial damage), cecum and colon (necrotic or ulcerative colitis, vascular congestion, and sub-serous hemorrhage), heart (myocardial hemorrhage), and brain and spinal cord (nonsuppurative encephalitis, proliferation of endothelial cells, perivascular cuffing, microgliosis, and focal necrosis). To confirm the presence of CSF antigen in tissues, IHC was performed using the EnVision™ peroxidase-conjugated polymer reagent (DAKO, Denmark). In brief, tissues were reacted with a primary antibody (mouse anti-CSFV) (WH303, Animal and Plant Health Agency, New Haw, Addlestone, UK), followed by EnVision™/HRP, rabbit/mouse (EVN) regent (DAKO, USA), and 3,3'-diamino-benzidine tetrahydrochloride (DAB). The presence of CSF antigen is denoted by a dark brown deposit in the tissue section.

4.2. Detection of Anti-CSF Antibodies

Seven pig farms with the Jeju LOM infection were selected to estimate how Jeju LOM strains were introduced into the farms and how they spread within the farms. The anti-CSF antibody-positive rates for each pig farm and antibody titer levels for pigs within farms were examined according to age. Blood samples were collected from 20 pigs in each group: sows, suckling pigs (10–20 days old), weaning pigs (40–60 days old), growing pigs (90–120 days old), and finishing pigs (150–180 days old). To detect CSF-specific neutralizing antibodies, a neutralizing peroxidase-linked assay (NPLA) was performed according to the standards manual of the World Organization for Animal Health [19]. For PK-15 cell staining, the monoclonal antibody 3B6 (Median Diagnostics, Chuncheon, Korea) was used to detect the CSF E2 protein.

4.3. Environmental Samples Taken from a Slaughterhouse

In 2017, 242 samples were obtained from a slaughterhouse in Jeju to investigate CSFV (Jeju LOM strain). These included 71 samples from the driver's foot floor, 71 from vehicle wheels, 74 from the vehicle's pig-holding compartment, and 26 from other sites. Real-time quantitative PCR (qRT-PCR) was performed to detect the CSF antigen copy number in fecal and environmental samples. The VDx® CSFV qRT-PCR (MEDIAN Diagnostic Co. Cat No. NS-CSF-31, Gangwon-do, Korea), which uses TaqMan probes, detects the CSFV 5' UTR with high specificity; it does not detect BVDV or border disease virus, which also belong to the *Pestivirus* genus. Briefly, the qRT-PCR program comprised the following steps: cDNA synthesis (50 °C, 30 min) and initial inactivation (95 °C, 15 min), followed by a two-step PCR comprising 42 cycles of denaturation (95 °C, 10 s) and extension (60 °C, 60 s). A peroxidase-linked immunosorbent assay (PLA) was used to confirm viability of Jeju LOM strains. Briefly, PK-15 cells (grown to 80% confluence in 24-well plates) were inoculated for 72 h at 37 °C with 10% tissue homogenates including the Jeju LOM strain in a minimum essential medium. The PK-15 cells were fixed in pre-chilled 80% acetone after 72 h and reacted with a 3B6 monoclonal antibody specific for CSFV E2. Subsequently, the PK-15 cells were reacted with biotinylated anti-mouse IgG (H + L) (VECTOR Laboratories, Cat No. BA-9200, Burlingame, CA, USA) and ABC solution (VECTOR Laboratories, Cat No. PK-4000, Burlingame, CA, USA). After staining with DAB peroxidase substrate (VECTOR Laboratories, Cat No. SK-4100, Burlingame, CA, USA) following the manufacturer's instruction, the PK-15 cells were observed under a microscope.

4.4. Horizontal Transmission between Pigs

To investigate the transmission probability of the Jeju LOM strain among pigs, 40-day-old CSF antigen- and antibody-negative pigs from two pig farms (n = 24, 12 per farm) were used. Group 1 comprised of pigs with a wasting disease (PRRSV or PCV2) and Group 2 comprised of pigs with specific non-disease. Six pigs from each group were inoculated intramuscularly with 2 mL ($10^{4.0}$TCID$_{50}$/mL) of the Jeju LOM strain JJ16LOM-YJK08, which is a representative strain circulating in Jeju between 2014 and 2018. After 24 h, the six pigs from each group were housed with non-injected pigs and observed for clinical signs and symptoms. Blood was collected every week for 45 days and tested in the NPLA assay and by qRT-PCR. The estimated reproduction number (R0) and confidence interval (CI) were calculated as described previously [20] using the following formula: R0 = −In((1−AR)/S0)/(AR−(1−S0)); CI = AR ± 1.96 $\sqrt{ARx(1 - AR)/n}$.

4.5. Genomic Analysis of Commercial LOM Vaccine Strains and Jeju LOM Strains

The complete genome sequences of seven commercial LOM vaccine strains (16LOM-GC00, 16LOM-JY00, 16LOM-KM00 and 16LOM-KR00 (collected from a market in 2016), 02LOM-JY00 (collected from a market in 2002), 88LOM-suri (isolated from LOM-850 strain in 1988), and LOM-850 (original master seed in 1987)) were examined. In addition, five Jeju LOM strains isolated from pigs on Jeju Island between 2004 and 2007, and 16 Jeju LOM strains isolated from pigs on Jeju Island between 2014 and 2018, were analyzed. Positive selection analysis of the complete ORF (N^{pro}, C, E^{rns}, E1, E2, P7, NS2, NS3, NS4A, NS4B, NS5A, and NS5B) was conducted using several models available in the BASEML and CODEML modules of the PAML 4.6 software package [21]. Different values of the non-synonymous/synonymous (dN/dS) ratio (the omega parameter), were considered in accordance with the user manual. A dN/dS ratio of <1 indicates a purifying selection, a dN/dS ratio = 1 suggests an absence of selection (i.e., neutral evolution), and dN/dS >1 indicates a positive selection. The Bayes empirical Bayes (BEB) calculation of the posterior probabilities of site classes was used to calculate the probability that a site is under positive selection pressure [22]. TempEst (formerly known as "Path-O-gen") is a tool for investigating the temporal signals and "clocklikeness" of molecular phylogenies. The contemporaneous trees (in which all sequences were collected at the same time) and dated-tip trees (in which sequences are collected at different dates) were analyzed using the TempEst v1.5.1 program, which is temporal signal estimator tool [23]. The genome sequences of the Jeju LOM strains (n = 21) and commercial LOM vaccine strains (n = 8) in this study were submitted to the GenBank under accession numbers MN558862–MN558889.

4.6. Maximum Clade Credibility Tree

Complete sequences for the E2 gene of 145 CSFV isolates available in the GenBank Database, including complete E2 gene sequences of 8 commercial LOM vaccine strains and 21 Jeju LOM strains, were used to generate a BEAST input file using BEAUti within the BEAST package v1.8.1 [24]. Rates of nucleotide substitution per site and per year, and the most recent common ancestor (tMRCA), were estimated using a Bayesian MCMC approach. Each dataset was simulated with the following options: generation = 100,000,000, burn-in of 10%, and ESSs > 200. The exponential clock and expansion growth population model in the BEAST program was used to obtain the best-fit evolutionary model. The resulting convergence was analyzed using Tracer 1.5 [25]. Trees were summarized as a maximum clade credibility (MCC) tree using TreeAnnotator 1.7.4 [26] and visualized using Figtree 1.4 [27]. For each tree node, estimated divergence times and 95% HPD intervals, which summarize statistical uncertainties, were indicated.

4.7. Statistical Analysis

All statistical analyses were performed using the GraphPad Prism software, version 6.0, for Windows. Data were analyzed using one-way analysis of variance, followed by Tukey's multiple-comparison test. Groups showing significant differences ($p < 0.05$) at the same time point are indicated by different letters.

Author Contributions: I.-S.C., B.-H.H., B.-K.P. and D-J.A. conceived the study; S.C., J.-H.K. and D.-J.A. designed the experiments; S.C., J.-H.K., K.-S.K., S.S., W.-C.K., H.-J.K., G.-N.P. and R.-M.C. performed the experiments; J.-H.K., W.-C.K. and H.-J.K. acquired samples; S.C., R.-M.C. and D.-J.A. drafted the manuscript. All authors read and approved the final version.

References

1. Becher, P.; Avalos Ramirez, R.; Orlich, M.; Cedillo Rosales, S.; Konig, M.; Schweizer, M.; Stalder, H.; Schirrmeier, H.; Thiel, H.J. Genetic and antigenic characterization of novel pestivirus genotypes: Implications for classification. *Virology* **2003**, *311*, 96–104. [CrossRef]
2. Rice, C.M. Flaviviridae: The viruses and their replication. In *Fundamental Virology*, 3rd ed.; Knipe, D.M., Howley, P., Eds.; Lippincott Raven: Philadelphia, PA, USA, 1996; pp. 931–959.
3. Paton, D.J.; McGoldrick, A.; Greiser-Wilke, I.; Parchariyanon, S.; Song, J.Y.; Liou, P.P.; Stadejek, T.; Lowings, J.P.; Björklund, H.; Belák, S. Genetic typing of classical swine fever virus. *Vet. Microbiol.* **2000**, *73*, 137–157. [CrossRef]
4. Edwards, S.; Fukusho, A.; Lefevre, P.C.; Lipowski, A.; Pejsak, Z.; Roehe, P.; Westergaard, J. Classical swine fever: The global situation. *Vet. Microbiol.* **2000**, *73*, 103–119. [CrossRef]
5. Morilla, A.; Carvajal, M.A. Experiences with classical swine fever vaccination in Mexico. In *Trends in Emerging Viral Infections of Swine*; Morilla, A., Yoon, K.J., Zimmerman, J.J., Eds.; Iowa State Press, Blackwell Publishing Company: Ames, IA, USA, 2002; pp. 159–164.
6. Pijoan, C.; Campos, M.; Ochoa, G. Effect of a hog cholera vaccine strain on the bactericidal activity of porcine alveolar macrophages. *Rev. Latinoam. Microbiol.* **1980**, *22*, 69–71. [PubMed]
7. Lim, S.I.; Song, J.Y.; Kim, J.; Hyun, B.H.; Kim, H.Y.; Cho, I.S.; Kim, B.; Woo, G.H.; Lee, J.B.; An, D.J. Safety of classical swine fever virus vaccine strain LOM in pregnant sows and their offspring. *Vaccine* **2016**, *34*, 2021–2026. [CrossRef] [PubMed]
8. Lim, S.I.; Jeoung, H.Y.; Kim, B.; Song, J.Y.; Kim, J.; Kim, H.Y.; Cho, I.S.; Woo, G.H.; Lee, J.B.; An, D.J. Impact of porcine reproductive and respiratory syndrome virus and porcine circovirus-2 infection on the potency of the classical swine fever vaccine (LOM strain). *Vet. Microbiol.* **2016**, *193*, 36–41. [CrossRef] [PubMed]
9. Kim, B.; Song, J.Y.; Tark, D.S.; Lim, S.I.; Choi, E.J.; Park, C.K.; Lee, B.Y.; Wee, S.H.; Bae, Y.C.; Lee, O.S.; et al. Feed comtaminated with classical swine fever vaccine virus (LOM strain) can induce antibodies to the virus in pigs. *Vet. Rec.* **2008**, *162*, 12–17. [CrossRef]
10. Wieringa-Jelsma, T.; Quak, S.; Loeffen, W.L. Limited BVDV transmission and full protection against CSFV transmission in pigs experimentally infected with BVDV type 1b. *Vet. Microbiol.* **2006**, *118*, 26–36. [CrossRef]
11. Kang, M.I. *Epidemiological Survey Report on the Detection of CSF Vaccine (LOM Strain) in Jeju Island*; National Veterinary Research Quarantine Service (NVRQS) Publishing: Anyang, Korea, 2005; pp. 1–137.
12. Tamura, T.; Sakoda, Y.; Yoshino, F.; Nomura, T.; Yamamoto, N.; Sato, Y.; Okamatsu, M.; Ruggli, N.; Kida, H. Selection of classical swine fever virus with enhanced pathogenicity reveals synergistic virulence determinants in E2 and NS4B. *J. Virol.* **2012**, *86*, 8602–8613. [CrossRef] [PubMed]
13. Tamura, T.; Nagashima, N.; Ruggli, N.; Summerfield, A.; Kida, H.; Sakoda, Y. Npro of classical swine fever virus contributes to pathogenicity in pigs by preventing type I interferon induction at local replication sites. *Vet. Res.* **2014**, *45*, 47. [CrossRef] [PubMed]
14. Wu, R.; Li, L.; Zhao, Y.; Tu, J.; Pan, Z. Identification of two amino acids within E2 important for the pathogenicity of chimeric classical swine fever virus. *Virus. Res.* **2016**, *211*, 79–85. [CrossRef] [PubMed]
15. Holinka, L.G.; Fernandez-Sainz, I.; Sanford, B.; O'Donnell, V.; Gladue, D.P.; Carison, J.; Lu, Z.; Risatti, G.R.; Borca, M.V. Development of an improved live attenuated antigenic marker CSF vaccine strain candidate with an increased genetic stability. *Virology* **2014**, *471*, 13–18. [CrossRef] [PubMed]

16. Risatti, G.R.; Holinka, L.G.; Fernandez Sainz, I.; Carrillo, C.; Lu, Z.; Borca, M.V. N-linked glycosylation status of classical swine fever virus strain Brescia E2 glycoprotein influences virulence in swine. *J. Virol.* **2007**, *81*, 924–933. [CrossRef] [PubMed]

17. Ishikawa, K.; Nagai, H.; Katayama, K.; Tsutsui, M.; Tanabayashi, K.; Takeuchi, K.; Hishiyama, M.; Saitoh, A.; Takagi, M.; Gotoh, K.; et al. Comparison of the entire nucleotide and deduced amino acid sequences of the attenuated hog cholera vaccine strain GPE- and the wild-type parental strain ALD. *Arch. Virol.* **1995**, *140*, 1385–1391. [CrossRef] [PubMed]

18. Larochelle, R.; Antaya, M.; Morin, M.; Magar, R. Typing of porcine circovirus in clinical specimens by multiplex PCR. *J. Virol. Methods* **1999**, *80*, 69–75. [CrossRef]

19. Drew, T. Classical swine fever (hog cholera). In *Manual of Diagnostic Tests and Vaccines for Terrestrial Animals: Mammals, Birds and Bees*, 6th ed.; Office International des Epizooties (OIE), Ed.; OIE: Paris, France, 2008; pp. 1092–1106.

20. Dietz, K. The estimation of the basic reproduction number for infectious diseases. *Stat. Methods Med. Res.* **1993**, *2*, 23–41. [CrossRef] [PubMed]

21. Yang, Z. PAML 4: Phylogenetic analysis by maximum likelihood. *Mol. Biol. Evol.* **2007**, *24*, 1586–1591. [CrossRef] [PubMed]

22. Thompson, J.D.; Gibson, T.J.; Plewniak, F.; Jeanmougin, F.; Higgins, D.G. The CLUSTAL_X windows interface: Flexible strategies for multiple sequence alignment aided by quality analysis tools. *Nucleic Acids Res.* **1997**, *25*, 4876–4882. [CrossRef] [PubMed]

23. Rambaut, A.; Lam, T.T.; Carvalho, L.M.; Pybus, O.G. Exploring the temporal structure of heterochronous sequences using TempEst. *Virus Evol.* **2016**, *2*, vew007. [CrossRef] [PubMed]

24. Drummond, A.J.; Suchard, M.A.; Xie, D.; Rambaut, A. Bayesian phylogenetics with BEAUti and the BEAST 1.7. *Mol. Biol. Evol.* **2012**, *29*, 1969–1973. [CrossRef] [PubMed]

25. Rambaut, A.; Drummond, A.J. Tracer v1.5. 2009. Available online: http://beast.bio.ed.ac.uk/Tracer (accessed on 20 November 2019).

26. Rambaut, A.; Drummond, A.J. TreeAnnotator v1.7.0. 2012. Available online: http://beast.bio.ed.ac.uk (accessed on 20 November 2019).

27. Rambaut, A. FigFree v.1.4.0. 2012. Available online: http://tree.bio.ed.ac.uk/software/figtree (accessed on 20 November 2019).

Adverse Effects of Classical Swine Fever Virus LOM Vaccine and Jeju LOM Strains in Pregnant Sows and Specific Pathogen-Free Pigs

SeEun Choe [1,†], Jae-Hoon Kim [2,†], Ki-Sun Kim [1], Sok Song [1], Ra Mi Cha [1], Wan-Choul Kang [3], Hyeun-Ju Kim [3], Gyu-Nam Park [1], Jihye Shin [1], Hyoung-Nam Jo [2], In-Soo Cho [1], Bang-Hun Hyun [1], Bong-Kyun Park [1,4] and Dong-Jun An [1,*]

[1] Viral Disease Division, Animal and Plant Quarantine Agency (APQA), Gimcheon, Gyeongbuk 39660, Korea; ivvi59@korea.kr (S.C.); kisunkim@korea.kr (K.-S.K.); ssoboro@naver.com (S.S.); rami.cha01@korea.kr (R.M.C.); changep0418@gmail.com (G.-N.P.); shinjibong227@gmail.com (J.S.); chois38@korea.kr (I.-S.C.); hyunbh@korea.kr (B.-H.H.); park026@korea.kr (B.-K.P.)
[2] College of Veterinary Medicine and Veterinary Medical Research Institute, Jeju National University, Jeju 63243, Korea; kimjhoon@jejunu.ac.kr (J.-H.K.); engle59@naver.com (H.-N.J.)
[3] Jeju Special Self-Governing Provincial Veterinary Research Institute, Jeju 63344, Korea; kwc1041@korea.kr (W.-C.K.); bluemouse@korea.kr (H.-J.K.)
[4] College of Veterinary Medicine, Seoul University, Gwanak-ro, Gwanak-gu, Seoul 08826, Korea
* Correspondence: andj67@korea.kr
† Authors contributed equally.

Abstract: In Jeju island of South Korea, a classical swine fever (CSF) non-vaccinated region, many pig farmers insisted on abortion and stillbirth in pregnant sows and high mortality of suckling/weaning piglets by circulating CSF virus from 2014 to 2018. We investigated whether CSF viruses isolated from pigs in Jeju Island (Jeju LOM) have recovered their pathogenicity by conducting experiments using pregnant sows and specific pathogen-free (SPF) pigs. The CSF modified live LOM vaccine (MLV-LOM) and Jeju LOM strains induced abortion and stillbirth in pregnant sows. Viral antigens were detected in the organs of fetuses and stillborn piglets in the absence of specific pathological lesions associated with the virulent CSF virus in both groups (MLV-LOM and Jeju LOM strain). However, antigen was detected in one newborn piglet from a sow inoculated with a Jeju LOM strain, suggesting that it may cause persistent infections in pigs. SPF pigs inoculated with the MLV-LOM or Jeju LOM strains were asymptomatic, but virus antigen was detected in several organ and blood samples. Virus shedding in both groups of animals was not detected in the feces or saliva until 21 days post inoculation. The serum concentration of the three major cytokines, IFN-α, TNF-α, and IL-10, known to be related to lymphocytopenia, were similar in both groups when the MLV-LOM or Jeju LOM strains were inoculated into SPF pigs. In conclusion, Jeju LOM strains exhibited most of the characteristics of the MLV-LOM in pigs and resulted in the same adverse effects as the MLV-LOM strain.

Keywords: CSFV; pathogenicity; MLV-LOM; SPF pig; Jeju LOM strain

---

1. Introduction

Classical swine fever virus (CSFV) is a small, enveloped virus with a positive-stranded RNA genome of approximately 12.5 kb in size and contains a single, large, open reading frame that encodes a 3898 amino acid (aa) polyprotein [1]. Classical swine fever (CSF) is a devastating disease, causing substantial economic losses through the death of valuable livestock. Major outbreak of CSF is now rare, but sporadic epizootic incidents still occur frequently, causing chronic, atypical forms of the disease. Virulent CSFV enters the host through the mucous membranes of the oral and nasal cavities, known to infect tonsil cells and then spread into whole body using the circulation (blood and lymph) systems [2]. When CSFV infects pregnant sows, vertical transmission to the fetus was reported, which means CSFV may infect the fetus via passing placental barrier and the affected fetus may carry persistent infection (PI) [2]. CSFV-infected sows, depending on the gestation stage, show mild clinical signs whereas infection may result in mummification or absorption of fetuses and ends pregnancy with abortions or stillbirth [3–7].

Acute CSFV infection may result in high fever, leukopenia, thrombocytopenia, and hemorrhages in various organs [8]. CSFV also caused multiple pathological lesions such as enlarged lymph nodes, hemorrhages, and petechiae on the serosal and mucosal surfaces of many organs including the lungs, kidneys, intestines, and urinary bladder [8]. Previous reports showed that acute CSF infection induces a so-called cytokine storm by aberrant levels of type I interferon (IFN) and proinflammatory mediators [8,9]. It has been shown that lymphocyte depletion is related to a strong IFN-α response [9] and lymphocytopenia is closely associated with interleukin IL-1α, IL-6, and tumor necrosis factor TNF-α responses [10]. Chronic CSFV infection known to cause pathological changes including atrophy of the thymus, depletion of the lymphoid organs, necrosis, and ulceration of the small intestine, colon, and ileocecal valve [8]. These clinical signs and lesions were also caused by many other swine pathogens [8]. Various non-specific clinical signs and lesions among animals may be due to the host factor and the virulence of the CSFV strain. In addition, age, breed and immune status of each animal often play a role in the outcome of disease [11–13].

Use of a CSF-modified live LOM (Low virulence strain of Miyagi) vaccine (MLV-LOM) in pigs in Korea since 1974 was shown to result in adverse effects, such as abortion and stillbirth, in naïve pregnant sows that had not produced CSF antibody [14]. When the MLV-LOM was inoculated into piglets already infected with immunosuppressive pathogens, the MLV-LOM induced vaccine-specific antibodies without any adverse effects. [15]. However, the MLV-LOM remained in the pigs' bodies for a longer time, reflecting the possibility that virus shedding and transmission might occur [15]. A previous report showed that oral administration of the MLV-LOM can induce immunity in pigs. [16].

The Korean government maintains a MLV-LOM policy for CSF control on the mainland but not on Jeju Island, where the MLV-LOM vaccine has not been used since 2000 [17]. In 2014, pregnant sows on 20 Jeju Island pig farms were inoculated to commercial swine erysipelas vaccine mixed with the MLV-LOM [17]. Administration of the vaccine was stopped immediately, but between 2015 and 2018, pigs on an additional 91 farms were found to have been transmitted to the virus [17]. Jeju farmers and some pig disease experts insisted on abortion and stillbirth of pregnant sows and high mortality of suckling/weaning piglets by Jeju LOM strain [17]. Therefore, the safety of the MLV-LOM was questioned and its reversion to pathogenicity suspected.

The main purpose of this study was to determine whether the Jeju LOM strains on Jeju Island exhibited pathogenic properties when inoculated into pregnant sows and specific pathogen-free (SPF) pigs. We also analyze the causes of MLV-LOM strain influx and spread in CSF non-vaccinated area.

2. Results

2.1. Viral Antigen Detection in Pregnant Pigs 3 Weeks Post Inoculation

One (no. 37-5952) of three pregnant sows in group 1 was autopsied three weeks post inoculation (wpi) with strain JJ16LOM-YJK08 (Jeju LOM), and CSFV RNA was detected in the tonsils by qRT-PCR. In addition, 17/20 (85%) fetuses of the same pregnant sow were positive for CSFV RNA by qRT-PCR (Table 1). CSFV RNA was detected in the heart of a pregnant sow (no. 51-2104) in group 2, which was inoculated with strain JJ16LOM-YYM02 (Jeju LOM), and 9/14 (64%) fetuses were CSFV RNA positive (Table 1). In a pregnant sow (no. LI-5534) in group 3, inoculated with strain 16LOM-KM00 (MLV-LOM), a tonsil sample was CSFV RNA positive, and 7/9 (78%) fetuses were positive for the CSFV RNA (Table 1). No histologic preparations of the three pregnant sows revealed lesions associated with CSF. Pathologic examination of the internal organs of 43 fetuses from the three sows showed no specific lesions, and no viral antigen was detected by the immunohistochemical (IHC) assay.

Table 1. Autopsy results for pregnant sows three three weeks after inoculation with the modified live (MLV)–LOM or Jeju LOM strains.

Group	Inoculum Strain	No. of Pregnant Sow	Day of Inoculation Post-Pregnancy	Day of Autopsy Post-Pregnancy	Antigen Detection in Organs from Pregnant Sows				Antigen Positive Fetuses/Total Fetuses (%)
					Tonsil	Heart	Lymph Node	Other Organs *	
G1	JJ16LOM-YJK08	37-5952	66	87	+	-	-	-	17/20 (85)
G2	JJ16LOM-YYM02	51-2104	64	85	-	+	-	-	9/14 (64.2)
G3	16LOM-KM00	LI-5534	67	88	+	-	-	-	7/9 (77.7)

* Lung, spleen, liver, kidney, ileum, brain, bladder.

2.2. Pathogenicity in Pregnant Pigs and Their Piglets

In group 1, inoculated with strain JJ16LOM-YJK08 (Jeju LOM), and group 2, inoculated with strain JJ16LOM-YYM02 (Jeju LOM), the total number of fetuses produced was 23 and 32, respectively. In group 1, nine fetuses were mummified, 13 were stillborn, and one was a live birth; in group 2, 11 were mummified, 15 were stillborn, and six were live births. The crown–rump (C-R) length range of fetuses was 5.0–28.5 cm for group 1 and 6.5–30.0 cm for group 2 (Table 2). The total number of fetuses in group 3 inoculated with strain 16LOM-KM00 (MLV-LOM) were 13, of which 12 were mummified and one was a live birth. The C-R length of fetuses ranged from 11.5 to 28 cm (Table 2). CSFV RNA detection in fetuses was 20/23 (86.9%) for group 1, 23/32 (71.8%) for group 2, and 12/13 (92.3%) for group 3 samples by qRT-PCR (Table 2). When strains JJ16LOM-YJK08 and JJ16LOM-YYM02 were used as inocula, CSFV RNA was detected in all samples (13/13 and 15/15, respectively) from stillborn fetuses, and all 12 mummified fetuses in group 3 contained CSFV RNA (Table 2). In addition, one out of eight live piglets tested from all groups (1–3) was CSFV RNA positive in organ samples (Table 2).

One weak-born piglet and one still-born fetus delivered from sow no. 34-5053 in group 1 exhibited necrosis, hemorrhage, severe vacuolation, and perivascular cuffing in the white matter of cerebellum, and one fetus also exhibited severe myocardial necrosis in the heart (Figure 1A,C). Three piglets from sow no. 62-0093 in group 2 were identified as non-suppurative encephalitis with hemorrhage and mineral deposition in the white matter of in the cerebellum. However, no specific lesions were observed in fetuses in the other groups (3 and 4). By IHC staining, viral antigens were detected in the internal organs group 1 weak born piglet and stillborn fetus (Figure 1B,D) and in the heart of one stillborn group 2 fetus. Seroconversions for CSF neutralizing antibodies in pregnant pigs were on average 7 log $_2$ for group 1, 6.5 log $_2$ for group 2, and 7 log $_2$ for group 3, when measured 3 wpi, and 7 log $_2$, 9.5 log $_2$, and 10 log $_2$ at delivery, respectively.

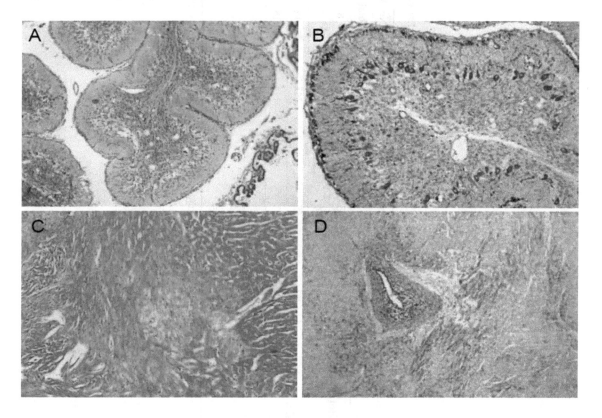

Figure 1. Severe vacuolation in the white matter of cerebellum of a weak born piglet (**A**); severe myocardial necrosis in the heart of a weak born piglet (**C**); and expression of LOM antigens in cerebellum (**B**) and heart (**D**) (A and C: H & E, × 200) and (B and D: IHC, × 200).

Table 2. Neonatal piglets from sows inoculated with MLV-LOM or Jeju LOM strains.

Group	Inoculum Strain	No. of Sow	* Day of Inoculation Post-Pregnancy (Days)	Total Period of Pregnancy (Days)	No. Viral Antigen Positive/No. of Offspring				** Positive Antigen/Test No. (%)	Crown-Rump (cm)
					Total	Mummified	Stillborn	Live		
G1	JJ16LOM-YJK08	102	65	113	8	6/6	2/2	-	8/8 (100)	19-28.5
		34-5053	66	114	15	0/3	11/11	***1/1	12/15 (80)	5-28
G2	JJ16LOM-YYM02	L1-6061	65	115	14	5/5	6/6	0/3	11/14 (78.5)	6.5-27.5
		62-0093	65	114	18	3/6	9/9	0/3	12/18 (66.6)	17-30
G3	16LOM-KM00	55-4424	65	114	7	7/7	-	-	7/7 (100)	11.5-17.5
		45-0502	64	113	6	5/5	-	0/1	5/6 (83.3)	16.5-28
G4	Control	720	65	114	17	-	0/2	0/15	0/17 (0)	25-30

* Inoculation concentration: $10^{3.5}TCID_{50}$/mL, 2ml/dose. ** Number positive for antigen by qRT-PCR. *** Antigen detection in the blood of a live neonatal suckling piglet.

2.3. Pathogenicity in SPF Pigs

The rectal temperatures of 22 SPF pigs did not exceed 40 °C until 14 days post inoculation (Figure 2A). CSF neutralizing antibodies for SPF pigs at 14 days post inoculation (dpi) were on average 5.9 $\log_2$ for group 1 inoculated with strain JJ16LOM-YJK08 (Jeju LOM), 6.4 $\log_2$ for group 2 inoculated with strain JJ16LOM-YJK08-F (Jeju LOM), and 6.0 $\log_2$ for group 3 inoculated with strain 16LOM-KO00 (MLV-LOM) (Figure 2B). In all groups, the neutralizing antibody titers showed a significant seroconversion ($p < 0.05$) when compared with uninoculated control group 4 at 14 dpi (Figure 2B). Virus-inoculated and uninoculated SPF pigs gained average weights of 2.02, 1.96, 2.22, and 2.45 kg in groups 1, 2, 3, and 4, respectively, during the observation period (14 days; Figure 2C). White blood cell (WBC) counts in the SPF pigs in groups 1, 2, 3, and 4 decreased to averages of 7142, 6300, 9868, and 13,400/µl at 4 dpi, respectively (Figure 2D). At 4 dpi, 6/10 SPF pigs (60%) in group 1 and 5/5 pigs (100%) in group 2 showed symptoms of temporary leukopenia (Figure 2D).

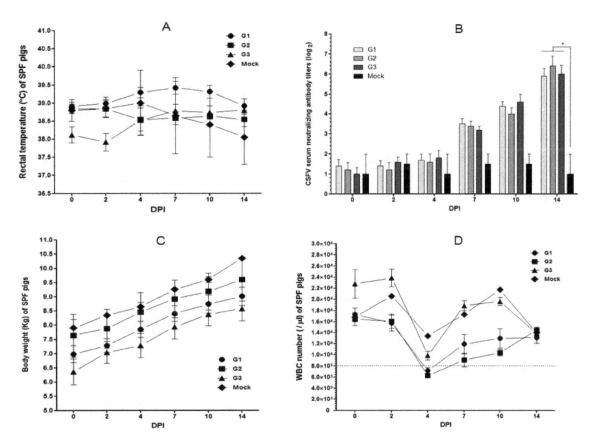

Figure 2. Changes in rectal temperature, neutralization antibodies, bodyweights, and white blood cell counts of specific pathogen-free pigs inoculated with the JJ16LOM-YJK08 in G1, JJ16LOM-YJK-F in G2, and 16LOM-KO00 in G3. Rectal temperature (**A**), neutralization antibodies (**B**), bodyweight (**C**), and white blood cells (**D**). Bars represent the mean ± standard error (SE) during animal experiment period. * $p < 0.05$ compared with neutralization antibody values among groups at 14 dpi (**B**). Below dotted line indicate leukopenia (**D**).

2.4. Histopathogenic Lesions and Virus Shedding in SPF Pigs

For group 1 SPF pigs, CSFV RNA was detected in 6/10 (60%) blood samples at 7 dpi, 8/10 (80%) at 10 dpi, and 3/10 (30%) at 14 dpi by qRT-PCR (Table 3). For group 2 pigs, CSFV RNA was detected in 4/5 (80%) blood samples at 7 dpi, 5/5 (100%) at 10 dpi, and 2/5 (40%) at 14 dpi. For group 3 SPF pigs, CSFV RNA was detected in only 2/5 (40%) blood samples tested at 10 dpi (Table 3). However, CSFV RNA was not detected in the saliva or feces of any of the SPF pigs tested (Table 3).

180

Diseases of Swine

Table 3. Detection of classical swine fever virus (CSFV) RNA in specific pathogen-free (SPF) pigs inoculated with the MLV-LOM or Jeju LOM strains.

Group	Inoculum Strain	No. of SPF Pigs	Sample	No. of CSFV RNA Positive Pigs/No. of Pigs Tested					
				* DPI0	DPI2	DPI4	DPI7	DPI10	DPI14
G1	JJ16LOM-YJK08	10	Blood	0/10	0/10	0/10	** 6/10	8/10	3/10
			Nasal	0/10	0/10	0/10	0/10	0/10	0/10
			Rectal	0/10	0/10	0/10	0/10	0/10	0/10
G2	JJ16LOM-YJK08-F	5	Blood	0/5	0/5	0/5	4/5	5/5	2/5
			Nasal	0/5	0/5	0/5	0/5	0/5	0/5
			Rectal	0/5	0/5	0/5	0/5	0/5	0/5
G3	16LOM-KM00	5	Blood	0/5	0/5	0/5	0/5	2/5	0/5
			Nasal	0/5	0/5	0/5	0/5	0/5	0/5
			Rectal	0/5	0/5	0/5	0/5	0/5	0/5
G4	Control	2	Blood	0/2	0/2	0/2	0/2	0/2	0/2
			Nasal	0/2	0/2	0/2	0/2	0/2	0/2
			Rectal	0/2	0/2	0/2	0/2	0/2	0/2

* DPI: days post-inoculation. ** CSFV RNA positive SPF pigs by the qRT-PCR.

By IHC staining, viral antigens were detected within the organs of 10 group 1 SPF pigs, specifically in 7/10 (70%) tonsil, 1/10 (10%) spleen, 1/10 (10%) ileum, and 2/10 (20%) submandibular lymph node samples (Figure 3, Table 4). In addition, SPF pigs in group 2 were positive in 3/5 (60%) tonsil samples only, while samples from group 3 SPF pigs contained antigens in all samples, i.e., 5/5 (100%) tonsil samples, 2/5 (40%) spleen samples, and 1/5 (20%) ileum sample (Table 4).

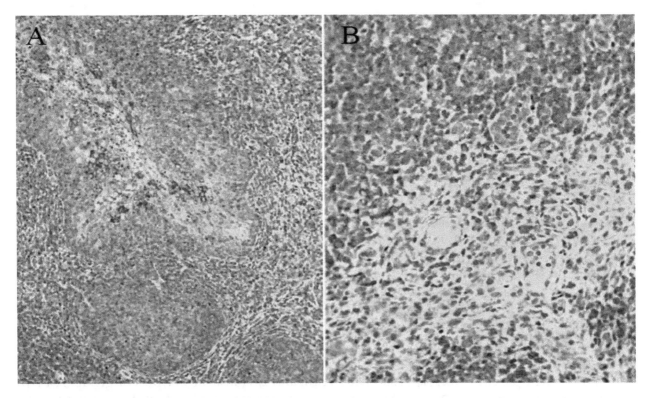

Figure 3. Immunohistochemical (IHC) results in SPF pigs. LOM antigens in the cryptal epithelium of tonsil (**A**) and solitary mono-nuclear cells in lymph node (**B**). Magnification × 200.

Table 4. Organs testing antigen positive after autopsy for SPF pigs inoculated with the MLV-LOM or Jeju LOM strains.

Group	Inoculum Strain	No. of SPF Pigs	Autopsy Day (DPI)	Antigen in Organs * of SPF Pigs (Copy Number (Log_{10}) by qRT-PCR/Score by IHC)											
				To	Sp	Lu	Ki	He	Li	Bl	Il	ML	SL	IL	Br
G1	JJ16LOM-YJK08	1	14	2.1/+	1.8/-	-	-	-	-	-	1.9/-	-	2.2/+	-	-
		2	14	2.5/++	2.0/-	-	-	-	-	-	1.4/-	1.6/-	1.8/-	-	-
		3	14	2.0/++	1.8/+	-	-	-	-	-	1.8/+	-	2.4/+	-	-
		4	14	2.3/+	-	-	-	-	-	-	1.7/-	-	1.8/-	-	-
		5	14	2.6/-	-	-	-	-	-	-	-	-	-	-	-
		6	21	-	-	-	-	-	-	-	-	-	-	-	-
		7	21	1.8/+	-	-	-	-	-	-	-	-	-	-	-
		8	21	-	-	-	-	-	-	-	-	-	-	-	-
		9	21	1.6/+	-	-	-	-	-	-	2.2/-	-	-	-	-
		10	21	2.7/+	-	-	-	-	-	2.0/V	-	1.6/-	-	-	-
G2	JJ16LOM-YJK08-F	1	21	-	-	-	-	-	-	-	-	-	-	-	-
		2	21	1.2/+	1.5/-	-	-	-	-	-	-	-	2.0/-	2.6/-	-
		3	21	-	-	-	-	1.8/-	-	-	-	-	-	-	-
		4	21	1.8/+	-	-	-	-	-	-	-	-	2.2/-	-	-
		5	21	2.3/+	-	-	-	-	-	-	-	-	1.9/-	-	-
G3	16LOM-KM00	1	14	1.8/+	1.9/-	-	-	-	-	-	1.7/-	-	1.6/-	-	-
		2	14	2.6/+	1.8/+	-	-	-	-	-	2.1/+	1.8/-	-	-	-
		3	14	2.4/+	1.3/+	-	-	-	-	-	-	-	-	-	-
		4	14	2.1/++	-	-	-	-	-	-	-	1.5/-	-	-	-
		5	14	2.7/+	-	-	-	-	-	-	-	-	-	-	-
G4	Control	1	14	-	-	-	-	-	-	-	-	-	-	-	-
		2	21	-	-	-	-	-	-	-	-	-	-	-	-

* To: tonsil, Sp: spleen, Lu: lung, Ki: kidney, He: heart, Li: liver, Bl: bladder, Il: ileum, ML: mesenteric lymph node, SL: submandibular lymph node, IL: inguinal lymph node, Br: brain.

2.5. Cytokine Concentrations in SPF Pigs Inoculated with the MLV-LOM and Jeju LOM Strains

The concentrations of IFN-α in sera were similar in SPF pigs in groups 1 (JJ16LOM-YJK08) and 3 (16LOM-KO11) at 4 dpi, but the concentration was higher in group 1 pigs at 7 dpi (Figure 4A). IL-10 was higher in group 1(JJ16LOM-YJK08) and 2 (JJ16LOM-YJK08-F) SPF pigs (Figure 4B) at 7 dpi. In addition, IL-1β concentrations were higher at 2 dpi in group 2 SPF pigs than in other groups (Figure 4C). The remaining cytokines (TNF-α, IL-6, IL-8, IL-12p40, IFNγ, and IL-4) showed no significant differences during the observation period between SPF pigs inoculated with the three strains (JJ16LOM-YJK08, JJ16LOM-YJK08-F, and 16LOM-KO11) (Figures 4D and 5A–E).

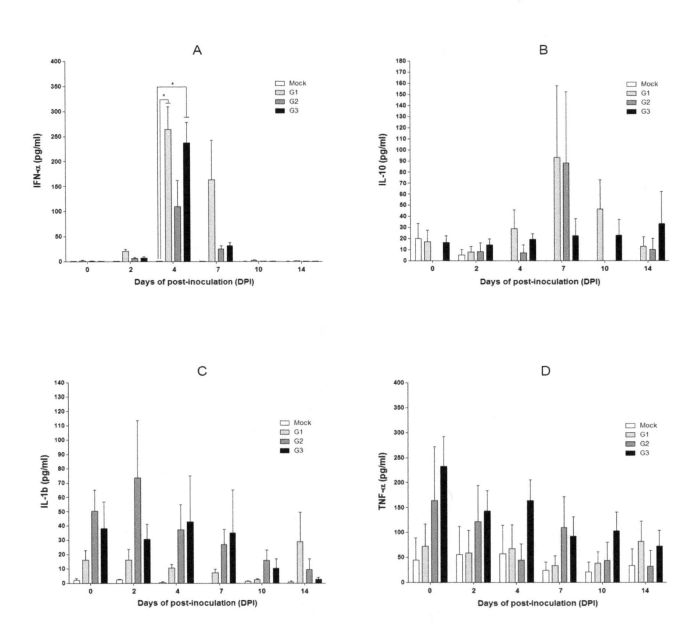

Figure 4. Cytokine concentrations in serum of SPF pigs over time post-infection. IFN-α (**A**), IL-10 (**B**), IL-1β (**C**), and TNF-α (**D**). Results are presented as mean ± standard deviation (SD) between 0 dpi and 14 dpi. Mock group is marked as the white column. G1 (JJ16LOM-YJK08), G2 (JJ16LOM-YJK08-F), and G3 (16LOM-KO11) are marked light grey, dark grey, and black, respectively. * $p < 0.05$ (A).

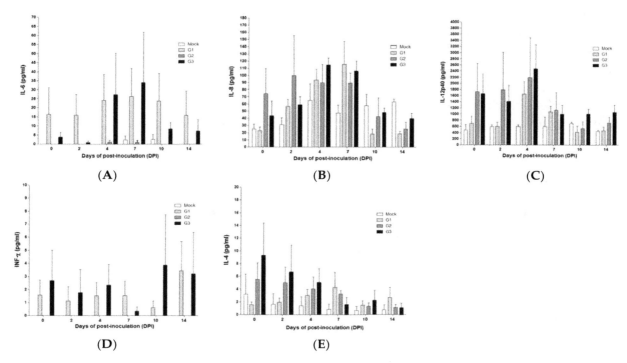

Figure 5. Cytokine levels in post-infection sera in SPF pigs. IL-6 (**A**), IL-8 (**B**), IL-12p40 (**C**), IFN-γ (**D**), and IL-4 (**E**). Results are presented as mean ± standard deviation (SD) between 0 dpi and 14 dpi. Mock group is marked as a white column. G1 (JJ16LOM-YJK08), G2 (JJ16LOM-YJK08-F), and G3 (16LOM-KO11) are marked light grey, dark grey, and black, respectively.

3. Discussion

The immunogenicity of the CSF MLV-LOM in pregnant sows was found to be excellent, but it was detected in some organs of their fetuses and sows, thus confirming that the MLV-LOM can pass through the placenta and infect fetuses [14]. In addition, the occurrence of stillborn or mummified fetuses suggests that the MLV-LOM may retain some pathogenicity in gestating pigs [14]. Interestingly, our results showed that the overall prevalence of infected fetuses was higher (92.3%) with the MLV-LOM than with the Jeju LOM strains (71.8–86.9%) isolated from Jeju Island. Histopathological examination revealed degeneration and necrosis of myocytes in the heart. Non-suppurative encephalitis and multifocal mineralizations in the brain only occurred in 9.1% (5/55) of fetuses delivered from sows inoculated with Jeju Island isolates. In addition, viral antigens were detected by the IHC test in 5.5% (3/55) of fetuses. One live piglet delivered from a sow inoculated with strain JJ16LOM-YJK08 exhibited severe vacuolar change with perivascular cuffing in cerebellum and myocardial degeneration, and a large amount of antigen was expressed in internal parenchymal organs. If the piglet had not been autopsied, it would have remained persistently infected and act as a carrier, steadily releasing the antigen. It has been shown that CSF infection occurs between 50 and 70 days of pregnancy, an immunotolerance phenomenon can be induced, and persistently infected offspring are born [3–7]. These piglets were healthy and survive for several months but die due to late onset form of CSF and they also shed high viral loads, which are enough for transmission to other pigs [3–7]. Recent studies have suggested that persistent infection can occur when newborn piglets are infected within the first 8 h of life, or even up to 48 h after birth [18,19].

In a previous report from 1990, safety tests with SPF pigs were conducted for the LOM-850 strain (the original MLV-LOM) and the LOM-suri strain cloned from LOM-850 [20]. Gross findings in SPF pigs inoculated with both strains were not observed, but all the groups showed mild lesions in the lymph nodes and bladder [20]. At necropsy, 10 days after vaccination, the redness of the lymph nodes was decreased, and bladder bleeding ceased [20]. In addition, IHC assay on SPF pigs at 21 days after vaccination were normal. Overall, gross and pathological findings decreased with time after vaccination and returned to normal at 21 days after vaccination [20]. In this study, we observed no specific clinical symptoms related to CSF in the pathogenicity tests on SPF pigs during the experimental period. However, CSFV RNA was detected in lymphoid organs such as tonsils, lymph nodes, spleen, and ileum, and showed a tendency to decrease in tissues with time post inoculation when assessed by qRT-PCR. When samples of SPF pig lymphoid organs were tested using the IHC stain, no lesions of lymphoid depletion, which are known to be characteristic of virulent CSFV infections, were observed. There was no specific high-temperature reaction in SPF pigs observed in this study, but transient leucopenia was observed in SPF pigs inoculated with strain JJ16LOM-JYK08 or JJ16LOM-JYK08-F at 4 dpi. However, the average WBC levels for these groups were 7142 and 6300/μl, which were not very low, and later, the WBC levels recovered.

Lymphocytopenia was well known as one of the typical characteristics of CSFV infections [8,21–23]. In general, lymphocytopenia, as well as blood coagulation disorder, are considered to be related to the upregulation of inflammatory cytokines, chemokines, and adhesion factors [24,25]. IFN-α is known to be involved in the induction of lymphocytopenia [9,10], and IL-10 is also known to related to general immunosuppression [26,27]. The concentration of IFN-α was highest at 4 dpi after strain LOM16-KO00 and JJ16LOM-YJK08 inoculation, but the difference between the two was not significant. The concentration of IL-10 at 7 dpi was higher in SPF pigs inoculated with strain JJ16LOM-YJK08 or JJ16LOM-YJK08-F than in those inoculated with LOM16-KO00. The recent study showed that TNF-α and IFN-α expressions in the sera of pigs infected with a moderately virulent CSFV increased, whereas concentrations in pigs following inoculation of the vaccine C-strain remained normal [28]. Generally, TNF-α is believed to be involved in the inflammatory response [28]. It has been also shown that an increase in TNF-α or IFN-α may induce the inflammatory response or apoptosis of lymphocytes after virulent CSFV infection [28]. In addition, TNF-α has been considered, alongside IL-1, IL-6, and IL-4, to be responsible for, among others, apoptosis in immune system cells, such as macrophages [10,29,30] and dendritic cells in lymphoid organs [27]. Several previous reports revealed that the increased expression of IL-8 after infection, without elucidation of its direct role in CSFV pathogenesis [24,25,31]. Our results suggest that TNF-α, IL-4, IL-6, and IL-8 showed no difference during the observation period between the three strains (JJ16LOM-YJK08, JJ16LOM-YJK08-F, and 16LOM-KO11).

Cytokine concentrations were at their maximum 2–3 days earlier in pigs infected with CSFV strains of moderate and high virulence when compared with those infected with a strain of low virulence [28]. These findings suggest that the C-strain vaccine virus replicates very slowly in some tissues, including tonsils, and therefore escape recognition by host antiviral responses. This slow virus (CSF vaccine strain) replication may have resulted in avoiding the untimely over-expression of IFNs and proinflammatory cytokines, and so indirectly protect immune cells and organs [28]. Based on previous suggestions, we assume that the MLV-LOM strain may share similarities with the C-strain vaccine virus because they are both live attenuated vaccine strains. In conclusion, the CSFV Jeju LOM strains showed no pathogenicity in SPF pigs but exhibited similarly to the MLV-LOM. The Jeju LOM strains produced similar adverse effects in the fetuses of pregnant sows to those of the MLV-LOM. Therefore, we suggest that the Jeju LOM strains are not pathogenic revertants of the MLV-LOM. Our epidemiologic results for CSFV (Jeju LOM) outbreak in Jeju from 2014 to 2018 indicated five major factors that may cause severe damage by Jeju LOM strain in Jeju pig farms of CSF non-vaccinated area. First, inoculation of MLV-LOM strain in pregnant sow (contraindication to vaccination policy); second, no stamping out for first Jeju LOM inoculated pregnant sow and their offspring suckling piglets; third, failure to clean and disinfect feces containing Jeju LOM strain in the pig farms; fourth, failure of disease prevention between slaughterhouse and pig farm; fifth, quarantine failure between mainland (South Korea) and Jeju island. Therefore, the MLV-LOM strain including Jeju LOM strain should never be inoculated in pregnant pigs without anti-CSF antibody. We suggest that MLV-LOM should be replaced quickly with CSF live marker vaccine with excellent safety and efficacy as a government CSF preventive policy.

4. Materials and Methods

4.1. Strains, Neutralization Antibody, IHC, and qRT-PCR

The MLV-LOM used was strain 16LOM-KM00. Three Jeju LOM isolates from Jeju Island were designated as strains JJ16LOM-YJK08, JJ16LOM-YJK08-F, and JJ16LOM-YYM02 [17]. A serum neutralization peroxidase-linked antibody (NPLA) assay to detect anti-CSFV antibody and a CSFV qRT-PCR and IHC to detect CSF antigen were analyzed using pig samples (serum and tissue) according to the previous paper [17].

4.2. Pregnant Pigs Inoculated with MLV-LOM and Jeju LOM Strains

Ten pregnant sows (64–67 days of gestation) were divided into three groups, and were inoculated with strain JJ16LOM-YJK08 (Jeju LOM) in group 1 (n = 3), strain JJ16LOM-YYM02 (Jeju LOM) in group 2 (n = 3), and strain 16LOM-KO00 (MLV-LOM) in group 3 (n = 3) with $10^{3.5}$ TCID$_{50}$/dose. Group 4 (n = 1) served as an uninoculated negative control. For groups 1–3, one pregnant sow from each group was autopsied at 3 wpi, and the remaining sows and their offspring piglets were autopsied after delivery. To investigate the presence of neutralizing antibodies, a NPLA was performed on the serum of sows collected before inoculation, 3 wpi, and at delivery (7 wpi). At 3 wpi, autopsies of pregnant sows and fetuses were tested for signs of CSF. At delivery, all piglets were examined for farrowing and the presence of antigen in their fetuses. The organs of their piglets were subjected to pathologic analysis.

4.3. SPF Pigs Inoculated with the MLV-LOM and Jeju LOM Strains

Twenty-two SPF pigs (on average 45–50 days old) were purchased from Optifarm company (Osong, Korea) and divided into four groups to allow comparison of the relative pathogenicity of the Jeju LOM and MLV-LOM. Group 1 animals (n = 10) were inoculated with strain JJ16LOM-YJK08 (Jeju LOM). Those in group 2 (n = 5) were inoculated with strain JJ16LOM-YJK-F (Jeju LOM). Those in group 3 (n = 5) were inoculated with a commercial vaccine strain (16LOM-KO00) (MLV-LOM), and group 4 pigs (n = 2) were mock as a negative uninoculated control. Clinical symptoms in SPF pigs were observed daily. Blood, saliva, and fecal swab samples were taken, and weight and temperature checks were performed before inoculation and at 2, 4, 7, 10, and 14 dpi for virus detection, leukocyte counts, weight and temperature changes, and seroconversion. At 14 dpi, five SPF pigs in group 1, five in group 3, and one in group 4 were autopsied to test for the presence of viruses within organs by qRT-PCR and IHC assays, and to note any lesions in tissues. The remaining SPF pigs were autopsied and collected samples (blood, saliva, and fecal) at 21 dpi.

4.4. Multiplex Immunoassay for SPF Pigs

The porcine cytokine and chemokine 9-plex Porcine ProcartaPlexTM Panel 1 (ThermoFisher Scientific, Cat no. EPX090-60829-901) was used to detect nine cytokines and chemokines (IFN-α, IFN-γ, TNF-α, IL-1β, IL-4, IL-6, IL-8, IL-10, and IL-12p40) in the sera from SPF pigs inoculated with MLV-LOM (16LOM-KO11) and Jeju LOM strains (JJ16LOM-YJK08 and JJ16LOM-YJK08-F). ProcartaPlex immunoassays are based on the principles of a sandwich ELISA, using two highly specific antibodies binding to different epitopes of one protein to quantitate all protein targets simultaneously using Luminex® 200™ (Luminex Co., TX, USA). In brief, serum fractions from blood collected in EDTA-containing tubes were obtained after centrifugation at 1000× g for 10 min at 20–25 °C. Magnetic beads were vortex-mixed for 30 s, 50 µl of the beads was added to each well, and then pig-specific universal assay buffer and sample were each added in 25 µl volumes to the wells. The plates were shaken at room temperature (RT) for 30 min, overnight at 4 °C in the dark, and then at RT for a further 30 min. Beads were then washed twice. Detection Antibody mix (25 µl) was added to the beads, and the beads were incubated with shaking at RT for 30 min and then washed twice. Streptavidin-PE (50 µl) was then added, and the beads were incubated with shaking at RT for 30 min and washed twice. Reading buffer (120 μl) was added, and incubation continued with shaking at RT for 5 min. The samples were read on Luminex® 200™ (Luminex Co., TX, USA).

4.5. Statistical Analysis

The data was analyzed by one-way ANOVA, which was followed by Tukey's multiple-comparison test using GraphPad Prism software (version 6.0). Results in groups are expressed as mean ± standard error (SE) and significant difference ($p < 0.05$) are indicated by an asterisk.

Author Contributions: Conceptualization, D.-J.A., B.-K.P., I.-S.C. and B.-H.H.; methodology, R.M.C., S.C., J.-H.K., K.-S.K., S.S., W.-C.K., G.-N.P., H.-N.J., J.S. and H.-J.K.; writing, R.M.C. and D.-J.A. All authors have read and agreed to the published version of the manuscript.

References

1. Thiel, H.J.; Collett, M.S.; Gould, E.A.; Heinz, F.X.; Houghton, M.; Meyers, G.; Purcell, R.H.; Rice, C.M. Family Flaviridae. In *Virus Taxonomy: Eighth Report of the International Committee on Taxonomy of Viruses*; Fauquet, C.M., Mayo, M., Maniloff, J., Desselberger, U., Ball, L.A., Eds.; Academic Press: San Diego, CA, USA, 2004; pp. 981–998.
2. Meyer, H.; Liess, B.; Frey, H.R.; Hermanns, W.; Trautwein, G. Experimental transplacental transmission of hog cholera virus in pigs. IV. Virological and serological studies in newborn piglets. *Zentralbl. Veterinarmed. B* **1981**, *28*, 659–668. [CrossRef]
3. von Benten, K.; Trautwein, G.; Richter-Reichhelm, H.B.; Liess, B.; Frey, H.R. Experimental transplacental transmission of hog cholera virus in pigs. III. Histopathological findings in the fetus. *Zentralbl. Veterinarmed. B* **1980**, *27*, 714–724. [CrossRef] [PubMed]
4. Stewart, W.C.; Carbrey, E.A.; Kresse, J.I. Transplacental hog cholera infection in susceptible sows. *Am. J. Vet. Res.* **1973**, *34*, 637–640. [PubMed]
5. Richter-Reichhelm, H.B.; Trautwein, G.; von Benten, K.; Liess, B.; Frey, H.R. Experimental transplacental transmission of hog cholera virus in pigs. II. Immunopathological findings in the fetus. *Zentralbl. Veterinarmed. B* **1980**, *27*, 243–252. [CrossRef]
6. Hermanns, W.; Trautwein, G.; Meyer, H.; Liess, B. Experimental transplacental transmission of hog cholera virus in pigs. V. Immunopathological findings in newborn pigs. *Zentralbl. Veterinarmed. B* **1981**, *28*, 669–683. [CrossRef]
7. Frey, H.R.; Liess, B.; Richter-Reichhelm, H.B.; von Benten, K.; Trautwein, G. Experimental transplacental transmission of hog cholera virus in pigs. I. Virological and serological studies. *Zentralbl. Veterinarmed. B* **1980**, *27*, 154–164. [CrossRef]
8. Sánchez-Cordón, P.J.; Romanini, S.; Salguero, F.J.; Nunez, A.; Bautista, M.J.; Jover, A.; Gomez-Villamos, J.C. Apoptosis of thymocytes related to cytokine expression in experimental classical swine fever. *J. Comp. Pathol.* **2002**, *127*, 239–248. [CrossRef]
9. Summerfield, A.; Alves, M.; Ruggli, N.; de Bruin, M.G.; McCullough, K.C. High IFN alpha responses associated with depletion of lymphocytes and natural IFN producing cells during classical swine fever. *J. Interferon Cytokine Res.* **2006**, *26*, 248–255. [CrossRef]
10. Sánchez-Cordón, P.J.; Núñez, A.; Salguero, F.J.; Pedrera, M.; Fernández de Marco, M.; Gómez-Villamandos, J.C. Lymphocyte apoptosis and thrombocytopenia in spleen during classical swine fever: role of macrophages and cytokines. *Vet. Pathol.* **2005**, *42*, 477–488. [CrossRef]
11. Moennig, V.; Floegel-Niesmann, G.; Greiser-Wilke, I. Clinical signs and epidemiology of classical swine fever: A review of new knowledge. *Vet. J.* **2003**, *165*, 11–20. [CrossRef]
12. Petrov, A.; Blohm, U.; Beer, M.; Pietschmann, J.; Blome, S. Comparative analyses of host responses upon infection with moderately virulent classical swine fever virus in domestic pigs and wild boar. *Virol. J.* **2014**, *11*, 134. [CrossRef] [PubMed]
13. Kaden, V.; Ziegler, U.; Lange, E.; Dedek, J. Classical swine fever virus: Clinical, virological, serological and hematological findings after infection of domestic pigs and wild boars with the field isolate "Spante" originating from wild boar. *Berl. Munch. Tierarztl. Wochenschr.* **2000**, *113*, 412–416. [PubMed]

14. Lim, S.I.; Song, J.Y.; Kim, J.; Hyun, B.H.; Kim, H.Y.; Cho, I.S.; Kim, B.; Woo, G.H.; Lee, J.B.; An, D.J. Safety of classical swine fever virus vaccine strain LOM in pregnant sows and their offspring. *Vaccine* **2016**, *34*, 2021–2026. [CrossRef] [PubMed]

15. Lim, S.I.; Jeoung, H.Y.; Kim, B.; Song, J.Y.; Kim, J.; Kim, H.Y.; Cho, I.S.; Woo, G.H.; Lee, J.B.; An, D.J. Impact of porcine reproductive and respiratory syndrome virus and porcine circovirus-2 infection on the potency of the classical swine fever vaccine (LOM strain). *Vet. Microbiol.* **2016**, *193*, 36–41. [CrossRef]

16. Kim, B.; Song, J.Y.; Tark, D.S.; Lim, S.I.; Choi, E.J.; Park, C.K.; Lee, B.Y.; Wee, S.H.; Bae, Y.C.; Lee, O.S.; et al. Feed comtaminated with classical swine fever vaccine virus (LOM strain) can induce antibodies to the virus in pigs. *Vet Rec.* **2008**, *162*, 12–17. [CrossRef]

17. Choe, S.; Kim, J.H.; Kim, K.S.; Song, S.; Kang, W.C.; Kim, H.J.; Park, G.N.; Cha, R.M.; Cho, I.S.; Hyun, B.H.; et al. Impact of a Live Attenuated Classical Swine Fever Virus Introduced to Jeju Island, a CSF-Free Area. *Pathogens* **2019**, *8*, 206. [CrossRef]

18. Cabezon, O.; Colom-Cadena, A.; Munoz-Gonzalez, S.; Perez-Simo, M.; Bohorquez, J.A.; Rosell, R.; Marco, I.; Domingo, M.; Lavin, S.; Ganges, L. Post-natal persistent infection with classical swine fever virus in wild boar: A strategy for viral maintenance? *Transbound. Emerg. Dis.* **2017**, *64*, 651–655. [CrossRef]

19. Munoz-Gonzalez, S.; Perez-Simo, M.; Munoz, M.; Bohorquez, J.A.; Rosell, R.; Summerfield, A.; Domingo, M.; Ruggli, N.; Ganges, L. Efficacy of a live attenuated vaccine in classical swine fever virus postnatally persistently infected pigs. *Vet. Res.* **2015**, *46*, 78. [CrossRef]

20. Kim, B.; Kim, Y.H.; Jin, Y.H.; Lee, O.S.; Choi, J.U.; Kim, C.G.; An, S.H.; Lee, J.J. Hog cholera live attenuated vaccine. III. Experiment of live attenuated LOM-Suri strain. *KRVS (Livestock health)* **1990**, *32*, 49–55.

21. Nielsen, J.; Lohse, L.; Rasmussen, T.B.; Uttenthal, Å. Classical swine fever in 6-and 11-week-old pigs: haematological and immunological parameters are modulated in pigs with mild clinical disease. *Vet. Immunol. Immunopathol.* **2010**, *138*, 159–173. [CrossRef]

22. Summerfield, A.; Hofmann, M.; McCullough, K.C. Immature granulocytic cells dominate the peripheral blood during classical swine fever and are targets for virus infection. *Vet. Immunol. Immunopathol.* **1998**, *63*, 289–301. [CrossRef]

23. Susa, M.; König, M.; Saalmuller, A.; Reddehase, M.J.; Thiel, H.J. Pathogenesis of classical swine fever: B-lymphocyte deficiency caused by hog cholera virus. *J. Virol.* **1992**, *66*, 1171–1175. [PubMed]

24. Bensaude, E.; Turner, J.L.; Wakeley, P.R.; Sweetman, D.A.; Pardieu, C.; Drew, T.W.; Wileman, T.; Powell, P.P. Classical swine fever virus induces proinflammatory cytokines and tissue factor expression and inhibits apoptosis and interferon synthesis during the establishment of long-term infection of porcine vascular endothelial cells. *J. Gen. Virol.* **2004**, *85*, 1029–1037. [CrossRef] [PubMed]

25. Graham, S.P.; Everett, H.E.; Johns, H.L.; Haines, F.J.; La Rocca, S.A.; Khatri, M.; Wright, I.K.; Drew, T.W.; Crooke, H.R. Characterisation of virus-specific peripheral blood cell cytokine responses following vaccination or infection with classical swine fever viruses. *Vet. Microbiol.* **2010**, *142*, 34–40. [CrossRef]

26. Jamin, A.; Gorin, S.; Cariolet, R.; Le Potier, M.F.; Kuntz-Simon, G. Classical swine fever virus induces activation of plasmacytoid and conventional dendritic cells in tonsil, blood, and spleen of infected pigs. *Vet. Res.* **2008**, *39*, 7. [CrossRef]

27. Suradhat, S.; Sada, W.; Buranapraditkun, S.; Damrongwatanapokin, S. The kinetics of cytokine production and CD25 expression by porcine lymphocyte subpopulations following exposure to classical swine fever virus (CSFV). *Vet. Immunol. Immunopathol.* **2005**, *106*, 197–208. [CrossRef]

28. Wang, J.; Sun, Y.; Meng, X.Y.; Li, L.F.; Li, Y.; Luo, Y.; Wang, W.; Yu, S.; Yin, C.; Li, S.; et al. Comprehensive evaluation of the host responses to infection with differentially virulent classical swine fever virus strains in pigs. *Virus Res.* **2018**, *255*, 68–76. [CrossRef]

29. Choi, C.; Hwang, K.K.; Chae, C. Classical swine fever virus induces tumor necrosis factor-alpha and lymphocyte apoptosis. *Arch. Virol.* **2004**, *149*, 875–889. [CrossRef]

30. Knoetig, S.M.; Summerfield, A.; Spagnuolo-Weaver, M.; McCullough, K.C. Immunopathogenesis of classical swine fever: role of monocytic cells. *Immunology* **1999**, *97*, 359–366. [CrossRef]

31. Tang, Q.; Guo, K.; Kang, K.; Zhang, Y.; He, L.; Wang, J. Classical swine fever virus NS2 protein promotes interleukin-8 expression and inhibits MG132-induced apoptosis. *Virus Genes* **2011**, *42*, 355–362. [CrossRef]

Apoptosis, Autophagy and Pyroptosis: Immune Escape Strategies for Persistent Infection and Pathogenesis of Classical Swine Fever Virus

Sheng-ming Ma, Qian Mao, Lin Yi, Ming-qiu Zhao and Jin-ding Chen *

College of Veterinary Medicine; South China Agricultural University; Guangzhou 510642, China; mashengming@stu.scau.edu.cn (S.-m.M.); maoqian@stu.scau.edu.cn (Q.M.); yilin@scau.edu.cn (L.Y.); zmingqiu@scau.edu.cn (M.-q.Z.)
* Correspondence: jdchen@scau.edu.cn

Abstract: Classical swine fever (CSF) is a severe acute infectious disease that results from classical swine fever virus (CSFV) infection, which leads to serious economic losses in the porcine industry worldwide. In recent years, numerous studies related to the immune escape mechanism of the persistent infection and pathogenesis of CSFV have been performed. Remarkably, several independent groups have reported that apoptosis, autophagy, and pyroptosis play a significant role in the occurrence and development of CSF, as well as in the immunological process. Apoptosis, autophagy, and pyroptosis are the fundamental biological processes that maintain normal homeostatic and metabolic function in eukaryotic organisms. In general, these three cellular biological processes are always understood as an immune defense response initiated by the organism after perceiving a pathogen infection. Nevertheless, several viruses, including CSFV and other common pathogens such as hepatitis C and influenza A, have evolved strategies for infection and replication using these three cellular biological process mechanisms. In this review, we summarize the known roles of apoptosis, autophagy, and pyroptosis in CSFV infection and how viruses manipulate these three cellular biological processes to evade the immune response.

Keywords: classical swine fever virus; apoptosis; autophagy; pyroptosis; pathogenesis

1. Introduction

Classical swine fever (CSF) is a serious porcine disease driven by the CSF virus (CSFV) that results in fever, leukopenia, abortion, hemorrhage, and high mortality: it has brought substantial economic losses to the world pig industry and has been classified as a class A infectious disease by the World Organization for Animal Health (OIE) [1,2]. CSFV is a single-stranded RNA flavivirus in the *Pestivirus* genus with a 12.3-kb genome and has a tropism for vascular endothelial cells and immune system cells [3]. This virus encodes a single 3898 amino acid polyprotein in its open reading frame (ORF), and this protein in turn undergoes processing to yield four structural proteins (C, E^{rns}, E1, and E2) and eight nonstructural proteins (N^{pro}, P7, NS2, NS3, NS4A, NS4B, NS5A, and NS5B) [4]. Infection with highly virulent CSFV strains leads to the occurrence of typical CSF, with hemorrhagic syndrome and immunosuppression as the main features [5,6]. Currently, treatment options for CSF are still limited; instead, prevention with vaccines against CSFV is usually used [7,8]. However, under immune selection pressure, CSFV has evolved and developed mechanisms that escape the host immune response, resulting in an outbreak of CSF or establishing persistent infection in an immune flock [9–11]. Although many studies have investigated the interaction mechanism between CSFV and the host, the pathogenesis and immune escape mechanism of CSFV still remain unclear [12–15]. It is still necessary to explore the pathogenic mechanisms of CSFV in order to develop specific drugs and vaccines for effective CSF prevention, control, and eradication.

The occurrence, development, and outcome of infectious diseases are the result of interaction between pathogens and hosts. In the long-term struggle between host and virus, the host initiates different forms of cellular biological processes to restrict viral replication [16–18]. However, in order to achieve persistent infection, viruses have evolved a variety of mechanisms to regulate cellular biological processes, thereby affecting the host inflammatory response and even cell survival, thus avoiding the host antiviral immune response [19–22]. Importantly, apoptosis, autophagy, and pyroptosis are fundamental biological processes in both normal physiology and pathology [23–26]. Apoptosis, as the most thoroughly characterized form of programmed cell death, is a physiological cell death that occurs when multicellular organisms respond to endogenous or exogenous stimuli [23,27]. Autophagy is a cell survival mechanism that involves the degradation and recycling of cytoplasmic components, including long-lived proteins, protein aggregates, damaged cytoplasmic organelles, and intracellular pathogens [28]. Different from other forms of cell death in morphology and mechanics, pyroptosis is a proinflammatory form of cell death regulated by the inflammasome and caspase-1 activation [29]. All of these three cellular biological processes are an important part of the process of growth and development and tissue remodeling and immune regulation, and they play an important and complex role in the immune response to virus infection [23–29].

Like other members of the family of Flaviviridae viruses, CSFV is dependent on host cells for viral replication [30]. In the long-term struggle with CSFV, the host has evolved complex anti-infective mechanisms to protect itself from infection, such as apoptosis, autophagy, and pyroptosis [31–34]. At the same time, CSFV has also evolved to exploit these three cellular biological processes using various strategies as well as effective escape mechanisms [31–34]. In this review, we summarize the known molecular mechanisms through which CSFV induces apoptosis, autophagy, and pyroptosis and the association of these three cellular biological processes with the pathogenesis of CSFV.

2. Apoptosis in the Pathogenesis of CSFV

Apoptosis, also known as programmed cell death of type I, is a physiological cell death that occurs when multicellular organisms respond to endogenous or exogenous stimuli [23,27,35]. Abnormal cell apoptosis often leads to disease. The virus-induced apoptosis of host cells is one of the important mechanisms of viral pathogenesis [22]. Apoptosis is the first line of defense against viral infection in host cells [16]. The host cells quickly start the apoptotic process under the stimulation of viruses and restrict the replication and transmission of viruses by quickly clearing the infected cells [16,22,36]. During virus infection, apoptosis can be triggered by diverse cellular signals, including the death receptor-mediated extrinsic pathway, the intrinsic mitochondrial pathway, the granzyme B-mediated pathway, and the endoplasmic reticulum stress-mediated pathway. When cells induce apoptosis, they destroy the intracellular environment of virus replication and expose virus particles to the cellular immune environment. The exposed virus particles are quickly phagocytized by macrophages. Meanwhile, dendritic cells recognize virus-infected cells and function as antigens, cross-presenting to trigger antivirus immune responses. However, the apoptosis of immune cells is beneficial for the virus to escape the monitoring of the host immune system [37,38]. In addition, some viruses or viral components delay or inhibit cell apoptosis through some cellular regulatory mechanisms, thus achieving persistent infection and survival in host cells [39,40].

CSFV is a typical immunosuppressive disease that greatly harms the hematopoietic and immune systems [41]. As a single-stranded enveloped RNA virus, CSFV has a strong affinity for vascular endothelial cells and immune system cells [31]. Leukopenia, in particular lymphopenia, is a characteristic early event during CSFV. Leukopenia involves leukocyte subpopulations in a disparate manner, with B-lymphocytes, helper T-cells, and cytotoxic T-cells being the most affected [42]. High titers of CSFV have been detected in bone marrow at the early stage of virus infection, which led to necrosis and the apoptosis of bone marrow hematopoietic cells and the apoptosis of bone marrow lymphocyte [43].

These lines of evidence indicate that the decrease in T-lymphocytes in peripheral blood is closely related to the damage of bone marrow lymphocyte apoptosis caused by CSFV. During CSFV infection, both mature peripheral and bone marrow neutrophils are affected, whereas immature neutrophils increase absolutely in the periphery, as do (coincidentally) immature myeloid progenitors in the bone marrow [44]. Further research has found granulocytopenia and disrupted bone marrow function to be a result of the death of hematopoietic cells as a consequence of interactions between viral and host mechanisms. In one study that used Terminal-deoxynucleoitidyl Transferase Mediated Nick End Labeling (TUNEL) staining and immunohistochemical analyses to examine apoptosis, researchers observed that the number of apoptotic cells was greater than the number of CSFV-infected cells, with many apoptotic and nonapoptotic cells being positive for tumor necrosis factor alpha (TNF-α) staining. This thus suggested that CSFV can drive apoptosis directly and indirectly. Moreover, one or more factors expressed by CSFV-infected macrophages (e.g., TNF-α) may induce apoptosis in uninfected bystander cells [31]. CSFV envelope glycoprotein E^{rns} is important for the pathogenesis of CSFV. There is evidence that E^{rns} inhibits the concanavalin A-induced proliferation of porcine lymphocytes, and indeed, the apoptosis of lymphocytes has been detected after incubation with E^{rns} [45,46]. It is also believed that CSFV-infected cells secrete a large number of extracellular viral glycoprotein E^{rns}, which induces apoptosis in adjacent noninfected CSFV cells. All these data suggest that the reduction of peripheral blood lymphocytes induced by CSFV infection may be the result of multiple mechanisms.

Interestingly, CSFV nonstructural protein N^{pro} and NS2 have also been shown to inhibit apoptosis. N^{pro} induces the proteasomal degradation of IRF3, thereby facilitating evasion of the interferon response, in addition to preventing the apoptotic death of cells in response to dsRNA, which may also be an important reason why CSFV infection in vitro cannot cause cytopathic effects [47]. Further investigations have showed that the interaction of N^{pro} and the antiapoptotic protein HAX-1 (HS-1-associated protein X-1) plays a prominent role in the regulation of apoptosis [48]. Moreover, CSFV NS2 activates the noncanonical nuclear factor-kappaB (NF-κB) transcription factor and induces endoplasmic reticulum stress in swine umbilical vein endothelial cells (SUVECs), thereby promoting the increased expression of interleukin (IL)-8 as well as of Bcl-2, which is an antiapoptotic protein [49,50]. SUVECs expressing green fluorescent protein (GFP)–NS2 were able to resist MG132-induced apoptosis [51]. This thus indicated that the mechanism for the CSFV NS2 protein inhibiting apoptosis may be an important process for the virus to achieve persistent infection.

In conclusion, the relationship between CSFV and apoptosis is complex. In the early stage of CSFV infection in some host cells, antiapoptotic effects are the main manifestation, which facilitate the replication of the virus in infected cells [47–50]. However, in the late stage of CSFV infection, apoptotic effects are predominant, which may be the defensive response of the body to viral infection or an important mechanism of severe damage to host tissue cells caused by viral infection [42–45].

3. Autophagy in the Pathogenesis of CSFV

Autophagy, also known as a cell survival mechanism, is a catabolic process that involves the degradation and recycling of cytoplasmic components, including long-lived proteins, protein aggregates, damaged cytoplasmic organelles, and intracellular pathogens [25,28]. During autophagy, cytoplasmic components are isolated by a membrane called the phagosome or isolation membrane, which expands to form a double-membrane vesicle called the autophagosome [51–53]. Autophagosomes can fuse with vesicles of the endocytic pathway to form amphisomes that eventually fuse with lysosomes where the sequestered material is degraded [25,52]. In eukaryotic cells, autophagy can be broadly classified as macroautophagy, microautophagy, and chaperone-mediated autophagy depending on the mechanism and molecular players involved in the targeting of a substrate to the lysosome [51]. Macroautophagy and microautophagy are relatively conservative in all eukaryotes, while chaperone-mediated autophagy generally occurs in higher eukaryotes [52]. In the presentation pathway, microautophagy and chaperone autophagy can directly present the target substance to lysosomes, while macroautophagy requires the formation of specific bilayer membrane complexes, which can be encapsulated and isolated for presentation [53,54]. Autophagy, as one of the innate immune mechanisms, can not only maintain cellular homeostasis, but also protect cells against the invasion of pathogenic microorganisms. Virus particles can be delivered to lysosomes for degradation [55]. In addition, autophagy can also activate cellular adaptive immunity by participating in antigen processing and presentation to major histocompatibility complex (MHC) class II molecules, thus affecting virus replication [56]. In *Sindbis virus* and *Tobacco mosaic virus* infections, autophagy successfully restricts intracellular pathogen replication and transmission [57,58]. Conversely, *human immunodeficiency virus type 1* and *herpes simplex virus type 1* can inhibit autophagy to facilitate replication [59,60]. Nevertheless, several viruses, such as *influenza A virus, dengue virus, hepatitis C virus*, and CSFV, have evolved strategies of replication using autophagic vesicles [32,61–63]. Autophagy is virus-specific; thus, understanding the interaction between autophagy and viral infection is essential to control disease transmission.

At present, several reports have shown that various Flaviviridae viruses, including the *Zika virus, dengue virus, West Nile virus, Japanese encephalitis virus*, and *hepatitis C virus*, activate and require some aspect of autophagy for robust viral replication [62–66]. CSFV, as an important member of the Flaviviridae family, has also been reported to manipulate autophagy during infection [32]. Pei et al. first performed the initial characterization of autophagy during CSFV infection in 2014 [32]. The authors showed that CSFV infection markedly elevated the number of double- and single-membrane vesicles in infected cells. These authors also showed that the virus infection not only induced both ATG12–ATG5 conjugation as well as the conversion of LC3-I to LC3-II, but also led to significant increases in ATG5 and BECN1 levels within cells infected with the CSFV virus. The authors also detected SQSTM1 degradation, indicating that CSFV infection enhanced autophagic flux and triggered a complete autophagic response. Moreover, CSFV resulted in increased CD63 and LC3 redistribution, with the colocalization of NS5A and E2 with LC3- and CD63-positive punctae. This thus suggested that these autophagosome-like structures may be necessary for the replication of CSFV. Conversely, no obvious changes in the expression level of autophagy marker proteins were present in mock- and UV-treated CSFV-infected cells. This thus suggested that UV irradiation disrupted the ability of CSFV to mediate autophagosome formation. They further showed that anti-E2 and anti-NS5A staining was primarily evident upon autophagosome-like vesicle membranes, suggesting that this is likely the site of CSFV replication. The authors also demonstrated that LC3 redistribution and the colocalization of LC3 and EGFP–NS5A occurred in pEGFP–NS5A-transfected cells. In addition, pEGFP–NS5A markedly increased the level of LC3-II and drove the degradation of SQSTM1. All of these findings not only enforced that CSFV replication is required for the induction of autophagy, but also suggested that NS5A is essential for the CSFV-mediated induction of autophagy. Importantly, these authors used autophagy regulators and shRNA to regulate the autophagic activities of CSFV-infected cells. The results explored that rapamycin treatment significantly upregulated viral E2 expression and resulted in increased CSFV yields, whereas 3-methyladenine (3-MA) treatment or shRNA-mediated knockdown of LC3 and BECN1 to inhibit autophagy reduced E2 protein levels and CSFV yields. The authors further found that modulating autophagy had a more significant impact on extracellular than intracellular virion yields. This thus indicated that autophagy is necessary both for viral replication and cytoplasmic virus relief.

Autophagy is divided into nonselective autophagy and selective autophagy according to the occurrence process. Under nutrient deficiency, cells maintain essential metabolic substances and energy by activating nonselective autophagy to degrade intracellular biomacromolecules and organelles [67]. On the contrary, selective autophagy usually occurs in the condition of adequate nutrition, which is a stress response of cells to remove damaged cells or overaccumulated proteins [68]. Mitophagy is a selective autophagy and an effective mitochondrial clearance mechanism in cells [69,70]. Many viral proteins can target mitochondria through their mitochondrial localization sequences during virus infection [71–73]. Damaged mitochondria caused by virus infection can be cleared up through mitophagy [69,70]. Previous studies have shown that CSFV infection induces the production of reactive oxygen species (ROS) in cultured host cells in vitro and leads to the disappearance of mitochondrial membrane potential in porcine peripheral blood lymphocytes, which is closely related to the reduction of mitochondrial numbers [74,75]. On this basis, Gou et al. performed a study to explore the mechanism of CSFV-induced mitophagy and the role of mitophagy in CSFV infection [34]. These authors showed that mitochondrial mass obviously decreased 36 h postinfection in PK-15 and 3D4/2 cells. Further, they treated cells with 3-MA, inhibiting phagophore formation and Bafilomycin A1 (BafA1), inhibiting the activity of vacuolar-type H+-ATPase before and during CSFV infection. These authors found that both autophagy inhibitors could invert the decline of mitochondrial mass induced by CSFV infection. Moreover, these authors observed that mitochondria were trapped by double-membrane vesicles in CSFV-infected cells, suggesting CSFV infection with CSFV-induced mitophagy. The Pink1/Parkin signaling pathway is one of the important mechanisms mediating the activation of mitophagy [76]. The authors also showed that the increased translocation of Pink1 and Parkin in purified mitochondria of CSFV-infected cells was observed. Meanwhile, CSFV upregulated the ubiquitination of MFN2 both in PK-15 and 3D4/2 cells. Among many mitochondrial membrane proteins, the ubiquitination degradation of the MFN2 protein has been proven to be closely related to the mitochondrial translocation of Parkin [77]. Further, PK-15 and 3D4/2 cells transfected with the GFP-LC3 plasmid were infected by CSFV and analyzed by confocal immunofluorescence assay. The data showed that the mitochondria conjunct with Parkin was trapped by GFP-LC3 puncta. The authors also utilized a tandem-tagged mRFP–GFP plasmid encoding a mitochondrial targeting signal sequence to assess mitophagy. This showed that CSFV-infected cells displayed greater red fluorescence protein (RFP) fluorescence, which indicated the degradation of mitochondria by lysosomes. Finally, the fusion of GFP–LC3, mitochondria, and lysosomes in PK-15 and 3D4/2 cells was analyzed by confocal microscopy, which proved that mitochondria wrapped by LC3 puncta were connected with lysosomes in CSFV-infected cells. In addition, these authors determined that CSFV N[pro] expression, RNA replication, and virus titers in the cells silenced endogenous Drp1 or Parkin through shRNA knockdown experiments. The results explored that knocking down Drp1 or Parkin suppressed CSFV replication, suggesting that CSFV promotes viral replication through mitochondrial division and mitophagy.

These above works indicate that CSFV infection not only results in autophagy in host cells, but also utilizes autophagy mechanisms for viral replication and virion release. Autophagy may be a pathogenic mechanism of CSFV to facilitate persistent viral infection.

4. Cross-Talk between Apoptosis and Autophagy in CSFV Pathogenesis

Autophagy and apoptosis are two main biological processes in cells, and there are significant differences between them in terms of metabolic pathways, morphological detection, and interaction with viruses. However, there is accumulating evidence that autophagy and apoptosis are closely related in function [78–80]. The activation of apoptosis requires the induction of an autophagy pathway, and autophagy can also protect cells by inhibiting apoptosis, which is conducive to the parasitism of pathogens in cells [81]. Studies have also shown that calpain, a molecule downstream of the apoptotic signal, can inhibit autophagy by degrading autophagy-associated proteins [82]. Therefore, it is necessary to assess how autophagy and apoptosis are linked in the context of viral infection to reveal the pathogenic mechanism of the virus.

It has been found that there are three relationships between autophagy and apoptosis in the process of inducing cell death, including collaboration, antagonism, and promotion [83]. Gou et al. found that autophagy and apoptotic signals were increased in the spleen of CSFV-infected piglets [84]. Interestingly, these autophagy-positive and apoptosis-positive cells were mainly distributed around splenic corpuscles. More importantly, CSFV caused LC3-II positive cells (about 40%) in pig spleen tissues, which simultaneously presented as TUNEL-positive. In vivo, the majority of apoptotic cells were found to be uninfected with CSFV. Similarly, some CSFV-infected cells did not exhibit signs of autophagy, and some cells that showed signs of autophagy were negative for CSFV infection, which implied a relation between autophagy and apoptosis in the spleen of pigs infected by CSFV. During the in vitro infection of CSFV, Pei et al. found that rapamycin-induced autophagy promoted cellular proliferation after virus infection, whereas shRNA-mediated inhibition of autophagy induced apoptosis in virus-infected cells, indicating that apoptosis is inhibited by CSFV-induced autophagy and thus contributes to virus propagation and persistent infection [85]. Interestingly, these authors also showed that the inhibition of autophagy with shRNA-based depletion of the essential autophagy proteins BECN1 and LC3 increased the expression of proapoptotic molecules, including Bax, cleaved-caspase3, and cleaved-PARP, and decreased the expression of antiapoptotic molecule Bcl-2 by upregulating the level of interferon-alpha (IFN-α), interferon-beta (IFN-β), tumor necrosis factor-related apoptosis inducing ligand (TRAIL), and factor associated suicide (FAS), indicating that apoptosis mediated by type I interferon is inhibited by CSFV-induced autophagy. Further, the authors analyzed the relationship between autophagy and retinoic acid inducible gene-I (RIG-I)-like receptor (RLR) signaling in CSFV infection and demonstrated that the expression level of RIG-I and melanoma differentiation-associated gene 5 (MDA5) were upregulated by silencing the gene expression of endogenous LC3 and BECN1, and the increased levels of type I interferon in autophagy-impaired cells were downregulated by silencing the gene expression of endogenous RIG-I and MDA5 during CSFV infection, suggesting that CSFV promotes type I interferon-induced apoptosis by upregulating the RLR signal. Moreover, silencing the gene expression of endogenous RIG-I and MDA5 upregulated CSFV-induced autophagic activities and increased the yield and titer of CSFV progeny, indicating that the RLR signal negatively regulates CSFV-induced autophagy. This work indicated that CSFV-induced autophagy inhibits cell apoptosis by downregulating RLR signaling-mediated levels of type I interferon production. Similarly, Gou et al. silenced endogenous Drp1 or Parkin through shRNA knockdown experiments and showed that CSFV enhanced the apoptosis of cells depleted of mitochondrial fission or mitophagy [33]. These studies demonstrate that CSFV-induced autophagy inhibits apoptosis and may be an important mechanism for persistent viral infection and immune escape.

5. Pyroptosis in the Pathogenesis of CSFV

Pyroptosis is a new form of programmed cell death that relies on the activation of caspase-1 and is accompanied by the release of a large number of proinflammatory cytokines [26]. Pyroptosis is closely linked with infectious disease occurrence, development, and immune regulation and plays an extremely important role in antagonizing and eliminating pathogenic infections and endogenous dangerous signals [29,86]. The morphological characteristics, mechanisms of occurrence and action, and factors involved in pyroptosis are significantly different from those of other cell death modes, such as apoptosis and necrosis [87]. Various viruses and viral components can induce pyroptosis. These viruses and viral components activate inflammatory corpuscles such as NLRP3, NLRC4, and NLRP1 and then cleave pro-caspase-1 into an active form [88,89]. Caspase-1 cleaves the gasdermin D (GSDMD) protein to form N- (GSDMD-N) and C- (GSDMD-C) terminal GSDMD fragments, in which GSDMD-N causes cell membrane perforation and cell charring [90,91]. On the other hand, caspase-1 cuts proforms of IL-1β and IL-18 into their mature forms, which reactivate and aggregate immune cells and induce the synthesis and release of other inflammatory cytokines (such as IL-6, IL-22, and IL-33), chemokines, and adhesion molecules, forming a "cascade effect", thus expanding the inflammatory response [92,93].

CSF is characterized by high fever ($\geq$40.5 °C) and multiple hemorrhages. The pathological damage caused by CSFV mainly includes vascular endothelial injury and a massive reduction of lymphocytes. Among these effects, damage to the vascular endothelium leads to an increase in vascular permeability, which in turn causes a series of inflammatory pathological syndromes. These series of syndromes suggest that the occurrence and development of CSF is closely related to a series of physiological, pathological, and immune response processes [12]. More importantly, the pathogenesis caused by CSFV infection is similar to that caused by a "cytokine storm", that is, the massive secretion disorder of related cytokines is closely related to disease progression [94,95]. The inflammatory pathological response is an important feature of CSFV infection, which plays a very important role in the pathogenesis of CSF [96].

Early researchers long believed that apoptosis is the main mechanism for lymphopenia syndrome during CSFV infection. However, pyroptosis has been shown to have several morphological characteristics similar to apoptosis, including damage to DNA, as well as positive annexin V and TUNEL staining [87]. Recently, Yuan et. performed animal experiments to investigate CSFV-induced pyroptosis in peripheral lymphoid organs [34]. The authors observed that CSFV infection can increase the proportion of TUNEL-positive cell frequencies in porcine peripheral lymphoid tissues. They also showed that CSFV infection promotes the cleavage of GSDMD to produce active GSDMD-N in the peripheral immune organs of pigs. Recent studies have shown that GSDMD cleavage is mediated by caspases, with the N-terminal fragments of this protein thereupon driving pyroptosis [90,91]. For further analysis, calcein AM/EthD-III staining was used to detect cell membrane damage in peripheral blood monocytes (PBMCs) with CSFV infection. The authors found that CSFV infection increased the proportion of cell membrane damage in PBMCs, and this depended on the activation of caspase-1. Consistently, CSFV infection also promotes the cleavage of GSDMD and stimulates IL-1β production in PBMCs. All of these data demonstrated that pyroptosis is involved in CSFV infection. In viral infection, the assembly of the NLRP3 inflammasome is an important mechanism for caspase-1 activation, pyroptosis, and inflammation [26,88]. Studies by Fan et al. showed that CSFV-infected porcine PBMCs caused the activation of an ATP-dependent K^+ ion channel and active NLRP3 inflammasome assembly, which led to caspase-1 activation and subsequent maturation and secretion of IL-1β, resulting in an inflammatory response [97]. Additional studies have showed that inhibiting the activation of the NLRP3 inflammasome can promote CSFV replication. These findings suggest that CSFV infection promotes the activation of NLRP3 inflammasome-mediated pyroptosis. In addition, studies have reported that *human immunodeficiency virus type 1* (HIV-1) infection causes a large reduction in CD4+ T cells, precisely because HIV-1 infection induces pyroptosis. It is noteworthy that only a small number of CD4+ T-cells are infected with HIV-1 [98]. Most cell death is caused by pyroptosis in infected cells. After the cells are damaged, the contents are released in large quantities, causing inflammation. The occurrence of this induces the death of the surrounding cells, the so-called "bystanders", which in turn creates a vicious circle that eventually leads to a significant reduction in CD4+ T-cells. In previous studies, some CSFV-infected peripheral lymphoid organs also showed positive TUNEL staining for cells that were not infected with CSFV, which likely occurred due to identical mechanisms through which HIV-1 infection causes bystander CD4+ T-cell death. These works suggest that CSFV-induced pyroptosis is an immune defense mechanism against the virus invading the body.

6. Conclusions and Future Directions

Apoptosis, autophagy, and pyroptosis are the fundamental biological processes that maintain normal homeostatic and metabolic function in eukaryotic organisms, and they play an important role in antiviral immunity [23–29]. In this review, we discussed the molecular mechanisms of these three cellular biological processes and their prominent role in the pathogenesis of CSFV. As described above and as concluded in Figure 1, in the case of CSFV infection, the host initiates apoptosis, autophagy, and pyroptosis through different signaling pathways to mediate the antiviral immune response. However, CSFV has evolved a variety of strategies to regulate these three cellular biological processes and evade the host immune response, thus achieving persistent infection in the host. Apoptosis, as an effective mechanism for eliminating pathogens, can be triggered by CSFV and its coding protein E^{rns} [45,46]. However, the apoptosis of immune cells is beneficial for CSFV to escape the monitoring of the host immune system [31,43–45]. Importantly, CSFV nonstructural protein N^{pro} and NS2 have been shown to inhibit apoptosis, which may be an important process for the virus to achieve persistent infection [48–50]. Autophagy is generally considered to be a cell survival mechanism. However, during CSFV infection, CSFV utilizes autophagy mechanisms for viral replication and virion release [32,34].

Moreover, CSFV-induced autophagy inhibits cell apoptosis by downregulating RLR signaling-mediated levels of type I interferon production, which may be an important mechanism for the immune escape of CSFV [85]. Pyroptosis is another important biological process of the antiviral immune response. The activation of NLRP3 inflammasome-mediated pyroptosis during CSFV infection may help explain why CSFV establishes a persistent infection in leukocytes [34,97]. Generally, apoptosis, autophagy, and pyroptosis can be observed throughout the occurrence and development of CSFV, and they play key roles in ultimate decisions of CSFV-infected cells' fates. Therefore, understanding the role of these three cellular biological processes in the pathogenesis of CSFV is important for the development of antiviral strategies. In recent years, although research on the interactions between CSFV and these three cellular biological processes has been deepening, the mechanisms are not yet fully clear.

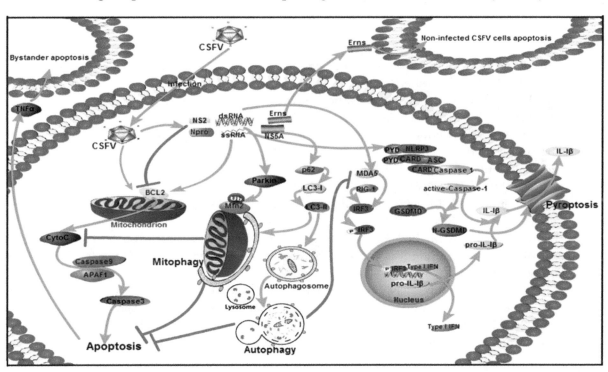

Figure 1. Apoptosis, autophagy, and pyroptosis in the pathogenesis of classical swine fever virus (CSFV). CSFV and its coding protein E^{rns} trigger apoptosis. The apoptosis of immune cells is beneficial for CSFV to escape the monitoring of the host immune system. Importantly, the CSFV nonstructural proteins N^{pro} and NS2 inhibit apoptosis, which may be an important process for the virus to achieve persistent infection. CSFV infection induces autophagy and mitophagy and utilizes their mechanisms for viral replication and virion release. Moreover, CSFV-induced autophagy inhibits cell apoptosis by downregulating retinoic acid inducible gene-I (RIG-I)-like receptor (RLR) signaling-mediated levels of type I interferon production, which may be an important mechanism for the immune escape of CSFV. CSFV infection promotes the activation of NLRP3 inflammasome-mediated pyroptosis, which may help explain why CSFV establishes a persistent infection in leukocytes.

Recently, increasing numbers of studies related to apoptosis, autophagy, and pyroptosis pathways have contributed to a wealth of knowledge and facilitated a better understanding of virus pathogenesis [23–29]. On this basis, and in accordance with the pathogenic characteristics of CSFV and the known roles of apoptosis, autophagy, and pyroptosis in CSFV infection, future research should mainly focus on revealing the molecular mechanism of these three cellular biological processes in the immune regulation of CSFV infection from different levels and perspectives. Meanwhile, more work should be contributed to the in-depth excavation of key molecules in different types of these three cellular biological process signaling pathways, applying these target molecules to vaccine development or drug design to control CSFV infection and potentially treat disease. Apoptosis, autophagy, and pyroptosis are three main cellular biological processes with significant differences in their molecular mechanisms. However, these three cellular biological processes are not independent biological processes, but have potential interaction mechanisms [25,82–84]. Therefore, in future studies, it is necessary to further reveal the mechanistic interplay between apoptosis, autophagy, and pyroptosis in CSFV infection and immunity in order to reveal the pathogenesis and immune escape mechanism of CSFV, which will have important guiding significance for the development of specific drugs and vaccines for CSF prevention, control, and eradication.

Author Contributions: Writing—original draft preparation, S.-m.M.; writing—review and editing, Q.M. and L.Y.; supervision and project administration, M.-q.Z. and J.-d.C. All authors contributed to the conception and design of the work.

References

1. Kleiboeker, S.B. Swine fever: Classical swine fever and african swine fever. *Vet. Clin. N. Am. Food Anim. Pract.* **2002**, *18*, 431–451. [CrossRef]
2. Lohse, L.; Nielsen, J.; Uttenthal, A. Early pathogenesis of classical swine fever virus (csfv) strains in danish pigs. *Vet. Microbiol.* **2012**, *159*, 327–336. [CrossRef] [PubMed]
3. Thiel, H.J.; Stark, R.; Weiland, E.; Rumenapf, T.; Meyers, G. Hog cholera virus: Molecular composition of virions from a pestivirus. *J. Virol.* **1991**, *65*, 4705–4712. [PubMed]
4. Armengol, E. Identification of t-cell epitopes in the structural and non-structural proteins of classical swine fever virus. *J. Gen. Virol.* **2002**, *83 Pt 3*, 551–560. [CrossRef]
5. Kosmidou, A.; Büttner, M.; Meyers, G. Isolation and characterization of cytopathogenic classical swine fever virus (csfv). *Arch. Virol.* **1998**, *143*, 1295–1309. [CrossRef]
6. Wang, J.; Sun, Y.; Xing-Yu, M.; Li, L.F.; Li, Y.; Luo, Y.; Wang, W.; Yu, S.; Yin, C.; Li, S.; et al. Comprehensive evaluation of the host responses to infection with differentially virulent classical swine fever virus strains in pigs. *Virus Res.* **2018**, *255*, 68–76. [CrossRef]
7. König, M.; Lengsfeld, T.; Pauly, T.; Stark, R.; Thiel, J.H. Classical swine fever virus: Independent induction of protective immunity by two structural glycoproteins. *J. Virol.* **1995**, *69*, 6479–6486.
8. Moormann, M.R.J.; Bouma, A.; Kramps, A.J.; Terpstra, C.; Smit, D.H.J. Development of a classical swine fever subunit marker vaccine and companion diagnostic test. *Vet. Microbiol.* **2000**, *73*, 209–219. [CrossRef]
9. Bensaude, E. Classical swine fever virus induces proinflammatory cytokines and tissue factor expression and inhibits apoptosis and interferon synthesis during the establishment of long-term infection of porcine vascular endothelial cells. *J. Gen. Virol.* **2004**, *85*, 1029–1037. [CrossRef]
10. Sun, J.; Shi, Z.; Guo, H.; Tu, C. Changes in the porcine peripheral blood mononuclear cell proteome induced by infection with highly virulent classical swine fever virus. *J. Gen. Virol.* **2010**, *91*, 2254–2262. [CrossRef]
11. Johns, H.L.; Bensaude, E.; La Rocca, S.A.; Seago, J.; Charleston, B.; Steinbach, F.; Drew, T.W.; Crooke, H.; Everett, H. Classical swine fever virus infection protects aortic endothelial cells from pipc-mediated apoptosis. *J. Gen. Virol.* **2010**, *91*, 1038–1046. [CrossRef] [PubMed]
12. Knoetig, S.M.; Summerfield, A.; Spagnuolo-Weaver, M.; Mccullough, K.C. Immunopathogenesis of classical swine fever. role of monocytic cells. *Immunology* **1999**, *97*, 359–366. [CrossRef] [PubMed]
13. Summerfield, A.; Mcneilly, F.; Walker, I.; Allan, G.; Knoetig, S.M.; Mccullough, K.C. Depletion of cd4(+) and cd8(high+) t-cells before the onset of viraemia during classical swine fever. *Vet. Immunol. Immunopathol.* **2001**, *78*, 3–19. [CrossRef]
14. Blome, S.; Meindl-Böhmer, A.; Nowak, G.; Moennig, V. Disseminated intravascular coagulation does not play a major role in the pathogenesis of classical swine fever. *Vet. Microbiol.* **2013**, *162*, 360–368. [CrossRef] [PubMed]
15. Chander, V.; Nandi, S.; Ravishankar, C.; Upmanyu, V.; Verma, R. Classical swine fever in pigs: Recent developments and future perspectives. *Anim. Health Res. Rev.* **2014**, *15*, 87–101. [CrossRef] [PubMed]
16. Nordén, R.; Nyström, K.; Aurelius, J.; Brisslert, M.; Olofsson, S. Virus-induced appearance of the selectin ligand slex in herpes simplex virus type 1-infected t-cells: Involvement of host and viral factors. *Glycobiology* **2013**, *23*, 310–321. [CrossRef]

17. Fuchs, Y.; Steller, H. Programmed cell death in animal development and disease. *Cell* **2011**, *147*, 7542–7758. [CrossRef]
18. Danthi, P. Viruses and the diversity of cell death. *Annu. Rev. Virol.* **2016**, *3*, 533. [CrossRef]
19. Jorgensen, I.; Rayamajhi, M.; Miao, E.A. Programmed cell death as a defence against infection. *Nat. Rev. Immunol.* **2017**, *17*, 151–164. [CrossRef]
20. Huska, J.D.; Hardwick, J.M. Programmed Cell Death and Virus Infection. *Ref. Mod. Biomed. Sci.* **2015**, *7*, 154–162.
21. Huysmans, M.; Saul, L.A.; Coll, N.S.; Nowack, M.K. Dying two deaths—Programmed cell death regulation in development and disease. *Curr. Opin. Plant Biol.* **2017**, *35*, 37–44. [CrossRef] [PubMed]
22. Carruthers, V.B.; Cotter, P.A.; Kumamoto, C.A. Microbial pathogenesis: Mechanisms of infectious disease. *Cell Host Microbe* **2007**, *2*, 214–219. [CrossRef] [PubMed]
23. Hengartner, M.O. The biochemistry of apoptosis. *Nature* **2000**, *407*, 770–776. [CrossRef] [PubMed]
24. Taylor, R.C.; Cullen, S.P.; Martin, S.J. Apoptosis: Controlled demolition at the cellular level. *Nat. Rev. Mol. Cell Biol.* **2008**, *9*, 231–241. [CrossRef]
25. Mizushima, N.; Komatsu, M. Autophagy: Renovation of cells and tissues. *Cell* **2011**, *147*, 728–741. [CrossRef]
26. Bergsbaken, T.; Fink, S.L.; Cookson, B.T. Pyroptosis: Host cell death and inflammation. *Nat. Rev. Microbiol.* **2009**, *7*, 99–109. [CrossRef]
27. Clarke, P.; Tyler, K.L. Apoptosis in animal models of virus-induced disease. *Nat. Rev. Microbiol.* **2009**, *7*, 144–155. [CrossRef]
28. Klionsky, D.J.; Emr, S.D. Autophagy as a regulated pathway of cellular degradation. *Science* **2000**, *290*, 1717–1721. [CrossRef]
29. Fink, S.L.; Cookson, B.T. Caspase-1-dependent pore formation during pyroptosis leads to osmotic lysis of infected host macrophages. *Cell. Microbiol.* **2000**, *8*, 1812–1825. [CrossRef]
30. Lange, A.; Blome, S.; Moennig, V.; Greiser-Wilke, I. Pathogenesis of classical swine fever—Similarities to viral haemorrhagic fevers: A review. *Berliner Und Münchener Tierärztliche Wochenschrift* **2011**, *124*, 36–47.
31. Choi, C.; Hwang, K.K.; Chae, C. Classical swine fever virusinduces tumor necrosis factor-α and lymphocyte apoptosis. *Arch. Virol.* **2004**, *149*, 875–889. [CrossRef] [PubMed]
32. Pei, J.; Zhao, M.; Ye, Z.; Gou, H.; Wang, J.; Yi, L.; Dong, X.; Liu, W.; Luo, Y.; Liao, M.; et al. Autophagy enhances the replication of classical swine fever virus in vitro. *Autophagy* **2014**, *10*, 93–110. [CrossRef] [PubMed]
33. Gou, H.; Zhao, M.; Xu, H.; Yuan, J.; He, W.; Zhu, M.; Ding, H.; Yi, L.; Chen, J. CSFV induced mitochondrial fission and mitophagy to inhibit apoptosis. *Oncotarget* **2017**, *8*, 24. [CrossRef] [PubMed]
34. Yuan, J.; Zhu, M.; Deng, S.; Fan, S.; Xu, H.; Liao, J.; Li, P.; Zheng, J.; Zhao, M.; Chen, J. Classical swine fever virus induces pyroptosis in the peripheral lymphoid organs of infected pigs. *Virus Res.* **2018**, *250*, 37–42. [CrossRef] [PubMed]
35. Clemens, M.J. Epstein-barr virus: Inhibition of apoptosis as a mechanism of cell transformation. *Int. J. Biochem. Cell Biol.* **2006**, *38*, 164–169. [CrossRef]
36. Clarke, P.; Debiasi, R.L.; Goody, R.; Hoyt, C.C.; Richardson-Burns, S.; Tyler, K.L. Mechanisms of reovirus-induced cell death and tissue injury: Role of apoptosis and virus-induced perturbation of host-cell signaling and transcription factor activation. *Viral Immunol.* **2005**, *18*, 89–115. [CrossRef]
37. Ross, M.E.; Caligiuri, M.A. Cytokine-induced apoptosis of human natural killer cells identifies a novel mechanism to regulate the innate immune response. *Blood* **1997**, *89*, 910–918. [CrossRef]
38. Whiteside, T.L. Apoptosis of immune cells in the tumor microenvironment and peripheral circulation of patients with cancer: Implications for immunotherapy. *Vaccine* **2002**, *20* (Suppl. S4), A46–A51. [CrossRef]
39. Roulston, A.; Marcellus, R.C.; Branton, P.E. Viruses and apoptosis. *Annu. Rev. Microbiol.* **1999**, *53*, 577. [CrossRef]
40. Jürg Tschopp Thome, M.; Hofmann, K.; Meinl, E. The fight of viruses against apoptosis. *Curr. Opin. Genet. Dev.* **1998**, *8*, 82–87.
41. Moennig, V. Introduction to classical swine fever: Virus, disease and control policy. *Vet. Microbiol.* **2000**, *73*, 93–102. [CrossRef]

42. Naniche, D.; Oldstone, M. Generalized immunosuppression: How viruses undermine the immune response. *Cell. Mol. Life Sci. CMLS* **2000**, *57*, 1399–1407. [CrossRef] [PubMed]

43. Zingle, K.; Summerfield, A.; Mccullough, K.C.; Inumaru, S. Induction of apoptosis in bone marrow neutrophil-lineage cells by classical swine fever virus. *J. Gen. Virol.* **2001**, *82*, 1309–1318.

44. Summerfield, A.; Knoetig, S.M.; Tschudin, R.; Mccullough, K.C. Pathogenesis of granulocytopenia and bone marrow atrophy during classical swine fever involves apoptosis and necrosis of uninfected cells. *Virology* **2000**, *272*, 50–60. [CrossRef] [PubMed]

45. Bruschke, C.J. Glycoprotein eˆ of pestiviruses induces apoptosis in lymphocytes of several species. *J. Virol.* **1997**, *71*, 6692–6696.

46. Meyers, G.; Saalmüller, A.; Büttner, M. Mutations abrogating the rnase activity in glycoprotein e of the pestivirus classical swine fever virus lead to virus attenuation. *J. Virol.* **2000**, *73*, 10224–10235.

47. Ruggli, N.; Summerfield, A.; Fiebach, A.R.; Guzylack-Piriou, L.; Tratschin, J.D. Classical swine fever virus can remain virulent after specific elimination of the interferon regulatory factor 3-degrading function of npro. *J. Virol.* **2008**, *83*, 817–829. [CrossRef]

48. Johns, H.L.; Doceul, V.; Everett, H.; Crooke, H.; Charleston, B.; Seago, J. The classical swine fever virus n-terminal protease npro binds to cellular hax-1. *J. Gen. Virol.* **2010**, *91*, 2677–2686. [CrossRef]

49. Tang, Q.; Guo, K.; Kang, K.; Zhang, Y.; He, L.; Wang, J. Classical swine fever virus ns2 protein promotes interleukin-8 expression and inhibits mg132-induced apoptosis. *Virus Genes* **2011**, *42*, 355–362. [CrossRef]

50. Tang, Q.H.; Zhang, Y.M.; Fan, L.; Tong, G.; Dai, C. Classic swine fever virus ns2 protein leads to the induction of cell cycle arrest at s-phase and endoplasmic reticulum stress. *Virol. J.* **2010**, *7*, 4. [CrossRef]

51. Hurley, J.; Schulman, B. Atomistic autophagy: The structures of cellular self-digestion. *Cell* **2014**, *157*, 300–311. [CrossRef] [PubMed]

52. Levine, B.; Kroemer, G. Autophagy in the pathogenesis of disease. *Cell* **2008**, *132*, 27–42. [CrossRef] [PubMed]

53. Jordan, T.X.; Randall, G. Manipulation or capitulation: Virus interactions with autophagy. *Microbes Infect.* **2012**, *14*, 126–139. [CrossRef] [PubMed]

54. Kuballa, P.; Nolte, W.M.; Castoreno, A.B.; Xavier, R.J. Autophagy and the immune system. *Annu. Rev. Immunol.* **2012**, *30*, 611–646. [CrossRef] [PubMed]

55. Chiramel, A.I.; Brady, N.R.; Bartenschlager, R. Divergent roles of autophagy in virus infection. *Cells* **2013**, *2*, 83–104. [CrossRef] [PubMed]

56. Paul, P.; Münz, C. Autophagy and mammalian viruses: Roles in immune response, viral replication, and beyond. *Adv. Virus Res.* **2016**, *95*, 149.

57. Yoshimori, T. How Autophagy Saves Mice: A Cell-Autonomous Defense System against Sindbis Virus Infection. *Cell Host Microbe* **2010**, *7*, 83–84. [CrossRef]

58. Xu, G.; Wang, S.; Han, S.; Xie, K.; Liu, Y. Plant bax inhibitor-1 interacts with atg6 to regulate autophagy and programmed cell death. *Autophagy* **2017**, *13*, 7. [CrossRef]

59. Zhou, D.; Spector, S.A. Human immunodeficiency virus type-1 infection inhibits autophagy. *AIDS* **2008**, *22*, 695–699. [CrossRef]

60. Tovilovic, G.; Ristic, B.; Siljic, M.; Nikolic, V.; Kravic-Stevovic, T.; Dulovic, M.; Milenkovic, M.; Knezevic, A.; Bosnjak, M.; Bumbasirevic, V.; et al. Mtor-independent autophagy counteracts apoptosis in herpes simplex virus type 1-infected u251 glioma cells. *Microbes Infect.* **2013**, *15*, 615–624. [CrossRef]

61. Zhou, Z.; Jiang, X.; Liu, D.; Fan, Z.; Hu, X.; Yan, J.; Wang, M.; Gao, G. Autophagy is involved in influenza a virus replication. *Autophagy* **2009**, *5*, 321–328. [CrossRef] [PubMed]

62. Heaton, N.S.; Glenn, R. Dengue virus and autophagy. *Viruses* **2011**, *3*, 1332–1341. [CrossRef] [PubMed]

63. Dreux, M.; Chisari, F.V. Impact of the autophagy machinery on hepatitis c virus infection. *Viruses* **2011**, *3*, 1342–1357. [CrossRef] [PubMed]

64. Chiramel, A.I.; Best, S.M. Role of autophagy in zika virus infection and pathogenesis. *Virus Res.* **2017**, *254*, 34–40. [CrossRef]

65. Vandergaast, R.; Fredericksen, B.L. West nile virus (wnv) replication is independent of autophagy in mammalian cells. *PLoS ONE* **2012**, *7*, e45800. [CrossRef]

66. Sharma, M.; Bhattacharyya, S.; Sharma, K.B.; Chauhan, S.; Asthana, S.; Abdin, M.Z.; Vratis, S.; Kalia, M. Japanese encephalitis virus activates autophagy through xbp1 and atf6 er stress sensors in neuronal cells. *J. Gen. Virol.* **2017**, *98*, 1027. [CrossRef]

67. Seglen, P.O.; Gordon, P.B.; Holen, I. Non-selective autophagy. *Semin. Cell Biol.* **1990**, *1*, 441.

68. Shaid, S.; Brandts, C.H.; Serve, H.; Dikic, I. Ubiquitination and selective autophagy. *Cell Death Differ.* **2013**, *20*, 21–30. [CrossRef]

69. Youle, R.J.; Narendra, D.P. Mechanisms of mitophagy. *Nat. Rev. Mol. Cell Biol.* **2011**, *12*, 9–14. [CrossRef]

70. Ding, W.X.; Yin, X.M. Mitophagy: Mechanisms, pathophysiological roles, and analysis. *Biol. Chem.* **2012**, *393*, 547–564. [CrossRef]

71. Kim, S.J.; Khan, M.; Quan, J.; Till, A.; Subramani, S.; Siddiqui, A. Hepatitis b virus disrupts mitochondrial dynamics: Induces fission and mitophagy to attenuate apoptosis. *PLoS Pathog.* **2013**, *9*, e1003722. [CrossRef] [PubMed]

72. Kim, S.J.; Syed, G.H.; Siddiqui, A.; Ou, J.H.J. Hepatitis c virus induces the mitochondrial translocation of parkin and subsequent mitophagy. *PLoS Pathog.* **2013**, *9*, e1003285. [CrossRef] [PubMed]

73. Kim, S.J.; Syed, G.H.; Khan, M.; Chiu, W.W.; Sohail, M.A.; Gish, R.G.; Siddiqui, A. Hepatitis c virus triggers mitochondrial fission and attenuates apoptosis to promote viral persistence. *Proc. Natl. Acad. Sci. USA* **2014**, *111*, 6413–6418. [CrossRef] [PubMed]

74. Summerfield, A.; Hofmann, M.A.; Mccullough, K.C. Low density blood granulocytic cells induced during classical swine fever are targets for virus infecion. *Vet. Immunol. Immunopathol.* **1998**, *63*, 289–301. [CrossRef]

75. He, L.; Zhang, Y.; Fang, Y.; Liang, W.; Lin, J.; Cheng, M. Classical swine fever virus induces oxidative stress in swine umbilical vein endothelial cells. *BMC Vet. Res.* **2014**, *10*, 279. [CrossRef]

76. Geisler, S.; Holmström, K.M.; Skujat, D.; Fiesel, F.C.; Rothfuss, O.C.; Kahle, P.J.; Springer, W. Pink1/parkin-mediated mitophagy is dependent on vdac1 and p62/sqstm1. *Nat. Cell Biol.* **2010**, *12*, 119–131. [CrossRef]

77. Sebastián, D.; Sorianello, E.; Segalés, J.; Irazoki, A.; Ruiz-Bonilla, V.; Sala, D.; Planet, E.; Berenguer-Llergo, A.; Muñoz, J.P.; Sánchez-Feutrie, M.; et al. Mfn2 deficiency links age-related sarcopenia and impaired autophagy to activation of an adaptive mitophagy pathway. *EMBO J.* **2016**, *35*, 1677–1693. [CrossRef]

78. Maiuri, M.C.; Zalckvar, E.; Kimchi, A.; Kroemer, G. Self-eating and self-killing: Crosstalk between autophagy and apoptosis. *Nat. Rev. Mol. Cell Biol.* **2007**, *8*, 741–752. [CrossRef]

79. Chen, Q.; Kang, J.; Fu, C. The independence of and associations among apoptosis, autophagy, and necrosis. *Signal. Transduct. Target. Ther.* **2018**, *3*, 18. [CrossRef]

80. Ouyang, L.; Shi, Z.; Zhao, S.; Wang, F.; Zhou, T.; Liu, B.; Bao, J.K. Programmed cell death pathways in cancer: A review of apoptosis, autophagy and programmed necrosis. *CellProlifer* **2012**, *90*, 487–498. [CrossRef]

81. Tylichová, Z.; Straková, N.; Vondráček, J.; Vaculová, A.H.; Kozubík, A.; Hofmanová, J. Activation of autophagy and ppary protect colon cancer cells against apoptosis induced by interactive effects of butyrate and dha in a cell type-dependent manner: The role of cell differentiation. *J. Nutr. Biochem.* **2017**, *39*, 145–155. [CrossRef] [PubMed]

82. Kuro, M.; Yoshizawa, K.; Uehara, N.; Lai, C.Y.; Kanematsu, S.; Miki, H.; Kimura, A.; Yuri, T.; Takahashi, K.; Tsubura, A. Calpain inhibition restores basal autophagy and suppresses apoptosis on mnu-induced photoreceptor cell injury in mice. *Invest. Ophthalmol Vis. Sci.* **2011**, *52*, 4352.

83. Eisenberg-Lerner, A.; Bialik, S.; Simon, H.U.; Kimchi, A. Life and death partners: Apoptosis, autophagy and the cross-talk between them. *Cell Death Differ.* **2009**, *16*, 966–975. [CrossRef] [PubMed]

84. Gou, H.; Zhao, M.; Fan, S.; Yuan, J.; Liao, J.; He, W.; Xu, H.; Chen, J. Autophagy induces apoptosis and death of t lymphocytes in the spleen of pigs infected with CSFV. *Sci. Rep.* **2017**, *7*, 13577. [CrossRef]

85. Pei, J.; Deng, J.; Ye, Z.; Wang, J.; Gou, H.; Liu, W.; Zhao, M.; Liao, M.; Yi, L.; Chen, J. Absence of autophagy promotes apoptosis by modulating the ros-dependent rlr signaling pathway in classical swine fever virus-infected cells. *Autophagy* **2016**, *2*, 1738–1758. [CrossRef]

86. Kesavardhana, S.; Kanneganti, T.D. Mechanisms governing inflammasome activation, assembly and pyroptosis induction. *Int. Immunol.* **2017**, *29*, 5. [CrossRef]

87. Fink, S.L.; Cookson, B.T. Apoptosis, pyroptosis, and necrosis: Mechanistic description of dead and dying eukaryotic cells. *Infect. Immun.* **2005**, *73*, 1907. [CrossRef]

88. Case, C.L. Regulating caspase-1 during infection: Roles of nlrs, aim2, and asc. *Yale J. Biol. Med.* **2011**, *84*, 333–343.

89. Miao, E.A.; Leaf, I.A.; Treuting, P.M.; Mao, D.P.; Dors, M.; Sarkar, A.; Warren, S.E.; Wewers, M.D.; Aderem, A. Caspase-1-induced pyroptosis is an innate immune effector mechanism against intracellular bacteria. *Nat. Immunol.* **2010**, *11*, 1136–1142. [CrossRef]

90. He, W.T.; Wan, H.; Hu, L.; Chen, P.; Wang, X.; Huang, Z.; Yang, Z.H.; Zhong, C.Q.; Han, J. Gasdermin d is an executor of pyroptosis and required for interleukin-1β secretion. *Cell Res.* **2015**, *25*, 1285–1298. [CrossRef]

91. Si, M.M.; Kanneganti, T.D. Gasdermin d: The long-awaited executioner of pyroptosis. *Cell Res.* **2015**, *25*, 1183.

92. Sahoo, M.; Ceballos-Olvera, I.; Barrio, L.D.; Re, F. Role of the inflammasome, il-1β, and il-18 in bacterial infections. *Sci. World J.* **2011**, *11*, 2037–2050. [CrossRef]

93. Fettelschoss, A.; Kistowska, M.; Leibundgutlandmann, S.; Beer, H.D.; Johansen, P.; Senti, G.; Contassot, E.; Bachmann, M.F.; French, L.E.; Oxenius, A. Inflammasome activation and il-1β target il-1α for secretion as opposed to surface expression. *Proc. Natl. Acad. Sci. USA* **2011**, *108*, 18055–18060. [CrossRef]

94. Summerfield, A.; Alves, M.; Ruggli, N.; Bruin, M.G.M.D.; Mccullough, K.C. High ifn-α responses associated with depletion of lymphocytes and natural ifn-producing cells during classical swine fever. *J. Interferon Cytokine Res.* **2006**, *26*, 248–255. [CrossRef] [PubMed]

95. Sánchez-Cordón, P.J.; Romanini, S.; Salguero, J.F.; Núnez, A.; Bautista, J.M.; Jover, A.; Gómez-Villamos, J.C. Apoptosis of thymocytes related to cytokine expression in experimental classical swine fever. *J. Compar. Pathol.* **2002**, *127*, 239–248. [CrossRef] [PubMed]

96. Sanchez-Cordon, P.J.; Nunez, A.; Salguero, F.J.; Carrasco, L.; Gómez-Villamandos, J.C. Evolution of T lymphocytes and cytokine expression in classical swine fever (CSF) virus infection. *J. Comp. Pathol.* **2005**, *132*, 249–260. [CrossRef] [PubMed]

97. Fan, S.; Yuan, J.; Deng, S.; Chen, Y.; Xie, B.; Wu, K.; Zhu, M.; Xu, H.; Huang, Y.; Yang, J. Activation of Interleukin-1β Release by the Classical Swine Fever Virus Is Dependent on the NLRP3 Inflammasome, Which Affects Virus Growth in Monocytes. *Front. Cell Infect. Microbiol.* **2018**, *8*, 225. [CrossRef] [PubMed]

98. Hazenberg, M.D.; Hamann, D.; Schuitemaker, H.; Miedema, F. T cell depletion in hiv-1 infection: How cd4+ t cells go out of stock. *Nat. Immunol.* **2000**, *1*, 285–289. [CrossRef] [PubMed]

Role of Wild Boar in the Spread of Classical Swine Fever in Japan

Satoshi Ito [1,2], Cristina Jurado [2], Jaime Bosch [2], Mitsugi Ito [3], José Manuel Sánchez-Vizcaíno [2], Norikazu Isoda [1,4,*] and Yoshihiro Sakoda [5,*]

[1] Research Center for Zoonosis Control, Hokkaido University, Kita 20, Nishi 10, Kita-ku, Sapporo, Hokkaido 001-0020, Japan; satoshi125@czc.hokudai.ac.jp
[2] VISAVET Center and Animal Health Department, University Complutense of Madrid, 28040 Madrid, Spain; cjdiaz@ucm.es (C.J.); jaimeboschlopez@gmail.com (J.B.); jmvizcaino@ucm.es (J.M.S.-V.)
[3] Akabane Animal Clinic, Co. Ltd., 55 Ishizoe, Akabane-cho, Tahara, Aichi-ken 441-3502, Japan; m-ito@oasis.ocn.ne.jp
[4] Global Station for Zoonosis Control, Global Institute for Collaborative Research and Education (GI-CoRE), Hokkaido University, Sapporo 001-0020, Japan
[5] Laboratory of Microbiology, Department of Disease Control, Faculty of Veterinary Medicine, Hokkaido University, Kita 18, Nishi 9, Kita-ku, Sapporo, Hokkaido 060-0018, Japan
* Correspondence: isoda@czc.hokudai.ac.jp (N.I.); sakoda@vetmed.hokudai.ac.jp (Y.S.)

Abstract: Since September 2018, nearly 900 notifications of classical swine fever (CSF) have been reported in Gifu Prefecture (Japan) affecting domestic pig and wild boar by the end of August 2019. To determine the epidemiological characteristics of its spread, a spatio-temporal analysis was performed using actual field data on the current epidemic. The spatial study, based on standard deviational ellipses of official CSF notifications, showed that the disease likely spread to the northeast part of the prefecture. A maximum significant spatial association estimated between CSF notifications was 23 km by the multi-distance spatial cluster analysis. A space-time permutation analysis identified two significant clusters with an approximate radius of 12 and 20 km and 124 and 98 days of duration, respectively. When the area of the identified clusters was overlaid on a map of habitat quality, approximately 82% and 75% of CSF notifications, respectively, were found in areas with potential contact between pigs and wild boar. The obtained results provide information on the current CSF epidemic, which is mainly driven by wild boar cases with sporadic outbreaks on domestic pig farms. These findings will help implement control measures in Gifu Prefecture.

Keywords: classical swine fever; spatio-temporal analysis; wild boar; transboundary diseases

1. Introduction

Classical swine fever (CSF) is caused by infection with the CSF virus (CSFV), which belongs to the genus *Pestivirus*, family *Flaviviridae*. CSF is described by the World Organisation for Animal Health as a highly contagious febrile disease with potential for high mortality that causes enormous economic loss in the pig industry worldwide [1]. CSFV is a positive-sense, single-stranded RNA virus with a genome of approximately 12.3 kb, comprising one large open reading frame that encodes a polyprotein and flanked by 5'-untranslated region (5'-UTR) and 3'-untranslated region [2]. During virus replication, the polyprotein is processed by cellular and viral proteases into four structural and nine nonstructural proteins [2]. Outbreaks of CSF have been reported over the past decade in Asia (Bhutan, Cambodia, China, India, Indonesia, the Republic of Korea, Lao PDR, Mongolia, Myanmar, Nepal, the Philippines, Thailand, Timor-Leste, and Vietnam), Europe (Latvia, Lithuania, the Russian Federation, Serbia, and

Ukraine), Africa (Madagascar), the Caribbean (the Dominican Republic, Guatemala, and Haiti), and Latin America (Bolivia, Colombia, Ecuador, and Peru) [3]. Based on the amino acid sequence of the 5'-UTR and E2, which is one of the structural region of the protein, CSFVs are classified into three genotypes (1, 2, and 3) and several subgenotypes (1.1–1.4, 2.1–2.3, and 3.1–3.4) [4,5]. The virulence of CSFV is categorized via a clinical score into highly virulent, moderately virulent, low virulent, and avirulent [6,7]. Although the CSFV genotype 2.1b isolated from the Republic of Korea was highly virulent, the same genotype isolated in Mongolia was moderately virulent [8,9]. Moreover, the recently classified CSFV genotype 2.1d from China was moderately virulent compared to different variants and antigenicity from field strains identified in China in the past [10].

No notifications of CSF were reported in Japan since 1992, and the country had an 11-year stretch of CSF-free status defined by the OIE Terrestrial Animal Health Code since 2007. However, CSF reemerged in Japan in September 2018 in Gifu Prefecture, which is located in the central part of the main island of Japan. Phylogenetic analysis revealed that the CSFV strain isolated in Japan in 2018 showed the highest identity in the complete E2 gene sequence with Chinese strains isolated between 2011 and 2015 and in the partial 5'-UTR sequence with strains isolated in China and Mongolia in 2014 and 2015 [11].

By the end of August 2019, a total of 39 CSFV outbreaks on pig farms in four prefectures and 1,071 cases in wild boar in seven prefectures have been reported [12]. Despite the implementation of intensive responses, including movement bans of domestic pigs, surveillance, and oral immunization of wild boar, new notifications of CSF cases in both wild boar and domestic pigs were being reported continually [13]. This might indicate that the pathogenic viruses were widely prevalent and persisted in wildlife around the affected area. As the Eurasian wild boar is also susceptible to CSFV, the circulation and persistence of CSFV among food animals and wildlife makes it difficult to carry out effective control measures for eradicating it in affected areas. Due to contact with infected animals and feeds contaminated with contagious pathogens in garbage dumped on the human sphere, naïve wild boar populations are often infected with CSFV [8,14–24]. Before the 1990s, CSF cases in wild boar were rare concerns as infection was detected rapidly due to the high virulence of circulating strains. However, disease detection appears delayed in the current epidemic due to infection with more moderately virulent strains [25]. As a consequence, there have been serious outbreaks of CSF in the wild boar population in Germany. During an outbreak of CSF in Germany from 1993 to 1998, an epidemiological field investigation confirmed that 59% of the primary cases in domestic pigs could be attributed to either direct or indirect contact with infected wild boar [17]. Virus characteristics and population size can both be considered critical factors for the persistence of CSFV, especially in wild boar populations [25]. It has been suggested that CSFV would be self-limiting within one year in populations of 2000 wild boar, whereas it will persist and become endemic in a larger population [26]. In addition, the population density of wild boar also has been suggested as being a potential factor for the persistence of CSF because more frequent turnover occurs in dense populations, which provides faster renewal of susceptible piglets that increases the chance that the virus will persist in the population [25]. Once the contagious viruses are transmitted to wildlife, specific control measures for wild boar will be needed to eradicate CSF in the affected area and to contain it more effectively.

The present study conducted a spatio-temporal analysis to obtain epidemiological information on current epidemics of CSF in Japan. Based on the official CSF reports on domestic pig farms and wild boar, notified in Gifu Prefecture from September 2018 to June 2019, we assessed the direction of the spread of the disease and identified areas with high densities of notifications. In addition, to identify spatio-temporal aggregation of notifications and to characterize land cover vegetation in areas of disease aggregation, a clustering analysis was conducted, and obtained clusters were then overlapped with quality habitat map. The obtained information can be used to develop more effective disease control measures for application in both domestic pigs and wild boar.

2. Results

2.1. Standard Deviational Ellipse Analysis

A standard deviational ellipse analysis was applied to describe the directional trend and dispersion of CSF notifications in the study area throughout the study period. The study covered the period between September 2018 and June 2019, which was divided into three stages (September–December, January–March, and April–June). Figure 1 illustrates standard deviational ellipses and CSF notifications between September 2018 and June 2019 (Figure 1). To indicate the potential explanation for the directional trend of the CSF outbreaks, the ellipses were overlaid on a map of snowfall area in Gifu Prefecture obtained from the National Land Information Division, Ministry of Land, Infrastructure, Transport and Tourism [27]. The findings showed that CSF notifications appeared to move northeast while spreading along the border of the snowfall area.

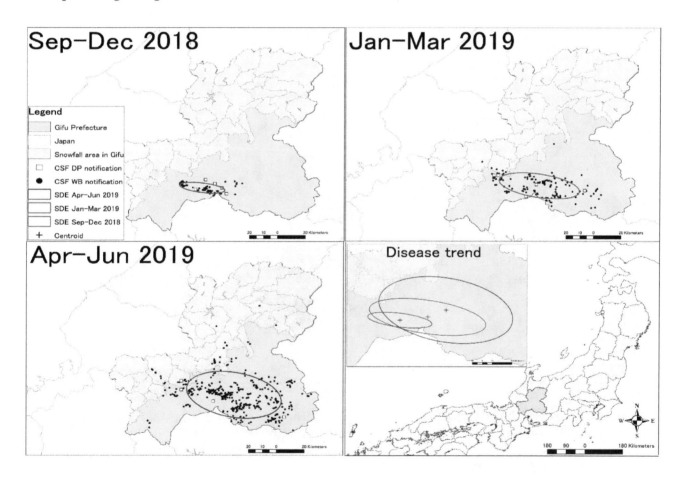

Figure 1. Directional distribution of classical swine fever (CSF) notifications from September 2018 to June 2019. Standard deviational ellipses (SDEs) identified between September and December 2018, between January and March 2019, and between April and June 2019. Ellipses were overlaid with CSF notifications distinguishing domestic pig (DP) (square) and wild boar (WB) (circle). Ellipses with centroids were combined to indicate the directional trend of the CSF outbreaks.

2.2. Multi-Distance Spatial Cluster Analysis

The multi-distance spatial cluster analysis was applied to explore the maximum distance between cases of CSF notifications. The results indicated that 23 km was the maximum distance of the significant spatial association between CSF notifications in Gifu Prefecture. The obtained maximum distance was used in the subsequent analyses.

2.3. Kernel Density Estimation Analysis

The kernel density estimation analysis was applied to describe the spatial distribution of the CSF notifications. The analysis showed that the highest density of CSF notifications was located in the southern part of Gifu Prefecture (Figure 2) with further expansion to the east. Among the 16 CSF-positive farms, 37.5% were located in areas with very high or high density of notifications, 31.25% in areas of medium density and 31.25% in areas of low density. Moreover, most of the non-affected domestic farms were located in areas with very low density of notifications (80%), followed by areas with low density (20%). The analysis revealed that CSF-positive farms were located in areas with higher density of notifications, whereas the non-affected farms tended to locate in areas with low density.

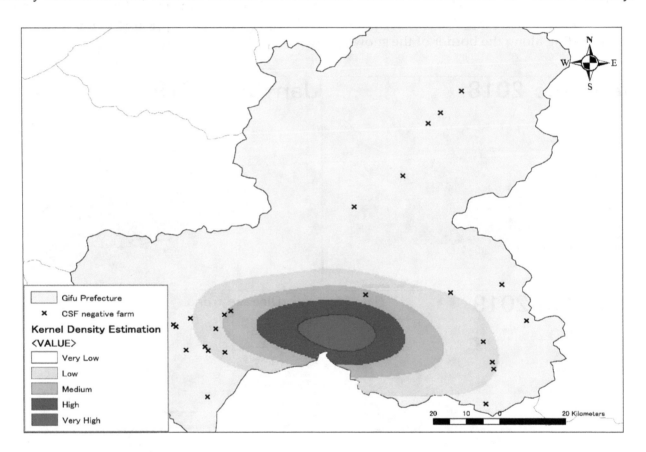

Figure 2. Density of CSF notifications in Gifu Prefecture. The heat map illustrates the estimated kernel density of CSF notifications (notifications/km^2) from very high (red) to very low (transparent). Each coloured area indicates the density of CSF notifications per square kilometer: very high (>0.400), high (0.300–0.399), medium (0.200–0.299), low (0.100–0.199), and very low (<0.100). The highest density of CSF notifications was located in the southern part of Gifu Prefecture. A very low density of CSF notifications was located in other areas of the prefecture. Locations of pig farms not affected by CSF are represented by crosses.

2.4. Space-Time Cluster Analysis

The space-time permutation analysis was applied to analyze the space-time patterns of the CSF notifications. The analysis identified two significant space-time clusters ($P < 0.05$) in Gifu Prefecture during the study period. Cluster 1, which had a radius of 12.12 km, covered 9 September 2018 to 13 January 2019, and contained 83 notifications, including 4 outbreaks on domestic pig farms. Cluster 2 had a radius of 19.79 km, spanning the period from 11 February 2019 to 19 May 2019, and contained 198 notifications, including three outbreaks in domestic pigs (Table 1).

Table 1. Observed and expected notifications, duration, start and end dates, and radius of each space-time cluster detected ($P < 0.05$) in CSF notifications in Gifu Prefecture.

Cluster	Observed Notifications	Expected Notifications	Duration (Days)	Start Date	End Date	Radius (km)
1	83	17.34	124	2018/9/9	2019/1/13	12.12
2	198	131.87	98	2019/2/11	2019/5/19	19.79

2.5. Quality of Available Habitat (QAH) Within Space-Time Cluster Area

In order to characterize the land cover vegetation within two significant space-time clusters, the clusters were overlaid with a QAH map. The results showed different patterns between cluster 1 and cluster 2 (Figure 3). In cluster 1, 50.6% of CSF notifications were reported in areas at QAH 1, while 31.3% were reported in areas at QAH 1.5, and 18.1% were reported in areas at QAH 2 (Table 2). In cluster 2, 22.7% of CSF notifications were reported in areas at QAH 1, 52.5% were reported in areas at QAH 1.5, 2.5% were reported in areas at QAH 1.75, and 22.2% were reported in areas at QAH 2 (Table 2).

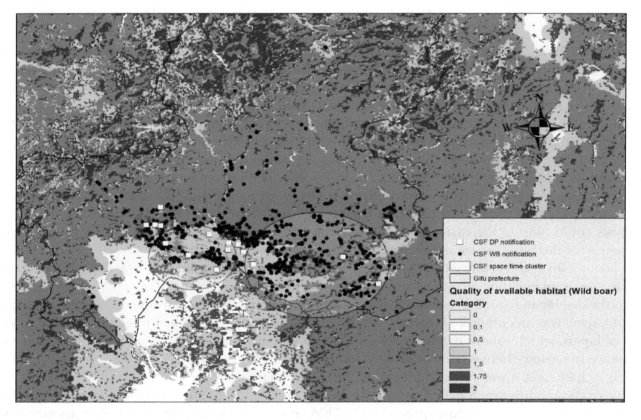

Figure 3. Locations of the significant space-time clusters of CSF. Notifications: ($P < 0.05$) in Gifu Prefecture overlaid on a map of the quality of available habitat (QAH) levels for wild boar. Graduated colors indicate the quality of habitat availability from darker colors (areas with better quality of habitat availability) to lighter colors (areas with worse quality of habitat availability).

The CSF notifications within clusters 1 and 2 occurred within habitats that included rainfed croplands (QAH 1), a closed (>40%) needle-leaved evergreen forest (>5 m) (QAH 1.5), a mosaic of cropland (50%–70%) and vegetation (grassland/shrubland/forest) (20%–50%) (QAH 1.75), a mosaic of vegetation (grassland/shrubland/forest) (50%–70%) and cropland (20%–50%) (QAH 2), closed (>40%) broadleaved deciduous forest (>5 m) (QAH 2), and closed to open (>15%) mixed broadleaved and needle-leaved forest (>5 m) (QAH 2).

Although different patterns of land cover vegetation were observed between clusters 1 and 2, nearly 50% of CSF notifications within cluster 1 and more than 75% within cluster 2 were notified in QAH 1.5–2, which provides the greatest opportunities for food and shelter for wild boar.

Table 2. Quality of availability habitats (QAH) of CSF notifications within the two identified space-time clusters.

QAH Category	Land Cover	Cluster 1			Cluster 2		
		DP (n)	WB (n)	Total (n) (%)	DP (n)	WB (n)	Total (n) (%)
1.0	Rainfed croplands	4	38	42 (50.6)	0	45	45 (22.7)
1.5	Closed (>40%) needleleaved evergreen forest (>5m)	0	26	26 (31.3)	3	101	104 (52.5)
1.75	Mosaic cropland (50–70%)/vegetation (grassland/shrubland/forest) (20–50%)	0	0	0 (0.0)	0	5	5 (2.5)
2.0	Mosaic vegetation (grassland/shrubland/forest) (50–70%)/cropland (20–50%)	0	0	0 (0.0)	0	14	14 (7.1)
2.0	Closed (>40%) broadleaved deciduous forest (>5m)	0	1	1 (1.2)	0	0	0 (0.0)
2.0	Closed to open (>15%) mixed broadleaved and needleleaved forest (>5m)	0	14	14 (16.9)	0	30	30 (15.2)
	Total	4	79	83 (100.0)		195	198 (100.0)

DP: domestic pig. WB: wild boar. n: the number of notifications.

3. Discussion

From 2018 until August 2019, all notifications of CSF outbreaks in Japan have been made in Gifu Prefecture as well as in the surrounding four prefectures. A total of 1110 notifications had been reported so far, with 1071 affecting wild boar and 39 affecting domestic pig farms. The continuous notification of CSF in the area might have been attributed to wide spread of the virus within wild boar populations favored by free animal movements, as well as to the emergence of epidemiologically related domestic pig farms. To prevent the disease spreading in wild boar, control measures including (i) fencing to restrict animal movements, (ii) hunting activities for active monitoring and to reduce susceptible populations, and (iii) disseminating baits for oral immunization, were implemented. However, the efficacy of these strategies has not been confirmed. Therefore, we conducted a spatio-temporal analysis to obtain epidemiological information of the spread of CSF in Gifu Prefecture. Results from this analysis could help to increase our understanding of the current CSF epidemic and to contribute strategies for the containment of the disease in domestic pigs and wild boar.

Japan is an island country that has achieved the status of freedom from several contagious animal diseases by implementing adequate control measures that take advantage of the country's geography. Nevertheless, Japan has imported outbreaks of contagious animal diseases from neighboring countries. In 2010, there was an outbreak of foot-and-mouth disease (FMD) in Miyazaki Prefecture in the southern part of Japan, which caused extensive losses in animal husbandry. According to the high degree of sequence homology between an original virus isolated in Japan and viruses that were circulating widely in East Asia, it was suspected that the FMD virus might have been introduced via movement of people or commodities from East Asia [28]. The high homology of genetic sequences between the CSF virus isolated in Japan and viruses prevailing in China suggests that the infectious CSF virus may have been introduced from China. Potential factors that could have contributed to disease introduction include easy access from the international airport to the affected area, which has regular and direct flights from China, and the relatively high population density of Chinese people in the affected area.

In the present study, standard deviational ellipse analysis was conducted to measure the standard distance of CSF notifications. Shifting the centroids of identified ellipses indicated that the disease notification has spread in a northeast direction. Overlaying the three identified ellipses with a map of snowfall area in Gifu Prefecture revealed that the disease spread along the border of the snowfall area. In the south of Gifu Prefecture, there is a widespread area of flat land with field crops or animal farms, residential areas, and forests surrounded by mountains to the north. As suggested by other authors [29,30], wild boar do not move to the snowfall or high mountain areas. Therefore, mountains could have acted as an effective geographical barrier to limit wild boar movements and guide the direction of the spread of CSF.

Another concern regarding the spread of the disease is the potential for it to jump to remote areas. During the epidemic, CSFV infections were confirmed on seven farms that were geographically distant from, but epidemiologically linked, to the farms affected by CSFV (i.e., run by the same owner, supported by the same husbandry company, etc.) [13]. Given the potential for transmission of the virus between pigs on any farms or from wild boar near that farm, the epidemiologically related farms may further expand the spread of disease. This "disordered" spread of disease could affect the accuracy of spatio-temporal analysis by overestimating the maximum distance of significant spatial association between notifications. During the FMD epidemic in Miyazaki, the disease was confirmed 70 km away from the zone of movement restriction, which could have been caused by vehicle transportation [28]. Unexpected occurrences of disease in epidemiologically related farms would require reviewing farm biosecurity measures, as well as disease monitoring protocols.

In the present study, the results of the multi-distance spatial cluster analysis revealed that the maximum distance of relationship between CSF notifications was 23 km. Because of the small number of CSF outbreaks on domestic pig farms, we estimated the maximum distance of the relationship between notifications of domestic pigs and wild boar. This assumption could have influenced our estimated distance resulting in overestimation due to long distance spread observed on domestic pig farms. Nevertheless, similar approaches have studied another transboundary animal disease, African swine fever (ASF), which shares hosts and most of the transmission mechanisms with CSF [31–33]. When comparing our results with other studies, the estimated distance (23 km) was similar to that obtained for notifications of ASF in domestic pigs (15 km) and wild boar (25 km) in Sardinia [32]. This finding may be useful for setting the range of effective surveillance and control zones in the affected area.

The application of cluster analysis to identify areas with significant spatio-temporal aggregation of the ASF outbreaks in Sardinia from 2004 to 2013 indicated four clusters, the largest of which had a radius of 30 km [33]. This does not correspond with the results of another report that identified one cluster with a radius of 3 km in the same area [32]. As discussed in Iglesias et al., methodological differences could have led to the discrepancy [32]. In present study, because of the small number of CSF outbreaks in pig farms, we could not identify the maximum distance for the relationship between notifications of CSF in pigs alone, but we were able to do it by considering pigs and wild boar together. The discordance between the findings of the two spatio-temporal analyses in Sardinia may suggest that by using mixed data for two species in the present study, we may have overestimated the distance of the spread of disease compared to true distance of transmission in each of the two species. However, we believe that this uncertainty would be acceptable for setting the monitoring area with high efficacy. Thus, these findings may be useful for setting the range of an effective surveillance and control zone.

Data on wild boar cases consisted of animals found dead and/or captured during surveillance activities. Many of wild boar were captured during active surveillance activities by setting traps and conducting hunting activities. Considering that most of the reported wild boar cases were located close to human habitats, the wild boar capture area may have been biased. Therefore, the disease could be wider spread in the area than what has been reported in official notifications, and the identified clusters could have had a shorter radius. Ideally, active virologic surveys should be intensively implemented to decrease the reporting biases by providing more samples to detect low levels of prevalence [34,35]. The Gifu Animal Health Administration has authorized hunting activities to reduce the number of susceptible, as well as potentially infected, individuals. Hunters are a critical group for implementing population control and proper disposal of wild boar carcasses.

According to the investigative report of the affected farms, there were some factors that might have increased the risk of CSFV introduction into affected farms, including (i) improper preparedness against invasion of wild or small animals into farms; (ii) imperfect clothing and boot changes in farms and pig pens, or disinfection of those materials; and (iii) inadequate vehicle disinfection [13].

To prevent contact among each of the hosts, in addition to raising awareness of disease among farmers and hunters, it is important to improve biosecurity measures in pig farms against CSFV as well as other infectious diseases.

Finally, we analyzed the QAH level of areas within the two identified clusters to characterize land cover vegetation in areas of disease aggregation. According to Bosch et al., a QAH 1 level corresponded to suitable areas for food or shelter for wild boar (mainly agricultural landscapes) [36]. In cluster 1, 50.6% of CSF notifications were reported in areas at QAH 1, whereas in cluster 2, 22.7% of CSF notifications were reported in areas at QAH 1. Considering that frequent direct and indirect contact is likely to occur between both hosts, contagious viruses in wild boar could be transmitted to pigs in the farms due to insufficient biosecurity in the affected farms since wild boar was the suspected source of infection on 80% of affected domestic pig farms in Gifu Prefecture during the studied epidemic [13,35]. On the other hand, almost 50% of CSF notifications within cluster 1 and over 75% within cluster 2 were associated with QAH 1.5–2, which mainly corresponded to natural landscapes. These natural areas provided the greatest opportunities for food and shelter for wild boar. In the case of ASF, it has been reported that wild boar can transmit the disease efficiently at local levels within their own population [32,36]. Furthermore, De la Torre et al. suggested that the spread of ASF in Europe was driven by contact between animals from different populations that moved short distances [37]. Although ASF is caused by another virus, given that wild boar play an important role in both diseases, it is plausible to assume that CSF also could have expanded through contact between individual wild boar. Therefore, it would be critical to control wild boar populations and manage wild boar carcasses adequately from the environment to reduce habitat contamination.

Interestingly, the QAH map could also identify routes of CSF introduction or spread, mediated by wild boar, through vegetation or travel corridors. Travel corridors are either unbroken vegetation corridors or patches of habitat that enable animals to travel securely from one habitat to another [36]. These patches of habitat and vegetation corridors could be used as strategic points of vaccination where oral baits could be placed. In Gifu Prefecture, the vegetation is composed mainly of broadleaved evergreen and broadleaved deciduous forests, which provide suitable habitat for wild boar [38,39]. Given that the composition of the vegetation in Gifu Prefecture is common throughout Japan, it is likely that the disease could spread similarly to other prefectures.

It should be noted that vegetation types and wild boar behavior could vary among geographical features. For example, mountains usually have gentle slopes in Germany, whereas Japanese mountains tend to have precipitous slopes [40]. These topographical differences may require different approaches for control of wild boar populations.

Almost one year has passed since the first notification of the CSF outbreak in Japan, and the spread of the disease has been confirmed mainly in wild boar. Fortunately, CSF outbreaks on domestic pig farms have been limited. Nevertheless, the potential risk of CSF introduction on farms could be high due to limited biosecurity, high number of wild boar cases in the area, and difficulties in implementing disease control measures in wildlife [13]. The results from this study provide information on the current epidemic, which may help improve current approaches for controlling CSF in Japan. Information on the direction and distance of disease spread could help with the implementation of control measures by modifying the area for control and surveillance zones or identifying specific locations for increasing efforts of oral immunization.

Given the potential risk of the ASF introduction from neighboring countries, we should summarize and disseminate the lessons learned from the current CSF outbreak to achieve the protection of ASF invasion or rapid containment of its occurrence even if it occurred.

4. Material and Methods

4.1. Data and Data Sources

Epidemiological data for the periods from 9 September 2018 to 25 June 2019 were provided by the Gifu Prefectural Government, which provided the dates and coordinates (latitude and longitude) of the notifications of CSF in domestic pigs and wild boar. A total of 743 CSF notifications, 16 outbreaks on domestic pig farms, and 727 cases in wild boar were confirmed by RT-PCR and/or ELISA tests in the laboratory [13]. As we focused on local transmission of CSFV, notifications of CSF in slaughterhouses or in facilities through which CSF-affected pigs had been transported were removed from the current study. Notifications of CSF in wild boar reported on the same day and location were regarded as one case.

4.2. Standard Deviational Ellipse Analysis

Standard deviational ellipse (SDE) analysis is a tool that provides the orientation and shape of a distribution, as well as its location, and dispersion or concentration of the data [41]. It requires a single point that is used to define the standard deviational ellipse. The analysis was conducted to describe the trend and spatial characteristics of CSF notifications in the study area in ArcGIS 10.6.1 software (ESRI Inc., Redlands, CA, USA) following an approach similar to Fonseca et al. and Lu et al. [42,43]. The ratio (R) of the long and short axes was used to identify the degree of clustering (R > 1) or dispersion (R = 1) [42,43]. To analyze temporal changes of CSF notifications, the study period was divided into three stages—(i) September to December 2018 (four months), (ii) January to March 2019 (three months), and (iii) April to June 2019 (three months).

4.3. Multi-Distance Spatial Cluster Analysis

A multi-distance spatial cluster analysis tool in ArcGIS software version 10.6.1 was used to identify the maximum distance of the relationships between CSF notifications according to the guide on the manufacture's website [44]. In brief, the tool uses a common transformation of Ripley's k function, wherein the expected result with a random set of events is equal to the input distance. The transformation L(d) is given by the following formula:

$$L(d) = \sqrt{\frac{A\sum_{i=1}^{N}\sum_{j=1,j\neq1}^{N}k(i,j)}{\pi N(N-1)}}$$

where A is the area, N is the number of events, d is the distance, and $k(i,j)$ is the weight, in which it is 1 when the distance between i and j is less than or equal to d and it is 0 when the distance between i and j is greater than d. To analyze the spatial pattern of CSF notifications, Observed K values were compared to the Expected K values of a completely random spatial distribution of CSF notifications with 999 simulations, which is equal to confidence levels of 99.9%.

The Diff K values contain the Observed K values minus the Expected K values. In the present analysis, the Expected K values that yield the highest Diff K values were applied as the maximum distance for relationships between notifications of CSF outbreaks in Gifu Prefecture.

4.4. Kernel Density Estimation Analysis

Kernel density estimation is a non-parametric estimator for describing the spatial extent of a series of events [45]. In the current study, the kernel density tool was applied to explore the influence of the CSF notifications in the study area by calculating the density of CSF notifications in ArcGIS 10.6.1. A radius of 23 km based on results obtained from Ripley's k function, was applied as the maximum distance for significant spatial association between CSF notifications. Kernel density estimation was divided into five categories according to the equal interval method.

4.5. Space-Time Cluster Analysis

A space-time permutation technique was applied to examine the presence of space-time clusters in Gifu Prefecture. The upper limit on the geographical size of the cluster was set as 23 km, the minimum time aggregation as seven days, and the maximum temporal cluster size as 50% of the total study period (default setting) [32]. A Monte Carlo process was implemented using 999 replications to test for the presence of candidate clusters ($P < 0.05$). Analyses were conducted in SaTScan software v9.6 (Kulldorff, Boston, MA, USA) [46].

4.6. QAH Within Space-Time Cluster Area

CSF notifications within significant space-time clusters were overlaid on a QAH map to characterize land cover vegetation in areas of disease aggregation. The QAH map developed by Bosch et al. [36] is a cartographic tool previously suggested as a potential tool for managing African swine fever. Briefly, it is a standardized distribution map based on global land cover vegetation (GLOBCOVER) that quantifies QAH for wild boar [47]. The QAH map provides seven levels of QAH, namely (i) 0, "absent"; (ii) 0.1, "unsuitable"; (iii) 0.5, "worst suitable area"; (iv) 1, "suitable areas for food or shelter"; (v) 1.5, "suitable areas for food and shelter, but used mainly for one or the other"; (vi) 1.75, "suitable areas for food and shelter, but mainly used for food"; and (vii) 2, "suitable areas for both food and shelter." In addition, the QAH map also differentiates between landscapes such as natural (mainly QAHs 2 and 1.5) and agricultural landscapes (QAHs 1.75 and 1), among others.

Author Contributions: Conceptualization, M.I., J.M.S.-V., and Y.S.; Methodology, S.I., C.J., and J.B.; Validation, S.I., C.J., J.B., and J.M.S.-V.; Formal Analysis, S.I., C.J., and J.B.; Data Curation, M.I., and Y.S.; Writing—Original Draft Preparation, S.I., and N.I.; Writing—Review and Editing, S.I., C.J., J.B., M.I., J.M.S.-V., and Y.S.; Supervision, M.I., J.M.S.-V., and Y.S.

Acknowledgments: We appreciate Gifu Prefectural Government cooperation in epidemiological data provision for the CSF outbreaks in Gifu Prefecture. C.J. is the recipient of a Spanish Government-funded PhD fellowship for the Training of Future Scholars (FPU) given by the Spanish Ministry of Education, Culture and Sports.

References

1. Edwards, S.; Fukusho, A.; Lefevre, P.C.; Lipowski, A.; Pejsak, Z.; Roehe, P.; Westergaard, J. Classical swine fever: The global situation. *Vet. Microbiol.* **2000**, *73*, 103–119. [CrossRef]
2. Lindenbach, B.D.; Murray, C.L.; Thiel, H.J.; Rice, C.M. *Fields Virology*, 6th ed.; Knipe, D.M., Howley, P.M., Eds.; Wolters Kluwer/Lippincott Williams & Wikins Health: Philadelphia, PA, USA, 2013.
3. OIE. World Animal Health Information System. Available online: http://www.oie.int/wahis_2/public/wahid.php/Diseaseinformation/Diseasetimelines (accessed on 7 September 2019).
4. Lowings, P.; Ibata, G.; Needham, J.; Paton, D. Classical swine fever virus diversity and evolution. *J. Gen. Virol.* **1996**, *77*, 1311–1321. [CrossRef] [PubMed]
5. Paton, D.J.; McGoldrick, A.; Greiser-Wilke, I.; Parchariyanon, S.; Song, J.Y.; Liou, P.P.; Stadejek, T.; Lowings, J.P.; Bjorklund, H.; Belak, S. Genetic typing of classical swine fever virus. *Vet. Microbiol.* **2000**, *73*, 137–157. [CrossRef]
6. Kameyama, K.I.; Nishi, T.; Yamada, M.; Masujin, K.; Morioka, K.; Kokuho, T.; Fukai, K. Experimental infection of pigs with a classical swine fever virus isolated in Japan for the first time in 26 years. *J. Veter Med. Sci.* **2019**, *81*, 1277–1284. [CrossRef] [PubMed]
7. Mittelholzer, C.; Moser, C.; Tratschin, J.D.; Hofmann, M.A. Analysis of classical swine fever virus replication kinetics allows differentiation of highly virulent from avirulent strains. *Vet. Microbiol.* **2000**, *74*, 293–308. [CrossRef]
8. Enkhbold, B.; Shatar, M.; Wakamori, S.; Tamura, T.; Hiono, T.; Matsuno, K.; Okamatsu, M.; Umemura, T.; Damdinjav, B.; Sakoda, Y. Genetic and virulence characterization of classical swine fever viruses isolated in Mongolia from 2007 to 2015. *Virus Genes* **2017**, *53*, 418–425. [CrossRef]

9.   Lim, S.I.; Kim, Y.K.; Lim, J.A.; Han, S.H.; Hyun, H.S.; Kim, K.S.; Hyun, B.H.; Kim, J.J.; Cho, I.S.; Song, J.Y.; et al. Antigenic characterization of classical swine fever virus YC11WB isolates from wild boar. *J. Vet. Sci.* **2017**, *18*, 201–207. [CrossRef]

10. Luo, Y.; Ji, S.; Liu, Y.; Lei, J.L.; Xia, S.L.; Wang, Y.; Du, M.L.; Shao, L.; Meng, X.Y.; Zhou, M.; et al. Isolation and Characterization of a Moderately Virulent Classical Swine Fever Virus Emerging in China. *Transbound. Emerg. Dis.* **2017**, *64*, 1848–1857. [CrossRef]

11. Postel, A.; Nishi, T.; Kameyama, K.I.; Meyer, D.; Suckstorff, O.; Fukai, K.; Becher, P. Reemergence of Classical Swine Fever, Japan, 2018. *Emerg. Infect. Dis.* **2019**, *25*, 1228–1231. [CrossRef]

12. Ministry of Agriculture, Forestry and Fisheries, Japan (MAFF). Update of Classical Swine Fever in Japan. Available online: http://www.maff.go.jp/j/syouan/douei/csf/index.html (accessed on 8 August 2019).

13. Ministry of Agriculture, Forestry and Fisheries, Japan (MAFF). *MId-Term Report: Epidemiological Investigation for Classical Swine Fever*; MAFF: Tokyo, Japan, 2019. (In Japanese)

14. Aoki, H.; Ishikawa, K.; Sakoda, Y.; Sekiguchi, H.; Kodama, M.; Suzuki, S.; Fukusho, A. Characterization of classical swine fever virus associated with defective interfering particles containing a cytopathogenic subgenomic RNA isolated from wild boar. *J. Vet. Med. Sci.* **2001**, *63*, 751–758. [CrossRef]

15. Bartak, P.; Greiser-Wilke, I. Genetic typing of classical swine fever virus isolates from the territory of the Czech Republic. *Vet. Microbiol.* **2000**, *77*, 59–70. [CrossRef]

16. David, D.; Edri, N.; Yakobson, B.A.; Bombarov, V.; King, R.; Davidson, I.; Pozzi, P.; Hadani, Y.; Bellaiche, M.; Schmeiser, S.; et al. Emergence of classical swine fever virus in Israel in 2009. *Vet. J.* **2011**, *190*, e146–e149. [CrossRef] [PubMed]

17. Fritzemeier, J.; Teuffert, J.; Greiser-Wilke, I.; Staubach, C.; Schluter, H.; Moennig, V. Epidemiology of classical swine fever in Germany in the 1990s. *Vet. Microbiol.* **2000**, *77*, 29–41. [CrossRef]

18. Jemersic, L.; Greiser-Wilke, I.; Barlic-Maganja, D.; Lojkic, M.; Madic, J.; Terzic, S.; Grom, J. Genetic typing of recent classical swine fever virus isolates from Croatia. *Vet. Microbiol.* **2003**, *96*, 25–33. [CrossRef]

19. Kim, Y.K.; Lim, S.I.; Kim, J.J.; Cho, Y.Y.; Song, J.Y.; Cho, I.S.; Hyun, B.H.; Choi, S.H.; Kim, S.H.; Park, E.H.; et al. Surveillance of classical swine fever in wild boar in South Korea from 2010-2014. *J. Vet. Med. Sci.* **2016**, *77*, 1667–1671. [CrossRef]

20. Pol, F.; Rossi, S.; Mesplede, A.; Kuntz-Simon, G.; Le Potier, M.F. Two outbreaks of classical swine fever in wild boar in France. *Vet. Rec.* **2008**, *162*, 811–816. [CrossRef]

21. Rajkhowa, T.K.; Hauhnar, L.; Lalrohlua, I.; Mohanarao, G.J. Emergence of 2.1. subgenotype of classical swine fever virus in pig population of India in 2011. *Vet. Q.* **2014**, *34*, 224–228. [CrossRef]

22. Schnyder, M.; Stark, K.D.; Vanzetti, T.; Salman, M.D.; Thor, B.; Schleiss, W.; Griot, C. Epidemiology and control of an outbreak of classical swine fever in wild boar in Switzerland. *Vet. Rec.* **2002**, *150*, 102–109. [CrossRef]

23. Zanardi, G.; Macchi, C.; Sacchi, C.; Rutili, D. Classical swine fever in wild boar in the Lombardy region of Italy from 1997 to 2002. *Vet. Rec.* **2003**, *152*, 461–465. [CrossRef]

24. Zhang, H.; Leng, C.; Feng, L.; Zhai, H.; Chen, J.; Liu, C.; Bai, Y.; Ye, C.; Peng, J.; An, T.; et al. A new subgenotype 2.1d isolates of classical swine fever virus in China, 2014. *Infect. Genet. Evol.* **2015**, *34*, 94–105. [CrossRef]

25. Moennig, V. The control of classical swine fever in wild boar. *Front. Microbiol.* **2015**, *6*, 1211. [CrossRef]

26. Rossi, S.; Fromont, E.; Pontier, D.; Cruciere, C.; Hars, J.; Barrat, J.; Pacholek, X.; Artois, M. Incidence and persistence of classical swine fever in free-ranging wild boar (Sus scrofa). *Epidemiol. Infect.* **2005**, *133*, 559–568. [CrossRef] [PubMed]

27. National Land Information DIvision, National Spatial Planning and Regional Policy Bureau, Ministry of Land, Infrastructure, Transport and Tourism, Japan. National Land Numerical Information Download Service. Available online: http://nlftp.mlit.go.jp/ksj/index.html (accessed on 21 August 2019).

28. Muroga, N.; Hayama, Y.; Yamamoto, T.; Kurogi, A.; Tsuda, T.; Tsutsui, T. The 2010 foot-and-mouth disease epidemic in Japan. *J. Vet. Med. Sci.* **2012**, *74*, 399–404. [CrossRef] [PubMed]

29. Tokida, K.; Maruyama, N. *Factor Affecting the Geographical Distribution of Japanese Wild Boars*; Japan Wildlife Research Center: Tokyo, Japan, 1980.

30. Takao, Y. *Wild Boars and the Protection of Farm Crops at the Foot of Mt. Hakusan in Gifu Prefecture, Japan*; Hakusan Nature Conservation Center: Kanazawa, Japan, 1997; pp. 57–66. (In Japanese)

31. Iglesias, I.; Munoz, M.J.; Montes, F.; Perez, A.; Gogin, A.; Kolbasov, D.; de la Torre, A. Reproductive Ratio for the Local Spread of African Swine Fever in Wild Boars in the Russian Federation. *Transbound. Emerg. Dis.* **2016**, *63*, e237–e245. [CrossRef] [PubMed]

32. Iglesias, I.; Rodriguez, A.; Feliziani, F.; Rolesu, S.; de la Torre, A. Spatio-temporal Analysis of African Swine Fever in Sardinia (2012–2014): Trends in Domestic Pigs and Wild Boar. *Transbound. Emerg. Dis.* **2017**, *64*, 656–662. [CrossRef]

33. Mur, L.; Atzeni, M.; Martinez-Lopez, B.; Feliziani, F.; Rolesu, S.; Sanchez-Vizcaino, J.M. Thirty-Five-Year Presence of African Swine Fever in Sardinia: History, Evolution and Risk Factors for Disease Maintenance. *Transbound. Emerg. Dis.* **2016**, *63*, e165–e177. [CrossRef]

34. Anonymous. Control and eradication of Classical Swine Fever in wild boar. *EFSA J.* **2009**, *932*, 1–18.

35. Artois, M.; Depner, K.R.; Guberti, V.; Hars, J.; Rossi, S.; Rutili, D. Classical swine fever (hog cholera) in wild boar in Europe. *Revue Scientifique Et Technique* **2002**, *21*, 287–303. [CrossRef]

36. Bosch, J.; Iglesias, I.; Munoz, M.J.; de la Torre, A. A Cartographic Tool for Managing African Swine Fever in Eurasia: Mapping Wild Boar Distribution Based on the Quality of Available Habitats. *Transbound. Emerg. Dis.* **2017**, *64*, 1720–1733. [CrossRef]

37. De la Torre, A.; Bosch, J.; Iglesias, I.; Munoz, M.J.; Mur, L.; Martinez-Lopez, B.; Martinez, M.; Sanchez-Vizcaino, J.M. Assessing the Risk of African Swine Fever Introduction into the European Union by Wild Boar. *Transbound. Emerg. Dis.* **2015**, *62*, 272–279. [CrossRef]

38. Ministry of Environment, Japan. Guideline for Developing the Specified Wildlife Conservation and Management Plan; Wild Boar. Available online: https://www.env.go.jp/nature/choju/plan/plan3-2a/index.html (accessed on 7 September 2019).

39. Gifu Prefecture. Nature Conservation. Available online: https://www.pref.gifu.lg.jp/kurashi/kankyo/shizenhogo/ (accessed on 7 September 2019). (In Japanese).

40. Geospatial Information Authority of Japan. World Topography (In Japanese). Available online: https://www.gsi.go.jp/CHIRIKYOUIKU/world_landform.html (accessed on 16 October 2019).

41. Yuill, R.S. The Standard Deviational Ellipse; An Updated Tool for Spatial Description. *Geogr. Ann. Ser. B* **1971**, *53*, 28–39. [CrossRef]

42. Fonseca, O.; Coronado, L.; Amaran, L.; Perera, C.L.; Centelles, Y.; Montano, D.N.; Alfonso, P.; Fernandex, O.; Santoro, K.R.; Frias-Lepoureau, M.T.; et al. Descriptive epidemiology of endemic Classical Swine Fever in Cuba. *Span. J. Agric. Res.* **2018**, *16*, e0506. [CrossRef]

43. Lu, Y.; Deng, X.J.; Chen, J.H.; Wang, J.Y.; Chen, Q.; Niu, B. Risk analysis of African swine fever in Poland based on spatio-temporal pattern and Latin hypercube sampling, 2014–2017. *BMC Vet. Res.* **2019**, *15*, 160. [CrossRef] [PubMed]

44. Environmental Systems Resaerch Institute. Multi-Distance Spatial Cluster Analysis (Ripey's K Function). Available online: https://pro.arcgis.com/en/pro-app/tool-reference/spatial-statistics/multi-distance-spatial-cluster-analysis.htm (accessed on 20 August 2019).

45. Bishop, C.M. *Pattern Recognition and Machine Learning*; Springer: New York, NY, USA, 2006.

46. Kulldorff, M.; Heffman, R.; Hartman, J.; Assuncao, R.; Mostashari, F. A space-time permutation scan statistic for disease outbreak detection. *PLoS Med.* **2005**, *2*, e59. [CrossRef] [PubMed]

47. Arino, O.; Ramos Perez, J.J.; Kalogirou, V.; Bontemps, S.; Defourny, P.; Van Bogaert, V. Global Land Cover Map for 2009 (GlobCover 2009). ESA UCL 2012. Available online: http://due.esrin.esa.int/page_globcover.php (accessed on 16 October 2019). [CrossRef]

Recent Advances in the Diagnosis of Classical Swine Fever and Future Perspectives

Lihua Wang [1,*]**, Rachel Madera** [1]**, Yuzhen Li** [1]**, David Scott McVey** [2]**, Barbara S. Drolet** [2] **and Jishu Shi** [1,*]

[1]   Department of Anatomy and Physiology, College of Veterinary Medicine, Kansas State University, Manhattan, KS 66506, USA; rachelmadera@vet.k-state.edu (R.M.); yuzhen@vet.k-state.edu (Y.L.)

[2]   United States Department of Agriculture, Arthropod-Borne Animal Diseases Research Unit, Center for Grain and Animal Health Research, Manhattan, KS 66502, USA; scott.mcvey@usda.gov (D.S.M.); barbara.drolet@usda.gov (B.S.D.)

*   Correspondence: lihua@vet.k-state.edu (L.W.); jshi@ksu.edu (J.S.)

Abstract: Classical swine fever (CSF) is a highly contagious viral disease of pigs, including wild boar. It is regarded as one of the major problems in the pig industry as it is still endemic in many regions of the world and has the potential to cause devastating epidemics, particularly in countries free of the disease. Rapid and reliable diagnosis is of utmost importance in the control of CSF. Since clinical presentations of CSF are highly variable and may be confused with other viral diseases in pigs, laboratory diagnosis is indispensable for an unambiguous diagnosis. On an international level, well-established diagnostic tests of CSF such as virus isolation, fluorescent antibody test (FAT), antigen capture antibody enzyme-linked immunosorbent assay (ELISA), reverse-transcription polymerase chain reaction (RT-PCR), virus neutralization test (VNT), and antibody ELISA have been described in detail in the OIE Terrestrial Manual. However, improved CSF diagnostic methods or alternatives based on modern technologies have been developed in recent years. This review thus presents recent advances in the diagnosis of CSF and future perspectives.

Keywords: classical swine fever; laboratory diagnosis; technologies; future perspectives

1. Introduction

Classical swine fever (CSF), a list-A disease classified by the World Organization for Animal Health (OIE), is considered as a transboundary animal disease by the Food and Agriculture Organization of the United Nations (FAO) [1]. The disease causes high morbidity and mortality in both feral and domestic pigs and can result in significant economic losses to the swine industry worldwide [2]. Currently, it is present in many countries in Asia, the Caribbean islands, Africa, and South and Central America (Figure 1). It is most likely to be introduced to CSF-free countries through inadvertent or deliberate importation of classical swine fever virus (CSFV) infected animals, animal products, and animal feed [2,3].

Classical swine fever virus (CSFV) is the etiologic agent of CSF and belongs to the genus *Pestivirus* in the *Flaviviridae* family [4]. The genome of CSFV is a positive single-strand RNA of about 12.3 kb. It contains untranslated regions at 5′ and 3′ ends and a single large open reading frame (ORF). The ORF codes four structural (C, E^{rns}, E1, and E2) and eight nonstructural viral proteins (N^{pro}, p7, NS2, NS3, NS4A, NS4B, NS5A, and NS5B) [5,6]. Based on the nucleotide sequences of 5′-non-translated region (5′-NTR) and glycoprotein E2, CSFVs are divided into three genotypes and 11 sub-genotypes (1.1–1.4, 2.1–2.3, and 3.1–3.4) [7–9]. As reported, CSFV genotype 2.1 and genotype 2.3 caused the more recent outbreaks in Europe [10]. Sub-genotypes 1.1, 2.1, 2.2, and 2.3 are prevalent in Asia [11], while sub-genotypes 3.1-3.4 are distributed in other separated geographic regions [1,12–14].

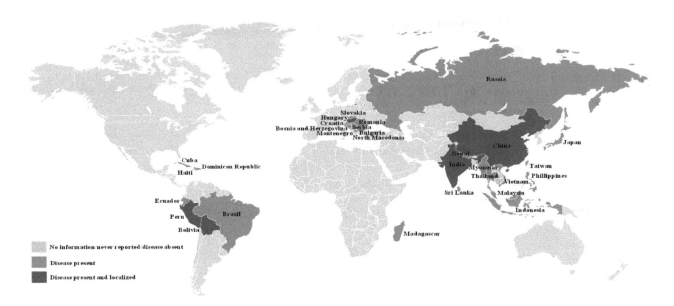

Figure1. Global distribution of classical swine fever (CSF) epidemics, 2020. Map based on data from CABI Invasive Species Compendium. Wallingford, UK: CAB International. In addition, we also incorporated the most current CSF epidemic information (disease present in Japan and Romania) from OIE, 2020. Names of countries with CSF are given in the map.

Traditional diagnostics for CSF include clinical signs, pathological findings, and antigen and antibody detection [15]. Although unique clinical and pathological observations such as "button" ulcers in the cecum and large intestine mucosa may be found exclusively in CSF, other clinical signs and pathological findings in pigs infected with CSFV are highly variable and are often similar to that of other viral diseases of pigs, such as African swine fever, pseudorabies, porcine dermatitis, and nephropathy syndrome (PDNS), post-weaning multisystemic wasting syndrome (PMWS), thrombocytopenic purpura, and various septicemic conditions [16]. Thus, laboratory diagnosis of CSF for detection of the specific CSFV antigen and antibody is indispensable [15,16]. The well-established diagnostic methods of CSF such as virus isolation, fluorescent antibody test (FAT), antigen capture antibody enzyme-linked immunosorbent assay (ELISA), reverse-transcription polymerase chain reaction (RT-PCR), virus neutralization test (VNT), and antibody ELISA (Table 1) have been widely used and well described in the OIE Terrestrial Manual [17]. Recently developed techniques and alternatives have made significant improvements in several key components of CSF diagnosis, including less sample and reagents required, less effort and time needed, increased detection efficiency (multiplexing), ease of performing and disposal, automation, and point of care (POC). This review provides an updated overview on laboratory diagnosis of CSF and future perspectives.

Table 1. Well-established CSF diagnostic methods and their application.

Method	Application	Advantages	Disadvantages
Virus Isolation	Confirmation of clinical cases; Making virus collections; May be used for individual animal freedom from infection prior to movement	"reference standard"; Very sensitive; Indicates active infection	Work intensive and time consuming; Requires specialized microscope and expertise
FAT [1]	Confirmation of clinical cases	Quick and direct visualization of antigens in tissue	Requires specialized equipment, expertise, and confirmatory test
Antigen-capture ELISA [2]	Population infection-free status; May be used for confirmation of clinical cases	Fast, does not require specialized equipment and suitable for herd screening	Low sensitivity; Cross-reactivity with other Pestiviruses
RT-PCR [3]	Confirmation of clinical cases; Prevalence of infection surveillance; May be used for population or individual animal freedom from infection prior to movement	Fast, sensitive, and specific	Specialized equipment; Possibility for false negative results due to sample degradation
VNT [4]	Individual animal infection-free status prior to movement; Prevalence of infection-surveillance; Immune status in individual animals or populations post-vaccination; Confirmation of clinical cases; May be used for population freedom from infection	Gold standard for sensitivity and specificity	Work intensive and time consuming; Requires specialized microscope and expertise
Antibody ELISA	Population freedom from infection; Individual animal freedom from infection prior to movement; Prevalence of infection-surveillance; Immune status in individual animals or populations post-vaccination	Fast, does not require specialized equipment and suitable for herd screening	Cross-reactivity with other Pestiviruses

Note: Table adapted from Table 1 in 2019 OIE Terrestrial Manual [17]; [1] Fluorescent antibody test; [2] Enzyme-linked immunosorbent assay; [3] Reverse-transcription polymerase chain reaction; [4] Virus neutralization test.

2. Antigen Detection

2.1. Virus Isolation

Virus isolation in cell culture is the oldest laboratory technique for detecting CSFV. Porcine kidney cell lines (PK-15 and SK-6) are often used for isolation of CSFV [17]. However, the use of other porcine cells including swine primary cells (pulmonary alveolar macrophages and peripheral blood mononuclear cells) may enhance the chances of obtaining different CSFVs with different growth characteristics. Since CSFV does not cause a cytopathic effect (CPE), the growth of CSFV in the cells is usually visualized by using immunological technologies with fluorescent or horseradish peroxidase (HRF)-conjugated antibodies [17–19].

The cell culture, virus propagation, and staining are labor intensive and time-consuming (weeks). In addition, skilled and experienced personnel and adequate facilities are needed for cell culture, handling CSFVs and accurate interpretation of the CPE. These disadvantages make virus isolation less attractive for mass surveillance or rapid diagnosis. However, virus isolation is still considered the "gold standard" for confirming CSF clinical cases and the only method for making virus collections (Table 1).

2.2. Fluorescence Antibody Test (FAT)

FAT is the commonly used staining method for CSFV detection. It utilizes fluorescein isothiocyanate (FITC) labeled antibodies to detect CSFV proteins in the slices of cryostat (frozen) tissues or fixed cells.

Anti-CSFV gamma-globulins prepared from specific pathogen-free pigs are recommended to be used. These globulins can ensure that most variant CSFVs will be captured. The differentiation of CSFV from other *pestiviruses* in FAT positive samples, especially bovine viral diarrhea virus (BVDV) and border disease virus (BDV), can be done using RT-PCR with genetic typing or virus isolation in cell culture with specific monoclonal antibody (mAb) typing [17,19].

The main advantages of FAT are that it is relatively easy and rapid to perform and allows direct visualization of the CSFVs in stained tissues. Therefore, it is useful for a first laboratory investigation in suspected clinical cases (Table 1). Several FITC conjugated anti-CSFV antibodies (polyclonal or monoclonal) for FAT are commercially available for research purposes, such as those from Creative Diagnostics, Bioss Inc., Biorbyt LLC, and so on. However, FAT requires highly specialized equipment (i.e., fluorescent microscope) and immunohistochemical staining expertise. It is only recommended to be used in laboratories that have the expertise of performing this technique.

The novel ViewRNA in situ hybridization method can detect CSFV RNA directly in infected cells [20]. Using RNA in an in situ hybridization method and specific probes of CSFV RNA, the relative location of CSFV RNA can be visualized in PK15 cells. The sensitivity of this method was three to four orders of magnitude higher than that of FAT. The specificity experiment showed that it was highly specific for CSFV (sub-genotypes 1.1, 2.1, 2.2, and 2.3) and without cross-reaction with other *pestiviruses* including BVDV, porcine parvovirus (PPV), porcine pseudorabies virus (PRV), and porcine circovirus II (PCV-2). This assay has the potential to be used for testing for CSFV in cells. However, it remains to be determined whether this method can be used to detect CSFV in swine tissues and it is still expensive and is not commercially available yet.

2.3. Antigen-Capture ELISA

Antigen-capture ELISA uses anti-CSFV antibodies on an ELISA plate to capture the CSFV proteins [21]. It has been developed for the rapid screening of large numbers of pigs with clinical suspicion of CSFV infection [15,17,21–23]. Commercial antigen-capture ELISA kits are available from several commercial vendors including IDEXX Laboratories, Thermo Fisher Scientific, MEDIAN Diagnostics, and so on. These kits are double-antibody-sandwich (DAS)-based ELISA for detecting CSFV E2 or E^{rns} protein in serum, blood, plasma, or tissue extracts (Table 2).

Antigen-capture ELISA is fast (provides results within 4 h), easy to perform, and does not require specialized equipment. It can be applied at a herd level for confirmation of clinical cases or determining infection-free population status (Table 1). However, its sensitivity and specificity are lower than most of the other diagnostics, especially the real-time RT-PCR. It is not recommended for testing individual animals and has been increasingly discouraged in recent years.

Table 2. List of representatives of commercially available CSF antigen-capture ELISA kits/reagents.

Name	Producer	Test Principle	Suitable Sample Materials	DIVA Potential	Web Site
IDEXX CSFV Ag Serum Plus	IDEXX Laboratories, Inc.	DAS ELISA test E^{rns}	Serum, plasma, tissue	Yes	https://www.idexx.com/en/livestock/livestock-tests/swine-tests/idexx-csfv-ag-serum-plus-test/
PrioCHECK™ CSFV Antigen ELISA kit	Thermo Fisher Scientific, Inc.	DAS ELISA test E2	Serum, blood, plasma, leukocyte concentrate, tissue extract	No	https://www.thermofisher.com/order/catalog/product/7610047?SID=srch-srp-7610047#/7610047?SID=srch-srp-7610047
VDPro®CSFV AG ELISA	MEDIAN Diagnostics Inc.	DAS ELISA test E2	Cell cultures, leukocyte concentrate, tissue extract	No	http://www.mediandiagnostics.com/eng/es-csf-02.php

Note: DAS, Double-antibody-sandwich; ELISA, enzyme-linked immunosorbent assay; DIVA, differentiate infected from vaccinated animals.

2.4. Real-Time Reverse Transcription Polymerase Chain Reaction (Real-Time RT-PCR)

Real-time RT-PCR has now replaced the traditional RT-PCR and has become an essential tool in the routine diagnosis of CSFV [24–26]. It is a suitable approach for confirmation of clinical cases and prevalence of infection surveillance for CSF (Table 1). Several commercial real-time RT-PCR kits are available for rapid and specific detection of CSFV RNA, including IDEXX RealPCR CSFV RNA Mix, virotype® CSFV RT-PCR Kit, CSFV dtec-RT-qPCR Test, ADIAVET™ CSF REAL TIME, CSFV genesig® Advanced and standard kits, and so on (Table 3). These kits use either SYBR green or TaqMan probe to detect the accumulation of amplicon during the exponential phase of the reaction, which can specifically and sensitively test the CSFV in serum, blood, plasma, viral culture, tissue, or swabs.

The disadvantages of real-time RT-PCR are its high cost and complexity due to simultaneous thermal cycling and fluorescence detection, false positives caused by laboratory contamination from polluted specimens or equipment, and false negatives caused by PCR inhibitors in the sample or degraded RNA [27]. The improved real-time RT-PCRs and advanced alternatives have been designed to help resolve these issues. One-step and automated RT-PCRs can reduce the risk of contamination [27–29]. The primer-probe energy transfer RT-PCR assay provides a higher specificity by analyzing the melting curve following PCR amplification [30,31]. The loop-mediated isothermal amplification (LAMP) assay can accumulate the CSFV amplicon under isothermal conditions [32–34]. The functionalized gold nanoparticles were developed as nanoflare probes for rapid detection of CSFV without nucleic acid amplification [35].

Multiplex real-time RT-PCR as a powerful technique has expanded exponentially in the diagnosis of CSF in recent years. It is quite useful and convenient for quick and accurate detection of different pathogens in mixed infections, which is common in swine production systems. Multiplex RT-PCR assays for rapid detection and genotyping of CSFVs [36,37], simultaneous detection, and differentiation of common swine viruses [38–41] have been developed. Additionally, multiplex combined high-throughput molecular diagnostic platform, user-friendly electronic microarray, magnetoelastic sensor, and microfluidic detection systems were developed as potential alternatives for detection and surveillance of CSFV infection [42–46]. These assays can save considerable time and effort without compromising robustness and sensitivity and can reduce the sample and reagent requirement as well.

Table 3. List of representatives of commercially available CSF Real-time RT-PCR kits/reagents.

Name	Producer	Test Principle	Suitable Sample Materials	Web Site
ADIAVET™ CSF REAL TIME	BioMérieux	Real-time RT-PCR test CSFV RNA	Serum, blood, viral culture, tissue	https://www.biomerieux-nordic.com/csfv-classical-swine-fever
CSFV dtec-RT-qPCR Test	Genetic PCR solutions™	Real-time RT-PCR test CSFV RNA	Serum, plasma, blood, viral culture, tissue	http://www.geneticpcr.com/index.php/en/pathogen-r-d-qpcr/classical-swine-fever-virus
CSFV genesig®Kits	Primerdesign™ Ltd	Real-time RT-PCR test CSFV RNA	Serum, plasma, blood, viral culture, tissue	https://www.genesig.com/products/9770-classical-swine-fever-virus
CSFV Real Time RT-PCR Kit	Creative Biogene	Real-time RT-PCR test CSFV RNA	Serum, plasma, tissue	https://www.creative-biogene.com/Classical-Swine-Fever-Virus-CSFV-Real-Time-RT-PCR-Kit-PDAS-AR002-1290596-88.html
Classical swine fever virus detection kits	Bioingentech Ltd	Real-time RT-PCR test CSFV RNA	Serum, blood, viral culture, tissue	https://www.kitpcr.com/pcr-kit/classical-swine-fever-virus-detection-kits/
IDEXX RealPCR CSFV RNA Mix	IDEXX Laboratories, Inc.	Real-time RT-PCR test CSFV RNA	Serum, plasma, blood, viral culture, tissue	https://www.idexx.com/en/livestock/livestock-tests/swine-tests/realpcr-csfv/
virotype®CSFV RT-PCR Kit	Indical Bioscience, GMBH	Real-time RT-PCR test CSFV RNA	Serum, plasma, blood, viral culture, tissue	https://www.indical.com/products/assays/

Note: RT-PCR, reverse-transcription polymerase chain reaction.

2.5. Next Generation Sequencing (NGS)

Next Generation Sequencing (NGS) is a highly sensitive method for generating sequence data and exploring the genetic characters of infectious agents. It has been extensively applied to metagenomics and whole-genome sequencing of infectious viral diseases of livestock [47,48]. By using NGS, researchers found that there might be a long-term persistence of genotype 2.3 CSFV strains in wild boar in Germany [49]. By analyzing NGS data of CSFV isolates of varying virulence in infected pigs, higher quasispecies diversity and more nucleotide variability were found in viral samples from pigs infected with the highly virulent isolates compared to samples of pigs infected with low and moderately virulent isolates [50]. Evolutionary changes in virus populations following the challenge of naïve and vaccinated pigs with the highly virulent CSFV strain were studied using the NGS technology and this study found that vaccination imposes a strong selective pressure on CSF viruses that subsequently replicate within the vaccinated animals [51].

The complete genome sequences obtained from NGS can provide detailed genetic information for construction of reliable phylogenetic relationships of CSFVs for monitoring the evolution and transmission patterns during field outbreaks or epidemics of CSF. One phylogenetic analysis using 58 CSFV complete genome sequences from different Asian countries indicated that the circulating Indian CSFV strains belong to different branches of the 1.1 sub-genotype [52]. These data combined those obtained from other different diagnostic tests can be used for meta-analysis of CSF prevalence, which is important for the investigation of CSF prevalence in different regions [52].

Currently, most of the NGS platforms are expensive to establish and require highly skilled molecular biologists and bioinformaticians. The implementation of NGS is still a challenge and cannot be used as a routine test for disease diagnosis due to cost and the time required [47,48]. However, with the novel and emerging sequencing technologies, cost-effective, user-friendly, and portable NGS will be developed and will act as an effective tool for CSF control and prevention.

3. Antibody Detection

3.1. Virus Neutralization Test (VNT)

VNT is the gold standard for sensitivity and specificity of antibody detection methods. It can be used for confirmation of clinical cases, prevalence of infection surveillance, evaluation of the immune status post-vaccination, and the efficacy of CSF vaccines (Table 1) [53–55]. However, VNT is a work-intensive and time-consuming procedure that requires cell culture and a high-containment laboratory that can handle infectious CSF virus. In addition, it cannot be automated, thus it is not suitable for mass analysis of samples [14,26,53–55].

More recently, alternatives have been developed to overcome the disadvantages of VNT. A neutralizing mAb-based competitive ELISA (cELISA) with emphasis on the replacement of VNT for C-strain post–vaccination monitoring was developed in our group. The test principle of this cELISA is that the neutralizing mAb can compete with C-strain vaccine induced neutralizing antibodies in pig serum to bind the capture antigen C-strain E2 protein. The established cELISA showed 100% sensitivity (95% confidence interval: 94.87 to 100%) and 100% specificity (95% confidence interval: 100 to 100%) when testing C-strain VNT negative pig sera ($n = 445$) and C-strain VNT positive pig sera ($n = 70$) and showed excellent agreement (Kappa = 0.957) with VNT when testing the pig sera ($n = 139$) in parallel. The inhibition rate of serum samples in the cELISA is highly correlated with their titers in VNT ($r^2 = 0.903$, $p < 0.001$). The C-strain antibody can be tested in pigs as early as 7 days post vaccination with the cELISA. This cELISA is a reliable, rapid, simple, safe, and cost-effective tool for sero-monitoring of C-strain vaccination at a population level [56]. In addition, another group developed a high-throughput VNT by using the recombinant CSFV possessing a small report tag and luciferase system. As reported, the VNT titers of the serum can be determined tentatively at 2 days post-infection (dpi) and are comparable to those obtained by conventional VNTs at 3 or 4 dpi. This system allows CSF virus growth to be easily and rapidly monitored and enabled the rapid and easy determination of the VNT titer using a luminometer, which could be a powerful tool to replace the conventional VNT as a high-throughput antibody test for CSFV infections [57].

3.2. Antibody ELISA

Antibody ELISA is the quickest, easiest, and most widely used technique for serological diagnosis and epidemiological investigation of CSF. It is suitable for herd or individual animal CSFV infection screening, prevalence of infection surveillance, and immune status checking in individual animals or populations post-vaccination (Table 1). The E2 protein is crucial for inducing an immune response in the host following CSFV infection [58]. Detection of E2 antibodies in the serum of animals is an easy and reliable method for monitoring CSFV infection during and after outbreaks and for testing coverage of immunization after vaccination [59–61].

Several commercial CSF antibody ELISA kits are available including those from Biocheck, Boehringer Ingelheim, Cusabio Technology LLC, IDEXX Laboratories, ID VET, Indical Bioscience, iNtRON Biotechnology, Median Diagnostics Inc., Thermo Fisher Scientific, and so on. Most of the commercial kits are indirect, competitive, or blocking ELISAs based on the detection of envelop glycoprotein E2 specific antibodies (Table 4). Limitations of these antibody ELISAs are lower specificity (i.e., cross-reactions with BVDV, BDV, and other *pestiviruses*) and inability to discriminate animals vaccinated with conventional attenuated vaccines or E2-based subunit vaccines.

Table 4. List of representatives of commercially available CSF antibody ELISA kits/reagents.

Name	Producer	Test Principle	Suitable Sample Materials	DIVA Potential	Web Site
BioChek CSFV E2 Antibody ELISA	Biochek	Indirect ELISA test E2 antibodies	Serum	No	https://www.biochek.com/swine-elisa/classical-swine-fever-antibody-test-kit/
Classical Swine Fever Virus Antibody(IgG) ELISA Kit	Cusabio Technology LLC	Indirect ELISA test CSFV antibodies	Serum	No	https://www.cusabio.com/ELISA-Kit/Classical-Swine-Fever-Virus-AntibodyIgG--ELISA-Kit-114911.html
IDEXX CSFV Ab	IDEXX Laboratories, Inc.	Blocking ELISA test CSFV antibodies	Serum, plasma	No	https://www.idexx.com/en/livestock/livestock-tests/swine-tests/idexx-csfv-ab-test/
ID Screen©Classical Swine Fever E2 Competition	ID VET	Competitive ELISA test E2 antibodies	Serum, plasma	No	https://www.id-vet.com/produit/id-screen-classical-swine-fever-e2-competition/
LiliF™ Classical Swine Fever virus Ab rapid test kit	iNtRON Biotechnology, Inc.	Lateral flow immuno-chromatographic assay test CSFV antibodies	Blood	No	https://intronbio.com: 6001/intronbioen/product/product_view.php?PRDT_ID=1891&page=1&Scate1=2&Scate2=2&Scate3=4&Scate4=16&Scate5=1&Scate6=-91-&Sword=
Pigtype CSFV Erns ELISA	Indical Bioscience, GMBH	Double-antigen ELISA test Erns antibodies	Serum, plasma	Yes	https://www.indical.com/products/assays/
PrioCHECK™ Porcine CSFV Ab 2.0 strip kit	Thermo Fisher Scientific, Inc.	Blocking ELISA (E2 antibodies)	Serum, plasma	No	https://www.thermofisher.com/order/catalog/product/7610600?SID=srch-srp-7610600#/7610600?SID=srch-srp-7610600
PrioCHECK™ CSFV Antibody ELISA kit	Thermo Fisher Scientific, Inc.	Blocking ELISA test E2 antibodies	Serum, plasma	No	https://www.thermofisher.com/order/catalog/product/7610046#/7610046
PrioCHECK™ CSFV Erns Antibody ELISA Kit	Thermo Fisher Scientific, Inc.	Blocking ELISA test Erns antibodies	Serum	Yes	https://www.thermofisher.com/order/catalog/product/7610370#/7610370
SVANOVIR®CSFV-Ab	Boehringer Ingelheim	Indirect ELISA test E2 antibodies	Serum	No	https://www.svanova.com/products/porcine/pp031.html
VDPro®CSFV AB C-ELISA	Median Diagnostics Inc.	Blocking ELISA test E2 antibodies	Serum	No	http://www.mediandiagnostics.com/eng/es-csf-02.php
VDPro® CSFV Erns Ab b-ELISA	Median Diagnostics Inc.	Blocking ELISA test Erns antibodies	Serum	Yes	http://www.mediandiagnostics.com/eng/es-csf-02.php
Classical Swine Fever Virus Antibodies Rapid Test Kit	Antibodies-online Inc	Sandwich GICA test CSFV antibodies	Blood, serum	No	https://www.antibodies-online.com/kit/5708730/Classical+Swine+Fever+Virus+Antibodies+Rapid+Test+Kit/

Note: GICA, Gold Immunochromatography Assay; ELISA, enzyme-linked immunosorbent assay.

4. Differentiation of Infected from Vaccinated Animals (DIVA) Diagnostic Methods

4.1. Genetic DIVA

The rationale of genetic DIVA (differentiation of infected from vaccinated animals) is the identification of genetic differences between vaccine strains and wild-type CSFVs. Both traditional RT-PCR and real-time RT-PCR (single-plex or multiplex)-based CSF genetic DIVA systems have been developed and evaluated [62–69]. Multiplex nested RT-PCR and real-time RT-PCR assays have been developed for differential detection of wild-type virus from C-strain vaccine [62–68]. A one-step RT-PCR using TaqMan minor-groove-binding (MGB) probes was developed to distinguish between attenuated Korean LOM and wild-type strains of CSFV in Korea [69]. A simple RT-PCR based on the T-rich insertions in CSFV genome was developed for rapid differentiation of wild-type and at least three attenuated lapinized vaccine strains [70]. The modified genotype 1.1 (including C-strain) real-time RT-PCR assay with a real-time RT-PCR assay that detects all known CSFV strains has been successfully used to distinguish C-strain vaccine from the circulating field strains that do not belong to genotype 1 [71].

The genetic DIVA approach facilitates a rapid and reliable differentiation of field virus infected from live attenuated virus vaccinated domestic pigs and wild boars. It is especially useful for detection of the infected animals that are incompletely protected by vaccination and will play a critical role for making decisions prior to and during cessation of a control strategy that employs vaccination with CSF live vaccines.

4.2. Serological DIVA

The ideal serological DIVA test has the ability to discriminate antibodies induced by CSFV infection from the vaccine-derived antibodies, so it can rule out CSFV infected pigs from vaccinated pigs [72]. This can be obtained by detection of specific antibodies against antigens or epitopes that are modified or lacking in a subunit or marker vaccine. It has been shown that antibodies to E^{rns} can be used as an indicator of CSFV infection in pigs and the E^{rns}-based ELISA can be used as a companion diagnostic test to identify CSFV-infected pigs vaccinated with the E2-based subunit or marker vaccines [73–76]. Currently, two E^{rns} ELISAs are commercially available and have been evaluated as accompanying DIVA diagnostic tools for E2 subunit vaccines, CP7_E2alf, or similar chimeric vaccines. One is prioCHECK CSFV E^{rns} (Thermo Fisher Scientific, Waltham, MA, USA); the other is pigtype CSFV E^{rns} Ab (Indical Bioscience, GMBH, Leipzig, Germany) (Table 4). Published data on their evaluations showed that prioCHECK CSFV E^{rns} has a sensitivity of 90–98% with sera from CSFV infected domestic pigs and a specificity of 89–96% with sera from vaccinated domestic pigs [77]. In combination with the marker vaccine "CP7_E2alf", pigtype CSFV E^{rns} Ab has a sensitivity of 90.2% and a specificity of 93.8% [78]. However, cross-reactivity with antibodies against other *pestiviruses* was observed for these two E^{rns} ELISAs [77,78]. Depending on the represented data, these two E^{rns} ELISAs are recommended to be used on a herd basis and not for diagnostic analysis on samples of single animals.

Additional approaches or alternatives are undergoing development or further optimization. These include the multiplex microsphere immunoassay [79], which is capable of discrimination within epitope-specific antibody populations [80] and the indirect E^{rns} antibody ELISA with *Pichia pastoris*-expressed E^{rns} [81]. Recently, our research group successfully generated a mAb against E^{rns}, which can specifically recognize C-strain, but not react with wild-type CSFVs or other viruses in the genus *Pestivirus*. A cELISA was developed in our group based on the strategy that the C-strain-specific mAb will compete with the C-strain vaccine-induced antibodies in pig serum to bind the capture antigen (C-strain E^{rns}) [unpublished data]. Different from the CSFV neutralizing monoclonal anti-E2 antibody based cELISA for sero-monitoring of C-strain vaccination at a population level [56], this novel anti-E^{rns} mAb-based cELISA is a valuable tool for measuring and differentiating immune responses to C-strain vaccination and/or infection in pigs. The data about the establishment and validation of this C-strain specific cELISA will be published separately at a later date. In brief, suitable tools for serological DIVA are available. However, there is room for improvement, especially with respect to cross-reactivity issues.

5. Point-of-Care (POC) Diagnostics

User-friendly, cost-effective, rapid, and reliable POC diagnostics (i.e., diagnosis of diseases directly on-site) are indispensable tools for immediate decisions of effective and evidence-based disease control strategies [82]. For example, dipstick tests are designed to use thin paper/plastic strips coated with specific antiviral antibodies to detect viral antigens in serum and other body fluids. Lateral flow assays (LFA) and microfluidic devices are two different and yet more complex technologies that are also based on the biochemical interaction of antigen–antibody. The principles for these three immunochromatographic assays are the same as sandwich ELISA and the major difference between them is that the immunological reaction is carried out on different platforms for different assays. POC studies in animal health management are rare compared to human and companion animal medicine. The immunochromatographic assay-based kits including Antigen Rapid Test Kit (Ring Biotechnology Co., Ltd., Beijing, China), LiliF™ CSFV antibody rapid test kit (iNtRON Biotechnology, Inc., Gyeonggi, South Korea), and CSFV Antibodies Rapid Test Kit (Antibodies-online Inc., Limerick, PA, USA) are commercially available for rapid testing of CSFV antigen or antibodies in the field. Laboratory-based assays, including the loop-mediated isothermal amplification, combined with a lateral flow dipstick assay [83], the immunochromatographic strip [84], and duplex lateral flow assay [85] have been investigated as potential CSF POC tools as well.

POC diagnostics showed advantages in rapidity and portability, which are the most important parameters considered by farmers and veterinarians [86]. It is foreseeable that as interests and needs of stakeholders increase and new portable POC technologies emerge, novel and applicable POC diagnostics will be developed for detection, control, and prevention of CSF in the field in the near future.

6. Future Perspectives

Although commercial and in-house diagnostics (antigen detection and antibody detection) of CSF are available, there is still room for improvement. The authors suggest that the following aspects should be considered: (i) Continuously improving the sensitivity, specificity, costs, speed, automation, and POC is necessary; (ii) Reference materials (serum bank, virus bank, and non-infectious molecular standards) should be produced and be accessible for validation of the developed CSF diagnostics; (iii) The development of DIVA diagnostics without cross-reaction with antibodies induced by other *pestiviruses* is critical.

The other emerging infectious diseases, such as the spreading of African swine fever in Asia and the ongoing pandemic of Coronavirus disease 2019 (COVID-19), may shift focus away from the CSF [87,88]. However, as long as CSF exists, it will remain a continuous threat to the pig industry worldwide. Therefore, international cooperation on surveillance and control of CSF becomes even more crucial, both currently and in the future. Researchers should continue to work on developing novel rapid and reliable diagnostics to facilitate the surveillance and control of CSF.

Author Contributions: Conceptualization: J.S., L.W., D.S.M. and B.S.D.; Data curation: L.W., R.M. and Y.L.; Investigation: L.W., R.M. and Y.L.; Supervision: J.S.; Writing–original draft: L.W.; Writing–review & editing: J.S., D.S.M. and B.S.D. All authors have read and agreed to the published version of the manuscript.

References

1.   Blome, S.; Staubach, C.; Henke, J.; Carlson, J.; Beer, M. Classical swine fever-an updated review. *Viruses* **2017**, *9*, 86. [CrossRef]

2. Brown, V.R.; Bevins, S.N. A review of classical swine fever virus and routes of introduction into the United States and the potential for virus establishment. *Front. Vet. Sci.* **2018**, *5*, 31. [CrossRef] [PubMed]

3. CABI. *Invasive Species Compendium*; CAB International: Wallingford, UK, 2020; Available online: www.cabi. org/isc (accessed on 29 May 2020).

4. Schirrmeier, H.; Strebelow, G.; Depner, K.; Hoffmann, B.; Beer, M. Genetic and antigenic characterization of an atypical pestivirus isolate, a putative member of a novel pestivirus species. *J. Gen. Virol.* **2004**, *85*, 3647–3652. [CrossRef] [PubMed]

5. Thiel, H.J.; Stark, R.; Weiland, E.; Rumenapf, T.; Meyers, G. Hog cholera virus: Molecular composition of virions from a pestivirus. *J. Virol.* **1991**, *65*, 4705–4712. [CrossRef] [PubMed]

6. Meyers, G.; Thiel, H.J.; Rümenapf, T. Classical swine fever virus: Recovery of infectious viruses from cDNA constructs and generation of recombinant cytopathogenic defective interfering particles. *J. Virol.* **1996**, *70*, 1588–1595. [CrossRef]

7. Lowings, P.; Ibata, G.; Needham, J.; Paton, D. Classical swine fever virus diversity and evolution. *J. Gen. Virol.* **1996**, *77*, 1311–1321. [CrossRef]

8. Paton, D.J.; Mcgoldrick, A.; Greiser-Wilke, I.; Parchariyanon, S.; Song, J.Y.; Liou, P.P.; Stadejek, T.; Lowings, J.P.; Björklund, H.; Belák, S. Genetic typing of classical swine fever virus. *Vet. Microbiol.* **2000**, *73*, 137–157. [CrossRef]

9. Deng, M.C.; Huang, C.C.; Huang, T.S.; Chang, C.Y.; Lin, Y.J.; Chien, M.S.; Jong, M.H. Phylogenetic analysis of classical swine fever virus isolated from Taiwan. *Vet. Microbiol.* **2005**, *106*, 187–193. [CrossRef]

10. Postel, A.; Moennig, V.; Becher, P. Classical swine fever in Europe-the current situation. *Berl. Munch. Tierarztl. Wochenschr.* **2013**, *126*, 468–475.

11. Postel, A.; Nishi, T.; Kameyama, K.I.; Meyer, D.; Suckstorff, O.; Fukai, K.; Becher, P. Reemergence of Classical Swine Fever, Japan, 2018. *Emerg. Infect. Dis.* **2019**, *25*, 1228–1231. [CrossRef]

12. Gomez-Villamandos, J.C.; Carrasco, L.; Bautista, M.J.; Sierra, M.A.; Quezada, M.; Hervas, J.; Chacón, M.F.; Ruiz-Villamor, E.; Salguero, F.J.; Sónchez-Cordón, P.J.; et al. African swine fever and classical swine fever: A review of the pathogenesis. *Dtsch. Tierarztl. Wochenschr.* **2003**, *110*, 165–169. [PubMed]

13. Paton, D.J.; Greiser-Wilke, I. Classical swine fever: An update. *Res. Vet. Sci.* **2003**, *75*, 169–178. [CrossRef]

14. Zhou, B. Classical swine fever in China—An update Minireview. *Front. Vet. Sci.* **2019**, *13*, 187. [CrossRef] [PubMed]

15. Greiser-Wilke, I.; Blome, S.; Moennig, V. Diagnostic methods for detection of Classical swine fever virus—Status quo and new developments. *Vaccine* **2007**, *25*, 5524–5530. [CrossRef] [PubMed]

16. Moennig, V.; Floegel-Niesmann, G.; Greiser-Wilke, I. Clinical signs and epidemiology of classical swine fever: A review of new knowledge. *Vet. J.* **2003**, *165*, 11–20. [CrossRef]

17. OIE Terrestrial Manual 2019. Available online: https://www.oie.int/fileadmin/Home/eng/Health_standards/ tahm/3.08.03_CSF.pdf (accessed on 29 May 2020).

18. Grummer, B.; Fischer, S.; Depner, K.; Riebe, R.; Blome, S.; Greiser-Wilke, I. Replication of classical swine fever virus strains and isolates in different porcine cell lines. *Dtsch. Tierarztl. Wochenschr.* **2006**, *113*, 138–142. [PubMed]

19. Chander, V.; Nandi, S.; Ravishankar, C.; Upmanyu, V.; Verma, R. Classical swine fever in pigs: Recent developments and future perspectives. *Anim. Health Res. Rev.* **2014**, *15*, 87–101. [CrossRef]

20. Zhang, Q.; Xu, L.; Zhang, Y.; Wang, T.; Zou, X.; Zhu, Y.; Zhao, C.; Chen, K.; Sun, Y.; Sun, J.; et al. A novel ViewRNA in situ hybridization method for the detection of the dynamic distribution of Classical Swine Fever Virus RNA in PK15 cells. *Virol. J.* **2017**, *14*, 81. [CrossRef]

21. Shannon, A.D.; Morrissy, C.; Mackintosh, S.G.; Westbury, H.A. Detection of hog cholera virus antigens in experimentally-infected pigs using an antigen-capture ELISA. *Vet. Microbiol.* **1993**, *34*, 233–248. [CrossRef]

22. Penrith, M.L.; Vosloo, W.; Mather, C. Classical swine fever (hog cholera): Review of aspects relevant to control. *Transbound. Emerg. Dis.* **2011**, *58*, 187–196. [CrossRef]

23. Moennig, V.; Becher, P. Pestivirus control programs: How far have we come and where are we going? *Anim. Health Res. Rev.* **2015**, *16*, 83–87. [CrossRef] [PubMed]

24. Dewulf, J.; Koenen, F.; Mintiens, K.; Denis, P.; Ribbens, S.; de Kruif, A. Analytical performance of several classical swine fever laboratory diagnostic techniques on live animals for detection of infection. *J. Virol. Methods* **2004**, *119*, 137–143. [CrossRef] [PubMed]

25. Depner, K.; Hoffmann, B.; Beer, M. Evaluation of real-time RT-PCR assay for the routine intra vitam diagnosis of classical swine fever. *Vet. Microbiol.* **2007**, *121*, 338–343. [CrossRef] [PubMed]

26. Postel, A.; Austermann-Busch, S.; Petrov, A.; Moennig, V.; Becher, P. Epidemiology, diagnosis and control of classical swine fever: Recent developments and future challenges. *Transbound. Emerg. Dis.* **2018**, *65*, 248–261. [CrossRef]

27. Espy, M.J.; Uhl, J.R.; Sloan, L.M.; Buckwalter, S.P.; Jones, M.F.; Vetter, E.A.; Yao, J.D.; Wengenack, N.L.; Rosenblatt, J.E.; Cockerill, F.R., 3rd; et al. Real-time PCR in clinical microbiology: Applications for routine laboratory testing. *Clin. Microbiol. Rev.* **2006**, *19*, 165–256. [CrossRef] [PubMed]

28. Lung, O.; Pasick, J.; Fisher, M.; Buchanan, C.; Erickson, A.; Ambagala, A. Insulated isothermal reverse transcriptase PCR (iiRT-PCR) for rapid and sensitive detection of classical swine fever virus. *Transbound. Emerg. Dis.* **2016**, *63*, e395–e402. [CrossRef]

29. Lung, O.; Fisher, M.; Erickson, A.; Nfon, C.; Ambagala, A. Fully automated and integrated multiplex detection of high consequence livestock viral genomes on a microfluidic platform. *Transbound. Emerg. Dis.* **2019**, *66*, 144–155. [CrossRef]

30. Liu, L.; Xia, H.; Belák, S.; Widén, F. Development of a primer-probe energy transfer real-time PCR assay for improved detection of classical swine fever virus. *J. Virol. Methods* **2009**, *160*, 69–73. [CrossRef]

31. Zhang, X.J.; Xia, H.; Everett, H.; Sosan, O.; Crooke, H.; Belák, S.; Widén, F.; Qiu, H.J.; Liu, L. Evaluation of a primer-probe energy transfer real-time PCR assay for detection of classical swine fever virus. *J. Virol. Methods* **2010**, *168*, 259–261. [CrossRef]

32. Chen, H.T.; Zhang, J.; Ma, L.N.; Ma, Y.P.; Ding, Y.Z.; Liu, X.T.; Chen, L.; Ma, L.Q.; Zhang, Y.G.; Liu, Y.S. Rapid pre-clinical detection of classical swine fever by reverse transcription loop-mediated isothermal amplification. *Mol. Cell. Probes* **2009**, *23*, 71–74. [CrossRef]

33. Yin, S.; Shang, Y.; Zhou, G.; Tian, H.; Liu, Y.; Cai, X.; Liu, X. Development and evaluation of rapid detection of classical swine fever virus by reverse transcription loop-mediated isothermal amplification (RT-LAMP). *J. Biotechnol.* **2010**, *146*, 147–150. [CrossRef] [PubMed]

34. Zhang, X.J.; Sun, Y.; Liu, L.; Belák, S.; Qiu, H.J. Validation of a loop-mediated isothermal amplification assay for visualised detection of wild-type classical swine fever virus. *J. Virol. Methods* **2010**, *167*, 74–78. [CrossRef] [PubMed]

35. Ning, P.; Wu, Z.; Li, X.; Zhou, Y.; Hu, A.; Gong, X.; He, J.; Xia, Y.; Guo, K.; Zhang, R.; et al. Development of functionalized gold nanoparticles as nanoflare probes for rapid detection of classical swine fever virus. *Colloids Surf. B Biointerfaces* **2018**, *171*, 110–114. [CrossRef] [PubMed]

36. Huang, Y.L.; Pang, V.F.; Pan, C.H.; Chen, T.H.; Jong, M.H.; Huang, T.S.; Jeng, C.R. Development of a reverse transcription multiplex real-time PCR for the detection and genotyping of classical swine fever virus. *J. Virol. Methods* **2009**, *160*, 111–118. [CrossRef]

37. Zheng, H.H.; Zhang, S.J.; Cui, J.T.; Zhang, J.; Wang, L.; Liu, F.; Chen, H.Y. Simultaneous detection of classical swine fever virus and porcine circovirus 3 by SYBR green I-based duplex real-time fluorescence quantitative PCR. *Mol. Cell. Probes* **2020**, *50*, 101524. [CrossRef]

38. Díaz de Arce, H.; Pérez, L.J.; Frías, M.T.; Rosell, R.; Tarradas, J.; Núñez, J.I.; Ganges, L. A multiplex RT-PCR assay for the rapid and differential diagnosis of classical swine fever and other pestivirus infections. *Vet. Microbiol.* **2009**, *139*, 245–252. [CrossRef]

39. Haines, F.J.; Hofmann, M.A.; King, D.P.; Drew, T.W.; Crooke, H.R. Development and validation of a multiplex, real-time RT PCR assay for the simultaneous detection of classical and African swine fever viruses. *PLoS ONE* **2013**, *8*, e71019. [CrossRef]

40. Shi, X.; Liu, X.; Wang, Q.; Das, A.; Ma, G.; Xu, L.; Sun, Q.; Peddireddi, L.; Jia, W.; Liu, Y.; et al. A multiplex real-time PCR panel assay for simultaneous detection and differentiation of 12 common swine viruses. *J. Virol. Methods* **2016**, *236*, 258–265. [CrossRef]

41. Zhao, Y.; Liu, F.; Li, Q.; Wu, M.; Lei, L.; Pan, Z. A multiplex RT-PCR assay for rapid and simultaneous detection of four RNA viruses in swine. *J. Virol. Methods* **2019**, *269*, 38–42. [CrossRef]

42. Xiao, L.; Wang, Y.; Kang, R.; Wu, X.; Lin, H.; Ye, Y.; Yu, J.; Ye, J.; Xie, J.; Cao, Y.; et al. Development and application of a novel Bio-Plex suspension array system for high-throughput multiplexed nucleic acid detection of seven respiratory and reproductive pathogens in swine. *J. Virol. Methods* **2018**, *261*, 104–111. [CrossRef]

43. Deregt, D.; Gilbert, S.A.; Dudas, S.; Pasick, J.; Baxi, S.; Burton, K.M.; Baxi, M.K. A multiplex DNA suspension microarray for simultaneous detection and differentiation of classical swine fever virus and other pestiviruses. *J. Virol. Methods* **2006**, *136*, 17–23. [CrossRef] [PubMed]

44. Erickson, A.; Fisher, M.; Furukawa-Stoffer, T.; Ambagala, A.; Hodko, D.; Pasick, J.; King, D.P.; Nfon, C.; Ortega Polo, R.; Lung, O. A multiplex reverse transcription PCR and automated electronic microarray assay for detection and differentiation of seven viruses affecting swine. *Transbound. Emerg. Dis.* **2018**, *65*, e272–e283. [CrossRef] [PubMed]

45. Guo, X.; Gao, S.; Sang, S.; Jian, A.; Duan, Q.; Ji, J.; Zhang, W. Detection system based on magnetoelastic sensor for classical swine fever virus. *Biosens. Bioelectron.* **2016**, *82*, 127–131. [CrossRef] [PubMed]

46. Fu, Y.; Li, W.; Dai, B.; Zheng, L.; Zhang, Z.; Qi, D.; Cheng, X.; Zhang, D.; Zhuang, D. Diagnosis of mixed infections with swine viruses using an integrated microfluidic platform. *Sens. Actuators B Chem.* **2020**, *312*, 128005. [CrossRef]

47. Van Borm, S.; Belák, S.; Freimanis, G.; Fusaro, A.; Granberg, F.; Höper, D.; King, D.P.; Monne, I.; Orton, R.; Rosseel, T. Next-generation sequencing in veterinary medicine: How can the massive amount of information arising from high-throughput technologies improve diagnosis, control, and management of infectious diseases? *Methods Mol. Biol.* **2015**, *1247*, 415–436.

48. Kumar, D.; Rao, P.P.; Hegde, N.R. Next-generation sequencing as diagnostic tool in veterinary research. *J. Anim. Res.* **2019**, *9*, 797–806. [CrossRef]

49. Leifer, I.; Hoffmann, B.; Höper, D.; Bruun Rasmussen, T.; Blome, S.; Strebelow, G.; Höreth-Böntgen, D.; Staubach, C.; Beer, M. Molecular epidemiology of current classical swine fever virus isolates of wild boar in Germany. *J. Gen. Virol.* **2010**, *91*, 2687–2697. [CrossRef]

50. Töpfer, A.; Höper, D.; Blome, S.; Beer, M.; Beerenwinkel, N.; Ruggli, N.; Leifer, I. Sequencing approach to analyze the role of quasispecies for classical swine fever. *Virology* **2013**, *438*, 14–19. [CrossRef]

51. Fahnøe, U.; Pedersen, A.G.; Johnston, C.M.; Orton, R.J.; Höper, D.; Beer, M.; Bukh, J.; Belsham, G.J.; Rasmussen, T.B. Virus adaptation and selection following challenge of animals vaccinated against classical swine fever virus. *Viruses* **2019**, *11*, 932. [CrossRef]

52. Malik, Y.S.; Bhat, S.; Kumar, O.R.V.; Yadav, A.K.; Sircar, S.; Ansari, M.I.; Sarma, D.K.; Rajkhowa, T.K.; Ghosh, S.; Dhama, K. Classical swine fever virus biology, clinicopathology, diagnosis, vaccines and a meta-analysis of prevalence: A review from the Indian Perspective. *Pathogens* **2020**, *9*, 500. [CrossRef]

53. Madera, R.; Gong, W.; Wang, L.; Burakova, Y.; Lleellish, K.; Galliher-Beckley, A.; Nietfeld, J.; Henningson, J.; Jia, K.; Li, P.; et al. Pigs immunized with a novel E2 subunit vaccine are protected from heterologous classical swine fever virus challenge. *BMC Vet. Res.* **2016**, *12*, 197. [CrossRef]

54. Madera, R.; Wang, L.; Gong, W.; Burakova, Y.; Buist, S.; Nietfeld, J.; Henningson, J.; Ozuna, A.G.C.; Tu, C.; Shi, J. Towards the development of a one-dose classical swine fever subunit vaccine: Antigen titration, onset and duration of immunity. *J. Vet. Sci.* **2018**, *19*, 393–405. [CrossRef] [PubMed]

55. Laughlin, R.C.; Madera, R.; Peres, Y.; Berquist, B.R.; Wang, L.; Buist, S.; Burakova, Y.; Palle, S.; Chung, C.J.; Rasmussen, M.V.; et al. Plant-made E2 glycoprotein single-dose vaccine protects pigs against classical swine fever. *Plant. Biotechnol. J.* **2019**, *17*, 410–420. [CrossRef] [PubMed]

56. Wang, L.; Mi, S.; Madera, R.; Ganges, L.; Borca, M.V.; Ren, J.; Cunningham, C.; Cino-Ozuna, A.G.; Li, H.; Tu, C.; et al. A neutralizing monoclonal antibody-based competitive ELISA for classical swine fever C-strain post-vaccination monitoring. *BMC Vet. Res.* **2020**, *16*, 14. [CrossRef]

57. Tetsuo, M.; Matsuno, K.; Tamura, T.; Fukuhara, T.; Kim, T.; Okamatsu, M.; Tautz, N.; Matsuura, Y.; Sakoda, Y. Development of a high-throughput serum neutralization test using recombinant pestiviruses possessing a small reporter tag. *Pathogens* **2020**, *9*, 188. [CrossRef] [PubMed]

58. Moser, C.; Ruggli, N.; Tratschin, J.D.; Hofmann, M.A. Detection of antibodies against classical swine fever virus in swine sera by indirect ELISA using recombinant envelope glycoprotein E2. *Vet. Microbiol.* **1996**, *51*, 41. [CrossRef]

59. Cheng, T.C.; Pan, C.H.; Chen, C.S.; Chuang, K.H.; Chuang, C.H.; Huang, C.C.; Chu, Y.Y.; Yang, Y.C.; Chu, P.Y.; Kao, C.H.; et al. Direct coating of culture medium from cells secreting classical swine fever virus E2 antigen on ELISA plates for detection of E2-specific antibodies. *Vet. J.* **2015**, *205*, 107–109. [CrossRef]

60. Clavijo, A.; Lin, M.; Riva, J.; Mallory, M.; Lin, F.; Zhou, E.M. Development of a competitive ELISA using a truncated E2 recombinant protein as antigen for detection of antibodies to classical swine fever virus. *Res. Vet. Sci.* **2001**, *70*, 1–7. [CrossRef]

61. Kumar, R.; Barman, N.N.; Khatoon, E.; Kumar, S. Development of single dilution immunoassay to detect E2 protein specific classical swine fever virus antibody. *Vet. Immunol. Immunopathol.* **2016**, *172*, 50–54. [CrossRef]

62. Li, Y.; Zhao, J.J.; Li, N.; Shi, Z.; Cheng, D.; Zhu, Q.H.; Tu, C.; Tong, G.Z.; Qiu, H.J. A multiplex nested RT-PCR for the detection and differentiation of wild-type viruses from C-strain vaccine of classical swine fever virus. *J. Virol. Methods* **2007**, *143*, 16–22. [CrossRef]

63. Zhao, J.J.; Cheng, D.; Li, N.; Sun, Y.; Shi, Z.; Zhu, Q.H.; Tu, C.; Tong, G.Z.; Qiu, H.J. Evaluation of a multiplex real-time RT-PCR for quantitative and differential detection of wild-type viruses and C-strain vaccine of Classical swine fever virus. *Vet. Microbiol.* **2008**, *126*, 1–10. [CrossRef] [PubMed]

64. Leifer, I.; Depner, K.; Blome, S.; Le Potier, M.F.; Le Dimna, M.; Beer, M.; Hoffmann, B. Differentiation of C-strain "Riems" or CP7_E2alf vaccinated animals from animals infected by classical swine fever virus field strains using real-time RT-PCR. *J. Virol. Methods* **2009**, *158*, 114–122. [CrossRef] [PubMed]

65. Liu, L.; Xia, H.; Everett, H.; Sosan, O.; Crooke, H.; Meindl-Böhmer, A.; Qiu, H.; Moennig, V.; Belák, S.; Widén, F. A generic real-time TaqMan assay for specific detection of lapinized Chinese vaccines against classical swine fever. *J. Virol. Methods* **2011**, *175*, 170–174. [CrossRef] [PubMed]

66. Zhang, X.J.; Han, Q.Y.; Sun, Y.; Zhang, X.; Qiu, H.J. Development of a triplex TaqMan real-time RT-PCR assay for differential detection of wild-type and HCLV vaccine strains of classical swine fever virus and bovine viral diarrhea virus 1. *Res. Vet. Sci.* **2012**, *92*, 512–518. [CrossRef] [PubMed]

67. Everett, H.E.; Crudgington, B.S.; Sosan-Soulé, O.; Crooke, H.R. Differential detection of classical swine fever virus challenge strains in C-strain vaccinated pigs. *BMC Vet. Res.* **2014**, *10*, 281. [CrossRef]

68. Widén, F.; Everett, H.; Blome, S.; Fernandez Pinero, J.; Uttenthal, A.; Cortey, M.; von Rosen, T.; Tignon, M.; Liu, L. Comparison of two real-time RT-PCR assays for differentiation of C-strain vaccinated from classical swine fever infected pigs and wild boars. *Res. Vet. Sci.* **2014**, *97*, 455–457. [CrossRef]

69. Cho, H.S.; Park, S.J.; Park, N.Y. Development of a reverse-transcription polymerase chain reaction assay with fluorogenic probes to discriminate Korean wild-type and vaccine isolates of Classical swine fever virus. *Can. J. Vet. Res.* **2006**, *70*, 226–229.

70. Pan, C.H.; Jong, M.H.; Huang, Y.L.; Huang, T.S.; Chao, P.H.; Lai, S.S. Rapid detection and differentiation of wild-type and three attenuated lapinized vaccine strains of classical swine fever virus by reverse transcription polymerase chain reaction. *J. Vet. Diagn. Investig.* **2008**, *20*, 448–456. [CrossRef]

71. Blome, S.; Gabriel, C.; Staubach, C.; Leifer, I.; Strebelow, G.; Beer, M. Genetic differentiation of infected from vaccinated animals after implementation of an emergency vaccination strategy against classical swine fever in wild boar. *Vet. Microbiol.* **2011**, *153*, 373–376. [CrossRef]

72. Schroeder, S.; von Rosen, T.; Blome, S.; Loeffen, W.; Haegeman, A.; Koenen, F.; Uttenthal, A. Evaluation of classical swine fever virus antibody detection assays with an emphasis on the differentiation of infected from vaccinated animals. *Rev. Sci. Tech.* **2012**, *31*, 997–1010. [CrossRef]

73. Lin, M.; Trottier, E.; Pasick, J. Antibody responses of pigs to defined E^{rns} fragments after infection with classical swine fever virus. *Clin. Diagn. Lab. Immunol.* **2005**, *12*, 180–186. [CrossRef]

74. Moormann, R.J.; Bouma, A.; Kramps, J.A.; Terpstra, C.; De Smit, H.J. Development of a classical swine fever subunit marker vaccine and companion diagnostic test. *Vet. Microbiol.* **2000**, *73*, 209–219. [CrossRef]

75. Langedijk, J.P.; Middel, W.G.; Meloen, R.H.; Kramps, J.A.; de Smit, J.A. Enzyme-linked immunosorbent assay using a virus type-specific peptide based on a subdomain of envelope protein Erns for serologic diagnosis of pestivirus infections in swine. *J. Clin. Microbiol.* **2001**, *39*, 906–912. [CrossRef] [PubMed]

76. de Smit, A.J. Laboratory diagnosis, epizootiology, and efficacy of marker vaccines in classical swine fever: A review. *Vet. Q.* **2000**, *22*, 182–188. [CrossRef] [PubMed]

77. Pannhorst, K.; Fröhlich, A.; Staubach, C.; Meyer, D.; Blome, S.; Becher, P. Evaluation of an Erns-based enzyme-linked immunosorbent assay to distinguish Classical swine fever virus-infected pigs from pigs vaccinated with CP7_E2alf. *J. Vet. Diagn. Investig.* **2015**, *27*, 449–460. [CrossRef] [PubMed]

78. Meyer, D.; Fritsche, S.; Luo, Y.; Engemann, C.; Blome, S.; Beyerbach, M.; Chang, C.Y.; Qiu, H.J.; Becher, P.; Postel, A. The double-antigen ELISA concept for early detection of E^{rns}-specific classical swine fever virus antibodies and application as an accompanying test for differentiation of infected from marker vaccinated animals. *Transbound. Emerg. Dis.* **2017**, *64*, 2013–2022. [CrossRef]

79. Xia, H.; Harimoorthy, R.; Vijayaraghavan, B.; Blome, S.; Widén, F.; Beer, M.; Belák, S.; Liu, L. Differentiation of classical swine fever virus infection from CP7_E2alf marker vaccination by a multiplex microsphere immunoassay. *Clin. Vaccine Immunol.* **2015**, *22*, 65–71. [CrossRef]

80. Bruderer, U.; van de Velde, J.; Frantzen, I.; De Bortoli, F. Discrimination within epitope specific antibody populations against classical swine fever virus is a new means of differentiating infection from vaccination. *J. Immunol. Methods* **2015**, *420*, 18–23. [CrossRef]

81. Luo, Y.; Li, L.; Austermann-Busch, S.; Dong, M.; Xu, J.; Shao, L.; Lei, J.; Li, N.; He, W.R.; Zhao, B.; et al. Enhanced expression of the Erns protein of classical swine fever virus in yeast and its application in an indirect enzyme-linked immunosorbent assay for antibody differentiation of infected from vaccinated animals. *J. Virol. Methods* **2015**, *222*, 22–27. [CrossRef]

82. Manessis, G.; Gelasakis, A.I.; Bossis, I. The challenge of introducing point of care diagnostics in farm animal health management. *Biomed. J. Sci. Tech. Res.* **2019**, *14*, 002601.

83. Chowdry, V.K.; Luo, Y.; Widén, F.; Qiu, H.J.; Shan, H.; Belák, S.; Liu, L. Development of a loop-mediated isothermal amplification assay combined with a lateral flow dipstick for rapid and simple detection of classical swine fever virus in the field. *J. Virol. Methods* **2014**, *197*, 14–18. [CrossRef] [PubMed]

84. Li, X.; Wang, L.; Shi, X.; Zhao, D.; Yang, J.; Yang, S.; Zhang, G. Development of an immunochromatographic strip for rapid detection of antibodies against classical swine fever virus. *J. Virol. Methods* **2012**, *180*, 32–37. [CrossRef] [PubMed]

85. Sastre, P.; Pérez, T.; Costa, S.; Yang, X.; Räber, A.; Blome, S.; Goller, K.V.; Gallardo, C.; Tapia, I.; García, J.; et al. Development of a duplex lateral flow assay for simultaneous detection of antibodies against African and Classical swine fever viruses. *J. Vet. Diagn. Investig.* **2016**, *28*, 543–549. [CrossRef]

86. Nannucci, L.; Barattini, P.; Bossis, I.; Woźniakowski, G.; Balka, G.; Pugliese, C. Point-of-service diagnostic technology for detection of swine viral diseases. *J. Vet. Res.* **2020**, *64*, 15–23. [CrossRef] [PubMed]

87. Dixon, L.K.; Sun, H.; Roberts, H. African swine fever. *Antivir. Res.* **2019**, *165*, 34–41. [CrossRef]

88. Arshad Ali, S.; Baloch, M.; Ahmed, N.; Arshad Ali, A.; Iqbal, A. The outbreak of coronavirus disease 2019 (COVID-19)-An emerging global health threat. *J. Infect. Public Health* **2020**, *13*, 644–646. [CrossRef]

PERMISSIONS

LIST OF CONTRIBUTORS

Elisa Crisci
Department of Population Health and Pathobiology, College of Veterinary Medicine, North Carolina State University, Raleigh, NC 27607, USA
Comparative Medicine Institute, North Carolina State University, Raleigh, NC 27607, USA

Lorenzo Fraile
Universitat de Lleida, 25198 Lleida, Spain

Maria Montoya
Centro de Investigaciones Biológicas, Consejo Superior de Investigaciones Científicas (CIB-CSIC), 28040 Madrid, Spain

Fabrizio Bertelloni, Mario Forzan, Barbara Turchi, Simona Sagona, Maurizio Mazzei, Antonio Felicioli, Filippo Fratini and Domenico Cerri
Department of Veterinary Science, University of Pisa, Viale delle Piagge 2, 56124 Pisa, Italy

Vincenzo Gervasi and Andrea Marcon
Wildlife Department, Istituto Superiore per la Protezione e la Ricerca Ambientale, 40064 Ozzano Emilia (BO), Italy

Silvia Bellini and Vittorio Guberti
Istituto Zooprofilattico della Lombardia ed Emilia-Romagna, 25124 Brescia, Italy

Madoka Tetsuo, Taksoo Kim and Masatoshi Okamatsu
Laboratory of Microbiology, Division of Disease Control, Faculty of Veterinary Medicine, Hokkaido University, Sapporo, Hokkaido 060-0818, Japan

Keita Matsuno
Laboratory of Microbiology, Division of Disease Control, Faculty of Veterinary Medicine, Hokkaido University, Sapporo, Hokkaido 060-0818, Japan
Global Station for Zoonosis Control, Global Institute for Collaborative Research and Education (GI-CoRE), Hokkaido University, Sapporo 001-0020, Japan

Takasuke Fukuhara and Yoshiharu Matsuura
Department of Molecular Virology, Research Institute for Microbial Diseases, Osaka University, Osaka 565-0871, Japan

Tomokazu Tamura
Department of Molecular Virology, Research Institute for Microbial Diseases, Osaka University, Osaka 565-0871, Japan

Department of Molecular Biology, Princeton University, Washington Road, Princeton, NJ 08540, USA

Norbert Tautz
Institute of Virology and Cell Biology, University of Lübeck, D-23562 Lübeck, Germany

Seong-In Lim
Virus Disease Division, Animal and Plant Quarantine Agency, Gimchen, Gyeongbuk-do 39660, Korea

Dae-Sung Yu
Division of Veterinary Epidemiological, Animal and Plant Quarantine Agency, Gimchen, Gyeongbuk-do 39660, Korea

Sung-Hyun Choi and Byung-Il Jung
Korea Pork Producers Association, Seocho-gu, Seoul 06643, Korea

Bong-Kyun Park
Viral Disease Division, Animal and Plant Quarantine Agency (APQA), Gimcheon, Gyeongbuk 39660, Korea
College of Veterinary Medicine, Seoul University, Gwanak-ro, Gwanak-gu, Seoul 08826, Korea

Genxi Hao and Huawei Zhang
State Key Laboratory of Agricultural Microbiology, Huazhong Agricultural University, Wuhan 430070, China
Laboratory of Animal Virology, College of Veterinary Medicine, Huazhong Agricultural University, Wuhan 430070, China

Huanchun Chen, Ping Qian and Xiangmin Li
State Key Laboratory of Agricultural Microbiology, Huazhong Agricultural University, Wuhan 430070, China
Laboratory of Animal Virology, College of Veterinary Medicine, Huazhong Agricultural University, Wuhan 430070, China
Key Laboratory of Development of Veterinary Diagnostic Products, Ministry of Agriculture, Wuhan 430070, China
Key Laboratory of Preventive Veterinary Medicine in Hubei Province, The Cooperative Innovation Center for Sustainable Pig Production, Wuhan 430070, China

Yu-Liang Huang, Kuo-Jung Tsai, Ming-Chung Deng, Hsin-Meng Liu and Chia-Yi Chang
Animal Health Research Institute, Council of Agriculture, Executive Yuan, 376 Chung-Cheng Road, Tansui, New Taipei City 25158, Taiwan

Chin-Cheng Huang
Council of Agriculture, Executive Yuan, No. 37 Nanhai Road, Taipei 10014, Taiwan

Fun-In Wang
School of Veterinary Medicine, National Taiwan University, No. 1, Section 4, Roosevelt Road, Taipei 10617, Taiwan

Norikazu Isoda
Unit of Risk Analysis and Management, Research Center for Zoonosis Control, Hokkaido University, Kita 20, Nishi 10, Kita-Ku, Sapporo 001-0020, Japan
Global Station for Zoonosis Control, Global Institute for Collaborative Research and Education (GI-CoRE), Hokkaido University, Sapporo 001-0020, Japan

Kairi Baba and Kohei Makita
Veterinary Epidemiology Unit, School of Veterinary Medicine, Rakuno Gakuen University, 582, Bunkyodai Midorimachi, Ebetsu 069-8501, Japan

Yi-Chia Li, Ming-Tang Chiou and Chao-Nan Lin
Animal Disease Diagnostic Center, College of Veterinary Medicine, National Pingtung University of Science and Technology, Pingtung 91201, Taiwan
Department of Veterinary Medicine, College of Veterinary Medicine, National Pingtung University of Science and Technology, Pingtung 91201, Taiwan

José Alejandro Bohórquez, Sara Muñoz-González, Marta Pérez-Simó, Iván Muñoz and Llilianne Ganges
OIE Reference Laboratory for Classical Swine Fever, IRTA-CReSA, 08193 Barcelona, Spain

Rosa Rosell
OIE Reference Laboratory for Classical Swine Fever, IRTA-CReSA, 08193 Barcelona, Spain
Departament d'Agricultura, Ramadería, Pesca, Alimentació I Medi Natural i Rural (DAAM), 08007 Generalitat de Catalunya, Spain

Liani Coronado
OIE Reference Laboratory for Classical Swine Fever, IRTA-CReSA, 08193 Barcelona, Spain
Centro Nacional de Sanidad Agropecuaria (CENSA), Mayabeque 32700, Cuba

Mariano Domingo
OIE Reference Laboratory for Classical Swine Fever, IRTA-CReSA, 08193 Barcelona, Spain
Servei de Diagnòstic de Patologia Veterinària (SDPV), Departament de Sanitat I d'Anatomia Animals, Universitat Autònoma de Barcelona, Bellaterra, 08193 Barcelona, Spain

Gyu-Nam Park
Viral Disease Division, Animal and Plant Quarantine Agency (APQA), Gimcheon, Gyeongbuk 39660, Korea

Van Phan Le and Thi Lan Nguyen
College of Veterinary Medicine, Vietnam National University of Agriculture, Hanoi 100000, Vietnam

Jae-Hoon Kim
College of Veterinary Medicine and Veterinary Medical Research Institute, Jeju National University, Jeju 63243, Korea

Yashpal Singh Malik, Sudipta Bhat, O. R. Shubhankar Sircar and Mohd Ikram Ansari
Division of Biological Standardization, ICAR-Indian Veterinary Research Institute, Izatnagar, Bareilly, Uttar Pradesh 243001, India

Vinodh Kumar
Division of Epidemiology, ICAR-Indian Veterinary Research Institute, Izatnagar, Bareilly, Uttar Pradesh 243122, India

Ajay Kumar Yadav
Animal Health, ICAR-National Research Centre on Pig (ICAR-NRCP), Guwahati, Assam 781015, India

Dilip Kumar Sarma
Department of Veterinary Microbiology, Assam Agricultural University, Khanapara, Guwahati 781022, India

Tridib Kumar Rajkhowa
College of Veterinary Sciences & Animal Husbandry, Central Agricultural University, Selesih, Aizawl, Mizoram 796001, India

Souvik Ghosh
Department of Biomedical Sciences, One Health Center for Zoonoses and Tropical Veterinary Medicine, Basseterre, West Indies

Kuldeep Dhama
Division of Pathology, ICAR-Indian Veterinary Research Institute, Izatnagar, Bareilly, Uttar Pradesh 243122, India

In-Soo Cho
Viral Disease Division, Animal and Plant Quarantine Agency (APQA), Gimcheon, Gyeongbuk 39660, Korea

Wan-Choul Kang and Hyeon-Ju Kim
Jeju Special Self-Governing Provincial Veterinary Research Institute, Jeju Island 63344, Korea

SeEun Choe, Ki-Sun Kim, Sok Song, Ra Mi Cha, Jihye Shin, Bang-Hun Hyun and Dong-Jun An
Viral Disease Division, Animal and Plant Quarantine Agency (APQA), Gimcheon, Gyeongbuk 39660, Korea

Hyoung-Nam Jo
College of Veterinary Medicine and Veterinary Medical Research Institute, Jeju National University, Jeju 63243, Korea

Sheng-ming Ma, Qian Mao, Lin Yi, Ming-qiu Zhao and Jin-ding Chen
College of Veterinary Medicine; South China Agricultural University; Guangzhou 510642, China

Satoshi Ito
Research Center for Zoonosis Control, Hokkaido University, Kita 20, Nishi 10, Kita-ku, Sapporo, Hokkaido 001-0020, Japan
VISAVET Center and Animal Health Department, University Complutense of Madrid, 28040 Madrid, Spain

Cristina Jurado, Jaime Bosch and José Manuel Sánchez-Vizcaíno
VISAVET Center and Animal Health Department, University Complutense of Madrid, 28040 Madrid, Spain

Mitsugi Ito
Akabane Animal Clinic, Co. Ltd., 55 Ishizoe, Akabane-cho, Tahara, Aichi-ken 441-3502, Japan

Yoshihiro Sakoda
Global Station for Zoonosis Control, Global Institute for Collaborative Research and Education (GI-CoRE), Hokkaido University, Sapporo 001-0020, Japan
Laboratory of Microbiology, Department of Disease Control, Faculty of Veterinary Medicine, Hokkaido University, Kita 18, Nishi 9, Kita-ku, Sapporo, Hokkaido 060-0018, Japan

Lihua Wang, Rachel Madera, Yuzhen Li and Jishu Shi
Department of Anatomy and Physiology, College of Veterinary Medicine, Kansas State University, Manhattan, KS 66506, USA

David Scott McVey and Barbara S. Drolet
United States Department of Agriculture, Arthropod-Borne Animal Diseases Research Unit, Center for Grain and Animal Health Research, Manhattan, KS 66502, USA

Index

A

Amino Acids, 45, 77-78, 160, 172

Antibody, 2, 12, 23, 25, 28, 32, 43-44, 49, 52-54, 56-58, 60-63, 65, 75, 79, 82, 85, 87-88, 102-105, 107-113, 115-116, 121-123, 125, 139, 142, 153, 156, 158, 170-171, 175, 179, 184-185, 213-214, 216, 220-221, 223-224, 227-229

Antibody Detection, 44, 63, 153, 214, 220, 224, 228

Apoptosis, 6-7, 10, 14, 16, 103, 109, 184, 186-190, 192-200

Autophagy, 103, 109, 188-199

B

Body Temperature, 69, 87, 161

Border Disease, 43-46, 53-54, 102, 143, 170, 216

Bovine Viral Diarrhea, 43-44, 53-55, 102, 128, 143-144, 216, 228

C

Cell Death, 14, 189, 192-194, 197-199

Cell Populations, 20, 22, 113, 123

Centrifugation, 75, 126, 185

Cerebellum, 162, 177, 183

Congestion, 132, 139, 153, 170

Cytokines, 5-7, 10-11, 13-16, 22, 24, 103, 174, 182, 184-187, 193, 196

D

Dilution, 29-30, 48, 53, 75, 88, 125, 228

Domestic Pigs, 27-28, 30-31, 33-34, 44-45, 49, 51, 56-59, 77, 89, 91-92, 97-101, 129, 137-138, 155, 161, 186, 202, 204, 206-207, 209, 212-213, 223

Dual Infections, 26, 77-79, 82, 110

E

Enteritis, 152-153, 163

F

Fecal Swabs, 78, 84-85, 87

Field Strains, 67, 202, 223, 228

Flaviviridae, 43, 45, 53-56, 67, 78, 88-89, 91, 102, 109, 130, 143-144, 157, 160, 172, 189, 191, 201, 213

Foetal Immune Response, 109, 112, 122, 124

G

Genetic Differences, 130, 169, 223

Genome Sequences, 141, 144, 165, 171, 220

Genotype, 2, 9, 19, 22-24, 33-34, 42, 56-58, 63, 67-68, 73-74, 77-80, 85-90, 110, 130-132, 135-136, 138-140, 142, 144-145, 147, 154-155, 159, 168, 202, 213, 220, 223

Gestation, 112-113, 118-119, 122, 124, 126, 155-156, 175, 185

H

Hemorrhages, 143, 151-153, 162, 175, 193

I

Ileum, 135-136, 176, 180-181, 184

Immune Status, 6, 151, 153, 175, 220-221

Infarction, 152, 169-170

Infected Sows, 113, 115-116, 118, 122, 175

Infectious Disease, 170, 188, 193, 197

Isolated Strains, 68-69, 73

L

Lesions, 17, 112-113, 116, 118, 122-124, 135-136, 138-139, 152-153, 160, 162, 168-170, 174-175, 177, 179, 183-185

Luciferase Activity, 45-50, 52-53

Lymph Nodes, 13, 18, 24, 74, 85, 87, 116, 135-137, 151-154, 162, 169-170, 175, 183-184

Lymphocytes, 5, 10, 13, 16-17, 20-21, 103, 135-137, 143, 153, 184, 186, 189-190, 192-193, 198-200

Lymphoid Tissues, 136, 138, 154, 194

M

Macrophages, 1-2, 5-7, 12, 14, 17-21, 23-25, 110-111, 135, 137, 162, 172, 184, 186, 189-190, 197

Modified Live Vaccines, 79, 161

Mucosal Surfaces, 151, 175

N

Nucleic Acid, 16, 108, 111, 150, 153, 218, 226

Nucleotide, 2, 23, 51, 57-58, 64, 68, 131, 138-140, 144-145, 147, 154, 165, 168-169, 171, 173, 213, 220

O

Omega Values, 165-166, 169

P

Pathogenicity, 24, 55, 57, 63, 67-69, 73-74, 76-77, 86, 89, 92, 97, 111, 130-132, 138-139, 160-161, 169, 172, 174-175, 177, 179, 183-185

Perivascular Cuffing, 135, 162, 170, 177, 183

Persistent Congenital Infection, 112-113, 122

Persistent Infection, 103, 107, 109, 111-113, 122-123, 127-128, 158, 169, 175, 183, 187-190, 193-195

Pestivirus, 43-45, 49, 52-53, 56, 67, 78, 91, 102, 109, 112, 124, 130, 143-144, 157-158, 160, 170, 172, 188, 196, 198, 201, 213, 223, 225-226, 228

Phylogenetic Analysis, 58-59, 64, 68-69, 75, 89, 97, 131, 141-142, 144, 146, 157, 173, 202, 220, 225

Phylogenetic Tree, 130-131, 133, 138-139, 144

Pneumonia, 1, 12, 25, 153, 162-163, 169

Pyroptosis, 103, 109, 188-189, 193-197, 199-200

R

Recombinant Viruses, 44-45, 47, 50

S

Serum Neutralization Test, 43-44, 48, 53, 156, 227

Spatio-temporal Analysis, 101, 201-202, 206-207, 212

Spleen, 13, 24, 74, 87, 116-117, 124, 135-137, 139, 152-155, 162-163, 169-170, 176, 180-181, 184, 186-187, 192-193, 199

Standard Deviational Ellipses, 91, 95, 201, 203

Subunit Vaccine, 102-103, 108, 110, 127, 227

Supernatants, 50, 52

Swine Kidney, 45-47

T

Tissue Culture, 75, 80, 161

Tonsil, 13, 87, 116-117, 124, 136-139, 162-163, 169, 174-176, 180-181, 187

Trans-placental Infection, 112-113, 118, 123

Trans-placental Transmission, 112, 122-124

U

Ulceration, 169, 175

Urinary Bladder, 113, 135-138, 151, 175

V

Vaccine Strain, 64, 85, 87, 107, 139, 154-155, 159-161, 166, 168-169, 172-173, 184-185, 187

Viral Antigens, 52, 136, 162, 174, 177, 180, 183, 224

Viral Loads, 78-79, 82, 84-88, 183

Viral Replication, 7, 25, 78, 112-113, 122-123, 189, 191-192, 194-195, 198

Virulence, 2, 9, 54-55, 67-68, 74-77, 90-91, 97, 100, 103, 111-113, 115-116, 119, 122-124, 127, 130, 132, 137-138, 140, 143, 153-155, 160-161, 172-173, 175, 184, 202, 210, 220

Virus Isolation, 44, 68, 72, 75, 139, 153, 213-214, 216

Virus Neutralization Test, 153, 213-214, 220

Virus Strains, 11, 23, 47, 80, 85, 139, 161, 187, 196, 225

Virus Titration, 52, 80, 87-88

W

Wild Boars, 27, 29, 31, 36-38, 40, 56-65, 92-93, 97, 99, 101, 128, 155, 186, 211-212, 223, 228

Wild-type Viruses, 47, 51, 228

Printed in the USA
CPSIA information can be obtained
at www.ICGtesting.com
JSHW051401091023
49903JS00006B/223

9 781647 404093